Basic Science of Nuclear Medicine

To all our families

Basic Science of Nuclear Medicine

Roy P. Parker

PhD FInstP
Professor of Medical Physics, The University of Leeds; Formerly
Senior Lecturer in Medical Physics, Institute of Cancer Research,
Royal Marsden Hospital, London.

Peter H. S. Smith

BA DPhil
Principal Physicist, Clwyd and Gwynedd Health
Authorities; Formerly Senior Physicist, Royal Marsden
Hospital, London

David M. Taylor

DSc FRSC MRCPath
Professor of Radiotoxicology, University of Heidelberg;
Director, Institute for Genetics and Toxicology,
Kernforschungszentrum Karlsruhe, FRG.
Formerly Senior Lecturer, Institute of Cancer Research, London.

Foreword by

W. V. Mayneord

CBE DSc LLD FRS
Emeritus Professor of Physics as Applied to Medicine,
University of London

SECOND EDITION

CHURCHILL LIVINGSTONE
EDINBURGH LONDON MELBOURNE AND NEW YORK 1984

CHURCHILL LIVINGSTONE
Medical Division of Longman Group Limited

Distributed in the United States of America by
Churchill Livingstone Inc., 1560 Broadway, New York,
N.Y. 10036, and by associated companies, branches
and representatives throughout the world.

First edition 1978
Second edition 1984

ISBN 0 443 02419 7

British Library Cataloguing in Publication Data

Parker, Roy P.
    Basic science of nuclear medicine.—2nd ed.
    1. Nuclear medicine
    I. Title   II. Smith, Peter H. S.
    III. Taylor, David M.
    616.07'575   R895

Library of Congress Cataloging in Publication Data

Parker, T. P. (Roy P.)
    Basic science of nuclear medicine.

    Includes index.
    1. Nuclear medicine.   I. Smith, Peter H. S.
    II. Taylor, David M. (David McIntyre)
    III. Title.
    [DNLM: 1. Nuclear medicine.   WN 440 P242b]
    R895.P3   1984   616.07'575   83-2099

Printed in Singapore by Selector Printing Co (Pte) Ltd

Foreword

Looking back over the history of medicine during this century one of the most striking features has been development arising from the discovery and utilisation of radiations from atomic nuclei. Initially confined virtually to the therapeutic use of radium the field has been transformed into a major branch of diagnostic medicine alongside the more classical therapeutic and diagnostic radiology using X-rays as their principal agent.

In the 1940s a very wide range of types of radioactive atoms became available, atoms which could be incorporated into molecules of particular biological and therefore medical interest. Vast new vistas were opened up in the visualisation of specific organs and systems of the body. Probably of even greater importance was a new ability to study the dynamics of physiological systems and organs in both health and disease, sometimes by incorporation into the human body of carefully chosen and prepared radiopharmaceutical compounds and sometimes by the study of appropriate compounds *in vitro*. Modern biochemistry and physiology (to say nothing of molecular biology) would be impossible without the techniques of radioactive labelling and detection.

To make effective and safe use of such techniques the practitioner of nuclear medicine requires to have knowledge of portions of a range of basic sciences such as radiation physics, biochemistry, organic chemistry, pharmacology and physiology, to say nothing of his usual acquaintance with anatomy. It happens, too, that since the emission of radiation from atomic nuclei is a random 'chance' event, to assess the significance of our observations we must resort to statistical argument, and must therefore add at least some elementary mathematical understanding to our armoury.

Hitherto these subjects have tended to be discussed in separate publications, so we welcome a text which brings together simple, clear expositions of the relevant and essential features of a number of scientific and technical skills interwoven and expounded with a wealth of practical examples likely to be met with in clinical practice. The student may have some elementary knowledge of a specific subject but it is salutary and necessary to be reminded that perhaps some other facet of knowledge is the important one in a particular instance. This book brings together the answers. It also emphasises very properly the hazards, both pharmaceutical and physical associated with these techniques, and gives clear practical advice about their assessment and avoidance.

This text will prove valuable to many practitioners and students of this exciting and rapidly developing branch of medicine.

W. V. Mayneord

Preface to the Second Edition

Books must follow sciences, not sciences books
Francis Bacon

During the six years since this book first appeared the science of nuclear medicine has continued to develop rapidly, thus in preparing the second edition extensive revision of the original text and the addition of several new chapters have been necessary.

The new edition retains the aim of the first, to present an integrated survey of the basic science of nuclear medicine in a manner which emphasises the relevance and importance of a sound understanding of the scientific principles upon which modern clinical radionuclide investigations are based.

Although the book covers most of the aspects of the basic science of nuclear medicine which are required by students preparing for the Diploma in Nuclear Medicine of the College of Radiographers and for the Master of Science in Nuclear Medicine of the University of London, it is not intended to be *the* text for these or any other specific courses. Rather it is intended to provide a general introduction for physicians, scientists, radiographers and technicians who are entering the field of nuclear medicine for the first time, and the presentation is designed to cater for the needs of readers with widely differing levels of previous training.

The format of the new edition retains the original five-part structure, but further chapters have been added to Parts II and III in order to cover new developments, especially in instrumentation, and to improve the general presentation of the various topics. In particular the original single chapter discussion of the basic principles of tracer techniques has been expanded into three chapters dealing with static and kinetic studies and radioimmunoassay; in Part III the developments in imaging techniques have been covered by the addition of three new chapters on emission tomography, dynamic imaging, and special techniques.

We conclude by thanking all those colleagues and students who have helped us by providing information, advice or suggestions or by pointing out errors or instances of lack of clarity of expression which they found in the first edition. We are particularly grateful to Miss Gillian Plummer for her help with the typescript, and to Mrs P. Taylor, BSc, MRSC, who once again accepted responsibility for the index. We also wish to express our appreciation of the patience and understanding shown by the publishers throughout the long period needed to complete this new edition.

Leeds,   R.P.P.
Bangor,   P.H.S.S.
Heidelberg,   D.M.T.
1984

Preface to the First Edition

Science is nothing but trained and organised common sense
T. E. Huxley

The rapid growth of nuclear medicine into a recognised medical speciality has created a world-wide need for physicians, radiographers and technicians who are well trained in radionuclide techniques. In recent years a number of text books on nuclear medicine have been published but none has presented a unified coverage of the scientific principles upon which it is based.

The aim of this book is to present an integrated survey of those aspects of physics, chemistry and related sciences which are essential to a clear understanding of the scientific basis of nuclear medicine. The book is based on the authors' personal experience in teaching students preparing for the Diploma in Nuclear Medicine of the College of Radiographers and the Master of Science in Nuclear Medicine of the University of London. It is intended, however, as a general introductory text for physicians, scientists, radiographers and technicians who are entering nuclear medicine or adjacent fields.

The approach adopted is to emphasise the relevance and importance of a sound understanding of the scientific principles underlying the use of radionuclide investigations in clinical practice. The use of mathematics has been reduced to a minimum in the main text but the more important mathematical concepts and derivations have been included in the appendices.

The subject matter is presented in five parts. Part I covers the basic physics of radiation and radioactivity; while Part II deals with radiation dosimetry, the biological effects of radiation and the principles of tracer techniques. The measurement of radioactivity and the principal aspects of modern instrumentation are presented in Part III. Those aspects of chemistry which are essential to a clear understanding of the preparation and use of radiopharmaceuticals are discussed in Part IV. The final section is concerned with the production of radionuclides and radiopharmaceuticals and with the practical aspects of laboratory practice, facilities and safety. A number of problems are included in Appendix 7 and suggestions for further reading are made in Appendix 8.

In conclusion, we wish to record our thanks to those colleagues and students who, by providing advice, comments and data, have helped us with the preparation of this manuscript. We are particularly indebted to Mrs Morag Perrott for producing the diagrams in the Medical Art Department of the Royal Marsden Hospital under the direction of Miss Lindsey Pegus; also to Mrs Louise Parkes and Mrs Betty Pycock who produced the typescript and Mrs Mary P. Taylor, B.Sc., M.R.I.C. who prepared the index. One of us (P.H.S.S.) is grateful to the Queensland Institute of Technology for secretarial assistance whilst he was Visiting Fellow during 1976. The patience and understanding of Miss Mary Emmerson of Churchill Livingstone throughout the prolonged gestation period of this book is greatly appreciated.

Royal Marsden Hospital,   R.P.P.
Sutton, Surrey   P.H.S.S.
1978   D.M.T.

Contents

1

Introduction

In broad terms nuclear medicine may be defined as the application of radionuclide techniques to the diagnosis and treatment of human disease. Although nuclear medicine has become a medical specialty only during the last fifteen or so years, radium-226 implants were first used for the treatment of tumours early this century and radioiodine was first used for the investigation of thyroid disease just prior to the Second World War.

Contemporary clinical radionuclide methods may be divided broadly into three groups. The largest division can be described as Diagnostic Procedures, such as organ imaging, in which a radionuclide, in a suitable chemical form, is administered to the patient and the distribution of radioactivity in the body is determined by an external radiation detector. In addition to producing a simple image of an organ or the whole body (Fig. 1.2), these techniques may also yield information on the function of some organs, for example, the kidneys or the heart (Fig. 1.3). Such functional examinations are becoming increasingly important, particularly in relation to cardiac and lung function studies. The second largest division of nuclear medicine, an area which is constantly expanding, does not involve administration of radionuclides to the patient but utilises radionuclide techniques to measure the concentrations of hormones, antibodies, drugs and other clinically important substances in samples of blood or tissues. The third broad classification of nuclear medicine, covering the therapeutic applications of radionuclides administered to patients, now represents only a small fraction of all nuclear medicine work and is primarily concerned with the treatment of thyroid disease. The main subdivisions of nuclear medicine are illustrated in Table 1.1.

Nuclear medicine is not the only investigatory technique involving radiation. Radiology is the oldest and nuclear magnetic resonance one of the newest. Ultrasonic techniques are becoming increasingly widespread in clinical departments, and in addition thermographic imaging has a specialised role to play. Computerised tomography was

1

Table 1.1 The major divisions of nuclear medicine

In vivo

Diagnostic: *Organ Imaging* e.g. Liver scan for the detection of a tumour.
                   Whole Body Imaging e.g. Skeletal survey for the detection of metastases.
                   Organ Uptake e.g. Determination of thyroid function using radioiodine.
                   Whole Body Retention e.g. Measurement of the absorption of orally administered Vitamin B-12
                   Dynamic Studies e.g. The investigation of cardiac function.
                   Body Spaces e.g. Measurement of plasma volume by isotope dilution analysis.

Therapeutic: *Treatment* e.g. Hyperthyroidism with iodine-131.

In vitro

Biochemical analysis: *Assay* of hormones, enzymes and other substances by radioimmunoassay, saturation analysis and related techniques.

originally developed for use with X-rays and has had a considerable impact on diagnostic radiology; similar techniques are now used in other imaging modalities, for example, nuclear medicine and nuclear magnetic resonance. All these investigative techniques provide clinical information of different types, as illustrated in Figures 1.1 to 1.7. Full information on other imaging modalities is given in specialist texts, but a summary is provided in Table 1.2.

Whereas the images produced by X-rays or ultrasound depend on the varying abilities of the body organs and tissues to transmit, absorb or scatter the incident radiation, nuclear medicine has an essentially functional basis as the image depends on the ability of the organ and tissue to concentrate the radionuclide. The distribution of any radioactive substance introduced into the body is dependent on physiological factors such as blood flow, vascular and extravascular fluid volumes, metabolic activity or the presence of phagocytic cells.

Table 1.2 Characteristics of different imaging modalities

Diagnostic radiology:	X-ray attenuation coefficients (predominantly density)
Nuclear medicine:	physiological function
Ultrasound:	mechanical and elastic properties
Thermography:	superficial temperature distribution
Nuclear magnetic resonance:	mobile proton distribution and environment

Thus the distribution of a radioactive substance in both space and time will be markedly dependent on its chemical properties. The radioactive substances used in nuclear medicine are generally called *radiopharmaceuticals*.

All nuclear medicine procedures can be regarded as requiring two essential components, a radiation detection system of adequate sensitivity and resolution and a radiopharmaceutical which will give an acceptable degree of localisation in the desired organ or tissue. Consequently, it is essential that everyone who is engaged in nuclear medicine should have a sound understanding of the basic physics of radioactivity and radiation detection systems as well as a knowledge of the chemistry of radiopharmaceuticals and of the mechanisms which underlie their localisation in specific organs or tissues.

These subjects, and related practical topics such as laboratory procedures, and radiation and other safety requirements, are discussed in the succeeding chapters of this book.

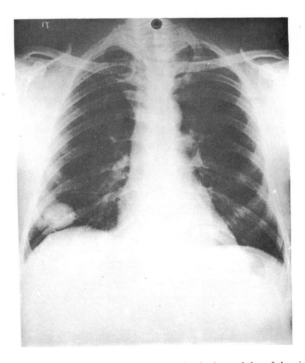

Fig. 1.1 Chest X-ray showing metastatic tumour in the lower lobe of the right lung. (Courtesy of Dr. J. S. Macdonald, Royal Marsden Hospital, London.)

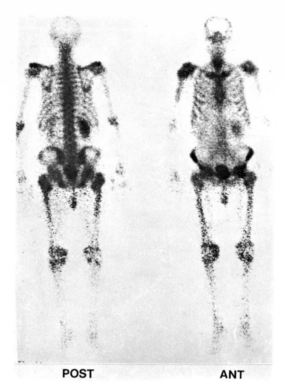

POST   **ANT**

Fig. 1.2 Whole body anterior (right) and posterior (left) images of a normal skeleton taken with a scanner after injection with 10 mCi of a Tc-99m labelled bone agent. (Courtesy of Internuclear Ltd., Swindon, England).

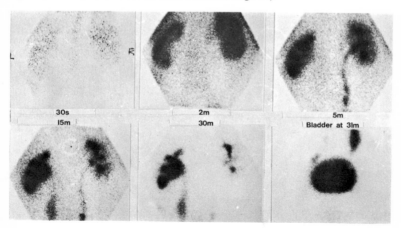

Fig. 1.3. Dynamic study, using a gamma camera, of the kidneys after injection of 10 mCi of Tc-99m DTPA. The times of the images after injection are indicated on the figure. Both kidneys are well perfused at 2 minutes and there is rapid transit of the radiopharmaceutical to dilated collecting systems and ureters. There is more retention of the radioactivity in the left kidney compared to the right. (Courtesy of Department of Nuclear Medicine, Guy's Hospital, London).

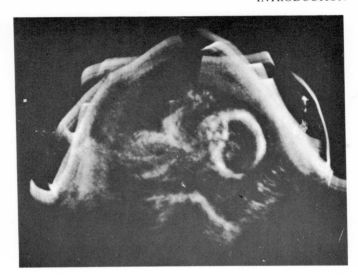

Fig. 1.4 Ultrasound scan of a transverse section through the abdomen showing foetus at 37 weeks gestation. (Courtesy of Dr. A. E. Joseph, Department of Nuclear Medicine and Ultrasound, Royal Marsden Hospital, London).

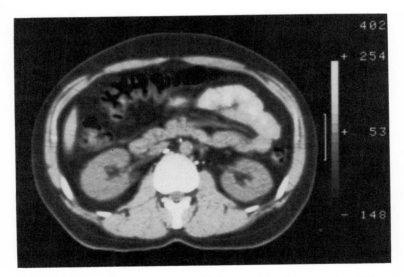

Fig. 1.5 A computerised axial tomographic image of the abdomen taken at the level of the kidneys. (Courtesy of Dr Janet Husband, CRC CT-Unit, Royal Marsden Hospital, Sutton, Surrey)

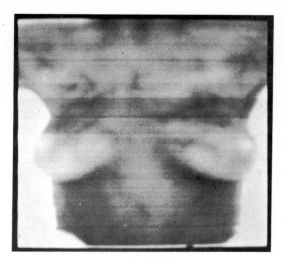

Fig. 1.6 Thermogram of normal breasts showing prominent vascularity where black represents warm tissue and white cold. (Courtesy of Dr C. H. Jones, Royal Marsden Hospital, London).

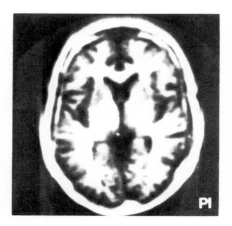

Fig. 1.7 A nuclear magnetic resonance (NMR) scan taken as a cross-section through the head. (Courtesy of Hammersmith Hospital, London and Picker International)

PART ONE

Basic physics

2

Radiation and matter

All the techniques discussed in Chapter 1 have involved radiation. In this book we are concerned with radiation emitted from radioactive substances. Two classes of radiation are emitted, particles and electromagnetic radiation. The former plays an important part in radionuclide therapy whilst the latter is the type principally involved in organ imaging.

2.1 Electromagnetic radiation

All electromagnetic radiation has the same nature and characteristics, only differing in energy. Separate names are used which indicate either the energy range or the mode of production. X-rays and gamma rays may have identical energy and differ only in the way they are produced. X-rays are produced when the energy of electrons changes and are normally generated by the bombardment of a target by high speed electrons, whilst gamma radiation originates from the nucleus of radioactive atoms. Other well known types of electromagnetic radiation are visible light, radio waves, infrared (used in thermography) and ultra violet. As can be seen from Figure 2.1, there is an enormous energy difference between high energy gamma or X-radiation and low energy radio waves. The standard unit for measuring energy is the joule (J) but the electron volt (eV) is still widely used. This is the amount of energy equal to the change in energy of one electronic charge when it moves through a potential of one volt. One eV approximately equals 1.6×10^{-19} J. For a full list of the basic units and their symbols see Appendix 3.

Electromagnetic radiation can be thought of in terms of 'packets of energy' called photons. For example, a 100 watt electric light bulb emits about 10^{20} visible light photons per second. Similarly when a radioactive substance gives off electromagnetic radiation it emits photons of a characteristic energy; however, far fewer protons are involved, and a nuclear medicine test may involve less than a million photons being emitted per second from the radioactive material used. Generally only a very small fraction of the photons emitted are

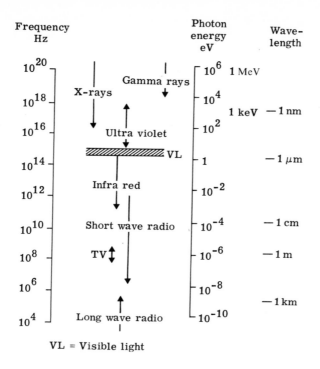

Fig. 2.1 The electromagnetic spectrum.

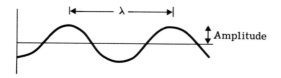

Fig. 2.2 Representation of wave motion of electromagnetic radiation.

detected and each photon is counted separately. Photons have no charge and in a vacuum they all, whatever their energy, travel with the velocity of light.

In some situations it is useful to think of electromagnetic radiation in terms of waves. This is most applicable when one is dealing with a very large number of photons, as in the case of visible light from an electric light bulb, rather than with individual high energy photons, such as encountered in dealing with gamma radiation. However, the two approaches are entirely complementary. A wave motion is characterised by the wavelength (λ), the distance from crest to crest, and frequency (ν), the number of oscillations of the wave per second (Fig. 2.2). The unit used to measure frequency is the hertz, equal to one cycle per second. The frequency and wavelength are linked by a fundamental constant—the velocity of light. Another one, Planck's constant, links frequency with energy. These relationships are set out in Table 2.1.

Table 2.1 Some fundamental characteristic properties and relationships used in discussing electromagnetic radiation

Characteristic properties:

Quantity	Unit	Symbol	Definition and conversion factors
Energy	joule	J	$\text{kg m}^2 \text{ s}^{-2}$
	electron volt	eV	$1 \text{ eV} \simeq 1 \cdot 6 \times 10^{-19} \text{ J}$
Frequency	hertz	Hz	s^{-1}
Wavelength	—	λ	m, μm or nm

Constants:

	Symbol	Value
Velocity of light	c	$3 \times 10^8 \text{ m s}^{-1}$
Planck's constant	h	$6 \cdot 6 \times 10^{-34} \text{ J s}$

Relationships:

Frequency and wavelength

$$\nu = \frac{c}{\lambda} \tag{2.1}$$

Energy and frequency

$$E = h\nu \tag{2.2}$$

Combining 2.1 and 2.2

$$E = \frac{hc}{\lambda}.$$

Inverse square law

$$I \propto \frac{1}{r^2}. \qquad \begin{aligned} I &= \text{intensity} \\ r &= \text{distance from source.} \end{aligned}$$

Worked example

A radioactive substance emits electromagnetic radiation of 0·51 MeV What is the energy in joules, the wavelength and frequency of the radiation?

$$E = 0\cdot51 \text{ MeV}$$

now
$$1 \text{ eV} \simeq 1\cdot6 \times 10^{-19} \text{ J}$$

$$\therefore \quad 0\cdot51 \text{ MeV} \simeq 0\cdot51 \times 10^6 \times 1\cdot6 \times 10^{-19} \text{ J}$$

$$= 0\cdot82 \times 10^{-13} \text{ J}.$$

To find frequency use equation 2.2 (Table 2.1)

$$E = hv$$

$$\therefore \quad v = \frac{E}{h} = \frac{0\cdot82 \times 10^{-13}}{6\cdot6 \times 10^{-34}} \text{ Hz}$$

$$= 0\cdot12 \times 10^{21} \text{ Hz}$$

To find wavelength use equation 2.1 (Table 2.1)

$$\lambda = \frac{c}{v} = \frac{3 \times 10^8}{0\cdot12 \times 10^{21}} = 2\cdot5 \times 10^{-12} \text{ m}$$

Check that the answers correspond with Figure 2.1.

Inverse square law

The intensity of a beam of electromagnetic radiation is the radiation energy flowing per second across a unit area perpendicular to the beam. If there is a point source of radiation the intensity in air will vary inversely as the square of the distance from that point. This is because the area through which the photons pass increases as the square of the distance and therefore the intensity must vary inversely as the square as shown diagrammatically in Figure 2.3.

2.2. Matter

Radiation emitted by radioactive substances may be wholly or partly composed of particles. In order to understand this type of radiation, the production of all types of radiation and their interaction with matter, it is necessary to know about the structure of matter and the basic particles from which it is composed and their properties.

Matter has the property of mass, that is, it interacts with other matter by means of gravitational force. In simple terms—you can weigh matter. It may be charged or neutral; if charged this charge may be positive or negative. Charged particles interact with each other via

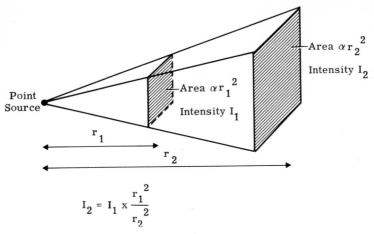

$$I_2 = I_1 \times \frac{r_1^2}{r_2^2}$$

Fig. 2.3 The intensity of radiation from a point-source varies inversely as the square of the distance.

the electrostatic force: unlike charges attract, like charges repel (Table 2.2).

There are two types of energy associated with matter, kinetic energy and potential energy. A body has kinetic energy due to its motion and this is equal to $\frac{1}{2}mv^2$, where m is its mass and v its velocity. Potential energy is due to the presence of gravitational attraction. A mass will fall to the earth when released; before this it has potential energy which is converted to kinetic energy as it falls. When it hits the ground the kinetic energy gained is itself converted to heat and sound energy. A charged body separated from another one of opposite

Table 2.2 Characteristic properties and interactions of matter

Characteristic properties:

Quantity	Name	Symbol	Definition
Mass	kilogram	kg	—
Electric charge	coulomb	C	sA

Interactions:

$$\text{Gravitational force} \propto \frac{m_1 m_2}{r^2}$$

$$\text{Electrostatic force} \propto \frac{q_1 q_2}{r^2}$$

where m_1 and q_1 are the mass and charge of particle 1 which interacts with another particle 2 of mass m_2 and charge q_2 at a distance r away.

charge will have electrostatic potential energy as well as gravitational potential energy.

Matter is made up of atoms and these in turn are composed of elementary particles. Many of these have been found but there are only four of importance to us. The particles which make up the nucleus are known collectively as nucleons and are of two types: protons, which carry a positive electrical charge, and neutrons which are uncharged. The third type of particle involved in the structure of the atom is the electron which carries a negative electrical charge equal in magnitude to the positive charge on the proton. Electrons are distributed outside the nucleus in orbits or shells and a more detailed discussion of the structure of the atom is given in the next chapter. A positron is identical to the electron except that it has a positive charge, opposite to that of the electron. It can be described as an 'anti-electron' and when it comes in contact with an electron both are annihilated. We shall see (Section 7.5) that this annihilation plays an important part in the production of 'annihilation radiation', a form of electromagnetic radiation.

The mass and charge of the elementary particles are often expressed in terms of the mass and charge of the proton (Table 2.3).

Table 2.3 The elementary particles

Particle		Charge		Mass	
		Coulombs	In terms of proton	kg	In terms of proton
Proton	} Nucleons	$+1.6 \times 10^{-19}$	$+1$	$1 \cdot 7 \times 10^{-27}$	1
Neutron		0	0	$1 \cdot 7 \times 10^{-27}$	1
Electron		$-1 \cdot 6 \times 10^{-19}$	-1	9×10^{-31}	1/1836
Positron		$+1 \cdot 6 \times 10^{-19}$	$+1$	9×10^{-31}	1/1836

2.3.   Radiation and matter

At the beginning of this century Albert Einstein showed that matter and radiation are not two completely separate entities, but are linked by his now famous equation:

$$E = mc^2 \qquad \begin{aligned} E &= \text{energy} \\ m &= \text{mass} \\ c &= \text{velocity of light.} \end{aligned}$$

The equation states that the mass of a particle or body is equivalent to a certain amount of energy, called the rest mass energy. The total energy of a body is therefore made up of:

Rest mass energy $(E = mc^2)$
Potential energy
Kinetic energy $(E = \frac{1}{2}mv^2)$ $v =$ velocity.

It was later shown that actual conversion could take place and matter be converted into energy. The converse, the transformation of energy in the form of radiation into mass, can also occur under special situations. This interconversion plays a major role in some of the phenomena underlying the practice of nuclear medicine. The whole of nuclear energy (Ch. 8) is based on it. One of the ways high energy gamma rays interact with matter is by transformation of the gamma ray energy into matter by creation of two particles (the phenomena of pair production—Ch. 7). In one mechanism of radioactive decay the atoms emit positrons which interact with electrons and mutually annihilate each other—their mass being converted into energy in the form of radiation (Ch. 5).

Worked example
What is the rest mass energy, in MeV, of an electron?

Mass of electron $= 9 \times 10^{-31}$ kg

Velocity of light $= 3 \times 10^8$ m s^{-1}

$$\therefore \quad E = 9 \times 10^{-31} \times (3 \times 10^8)^2 = 81 \times 10^{-15} J$$

Now $1\,eV = 1 \cdot 6 \times 10^{-19}$ J

$$\therefore \quad E = 0 \cdot 51 \text{ MeV}.$$

Photons or waves?
Electromagnetic radiation can be described in terms of photons or waves. When dealing with the relatively high energy electromagnetic radiation encountered in nuclear medicine the photon description is usually the most appropriate. Photons have particle-like properties but they do not have mass in the same sense that a stationary electron or other particle of matter has mass.

2.4. Conclusion

The fundamental properties of radiation and matter have been summarised in this Chapter. It has been shown that under certain circumstances matter can be created from electromagnetic radiation and vice versa. Some texts are recommended in Appendix 8 for those who wish to study the subject in more detail.

3

Atomic and nuclear structure

3.1. The atom

Over the centuries chemists have found that matter can be broken down into a limited number of substances—the chemical elements. There are just over a hundred elements and the basic unit or 'building block' is the atom.

The atom is composed of three elementary particles: the proton, the neutron and the electron (Table 2.3). The protons and neutrons (the nucleons) make up a small central nucleus whilst the electrons circle about this nucleus in orbits, called shells. The nucleus is extremely small compared with the overall size of the atom—the nucleus has a diameter of the order of 10^{-14} m compared with 10^{-10} m for the atom. This is equivalent to a football in the middle of a stadium.

The nucleus will be positively charged due to the protons, creating an attractive electrostatic force between the nucleus and the electrons arranged in orbits at different radii from the nucleus. A helpful analogy is the solar system with the earth and other planets (the electrons) circling around the sun (the nucleus) (Fig. 3.1). In the case of the solar system the forces involved are gravitational, but these play no role in the binding of the atom or nucleus. This is because the electrostatic force is far stronger. It should be remembered that the atom is a three-dimensional structure (Fig. 3.2) and that representations are highly schematic.

Unlike the solar system there are two restrictions on the atom, one is that there are a limited number of shells allowed and the other is that the total number of electrons in a shell is restricted. The shells are known by the letters K, L, M, etc. (Fig. 3.1) and the maximum number of electrons in these shells are 2, 8, 18. In heavy atoms several of the shells may be only partly filled.

The simplest atom is that of hydrogen, which has one proton and one electron in the K-shell. Helium has two protons, two neutrons and a filled K-shell. Lithium has three protons, four neutrons, two

THE ATOM   THE SOLAR SYSTEM

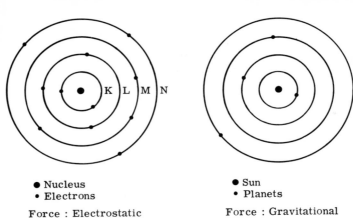

- Nucleus   ● Sun
- Electrons   • Planets

Force : Electrostatic   Force : Gravitational

Fig. 3.1 Comparison between the atom and the solar system.

electrons in the K-shell and one in the L-shell. These are illustrated in Figure 3.3.

The atom of each element has a definite number of protons in the nucleus—the atomic (or proton) number (symbol Z) and, since in its ground state the atom is electrically neutral, it is this number which determines the electronic structure of the atom and hence the chemical properties. The number of neutrons is given by the neutron number (N) and the total number of nucleons is called the atomic mass number (A). Some examples are shown in Table 3.1 with the notation used to characterise an atom.

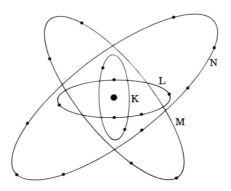

Fig. 3.2 Representation of the atom.

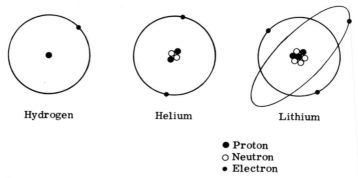

Hydrogen   Helium   Lithium

● Proton
○ Neutron
● Electron

Fig. 3.3 The atoms $^1_1$H, $^4_2$He and $^7_3$Li.

Potential and kinetic energy of electrons in shells
An electron separated from a positive nucleus will have electrostatic potential energy (Section 2.2). As it approaches and goes into orbit round the nucleus some of the energy is converted into kinetic energy and some is given off in the form of electromagnetic radiation—X-rays. The electrons in each shell of an atom have definite potential and kinetic energies due to their rotation around the nucleus.

Energy of electron = Potential energy + Kinetic energy.

Potential energy is normally, arbitrarily, taken as zero at infinity and so the potential energy of an electron in a shell is negative. This convention is confusing as it is the opposite of what one might expect. The potential energy is numerically greater than the kinetic energy and therefore the total energy will have a negative sign.

Table 3.1 The atomic and mass number of a selection of atoms

Element	Z	N	A	Symbol
Hydrogen	1	0	1	$^1_1$H
Helium	2	2	4	$^4_2$He
Oxygen	8	8	16	$^{16}_8$O
Copper	29	34	63	$^{63}_{29}$Cu
Lead	82	126	208	$^{208}_{82}$Pb
Uranium	92	146	238	$^{238}_{92}$U

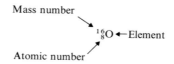

Mass number
$^{16}_8$O ← Element
Atomic number

Binding energy. The energy of an electron in a shell is often described in terms of its binding energy. This is the energy required to remove the electron from the atom. Numerically it will be equal to the total energy but of opposite sign.

For hydrogen:

K-shell electron.

Potential energy (PE) $= -26\,\mathrm{eV}$ (negative by definition—see above)

Kinetic energy (KE) $= +12 \cdot 5\,\mathrm{eV}$

$\therefore$ Total energy $= \mathrm{PE} + \mathrm{KE} = (-26) + 12 \cdot 5$
$= -13 \cdot 5\,\mathrm{eV}$

and Binding energy $= +13 \cdot 5\,\mathrm{eV}.$

The higher the atomic number of the atom the greater the binding energy of the electrons, varying for the *K*-shell as the square of the atomic number. The energy of electrons in outer shells is complicated by the interactions between electrons. Another effect of increasing atomic number is to reduce the radius of the shells.

Energy levels. The energy levels of electrons in two atoms, carbon and lead, are illustrated in Figure 3.4. Carbon is a relatively light atom and a major constituent of the body. Lead is the heaviest atom commonly encountered and widely used for collimation and in radiation protection. It will be noticed that the energy of the shells falls off rapidly with shell number, a result of the increasing radius and the 'screening' effect of the inner shell electrons on the nuclear charge seen by the outer electrons.

Ionization. This is the removal of an electron from an atom leaving it in a charged state

$$A \rightarrow A^+ + e^-.$$

Excitation. This occurs when energy is given to an atom sufficient to raise an electron to a lower binding energy shell but not sufficient for it to escape completely from the atom. An electron might be excited from the K to O shell for example

$$A \rightarrow A^*.$$

3.2.   Characteristic radiation

When an atom is ionized by removing an electron from an inner shell a vacancy will be left. Three mechanisms can cause a vacancy in an inner shell: the photoelectric effect, internal conversion and electron capture. These three processes will be discussed in detail in Chapters 5

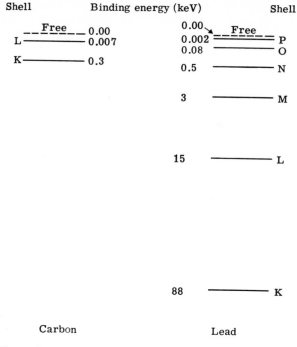

Fig. 3.4   Electronic energy levels of carbon and lead. Only principal shells are shown.

and 7. The vacancy is filled by an electron from a shell with a lower binding energy. This in turn creates a vacancy and the process will be repeated until an electron from outside the atom is captured (Fig. 3.5).

When each electron changes level it will change its energy and the binding energy difference between the shells is released in the form of an X-ray. Each atom has a unique set of energy levels and so the energy of the several X-rays emitted following a vacancy occurring in an inner shell will be characteristic of the atom.

In Figure 3.5 the vacancy in the K-shell is filled by an electron from the L-shell, giving rise to an X-ray known as an K_α X-ray. This occurs the majority of times but in about 20 per cent of cases it would be filled by an electron directly from the M-shell (K_β X-ray). Similarly the vacancy created in the L-shell is normally filled from the M shell (L_α X-ray) but sometimes from the N-shell (L_β X-ray).

3.3.   Chemical binding

The inner shells have fairly high energies—typically in the keV range. The outer electrons have energies of a few eV (Fig. 3.4) and it is these

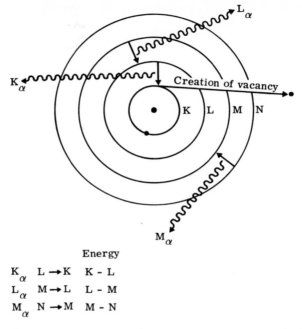

Energy		
K_α	$L \rightarrow K$	$K - L$
L_α	$M \rightarrow L$	$L - M$
M_α	$N \rightarrow M$	$M - N$

Fig. 3.5 Production of characteristic X-rays after creation of a vacancy in the K-shell.

outer electrons which are involved in the chemical binding of one atom to another. The inner electrons play no part in bonding as they have complete shells. This is discussed in further detail, together with the different types of chemical bonds, in Chapter 30.

3.4.   Modern concepts of the structure of the atom

The model of the atom which has been described was first put forward by Rutherford and modified by Niels Bohr in 1913. The electrons are thought of as discrete charged particles moving around the atom in well defined orbits at specific distances from the nucleus.

This concept is oversimplified. One is trying to describe the atom in terms appropriate to our day to day experience. It is not really surprising that these terms are incapable of describing something as small as the atom and which is governed by quantum-mechanical laws, such as those defining the radius of the orbits, which are only manifest at the atomic level.

It is more correct to think of the radius of a particular orbit as the average distance of an electron from the nucleus. At this distance from the nucleus the electron is most probably located, but it can be found either nearer the nucleus or further away. This can be visualised by thinking of the electron as 'smeared out' with the degree of blackness indicating the probability of an electron being at a particular place (Fig. 3.6). This approach helps to explain how the K-shell electron can interact with the nucleus in certain phenomena (electron capture and internal conversion, Ch. 5). There is a small, but definite, probability that the K-shell electron will actually be in the nucleus. This will be greater in atoms of high atomic number as the K-shell radius is smaller due to the larger electrostatic attraction.

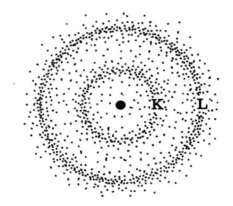

Fig. 3.6 Representation of shells of an atom of sodium.

3.5.   The structure of the nucleus

Nuclear force

The nucleus is very small and contains both neutrons and protons. Protons have a positive charge and there is therefore an electrostatic repulsive force between them. How does the nucleus stay together— why don't the protons fly apart? The neutrons, with no charge, and protons are bound together by a much stronger force, the nuclear force. This is an attractive force between proton and proton, neutron and neutron, and proton and neutron. It has a very short range, extending over only a few inter-nucleon separations, and is therefore entirely confined to the nucleus.

When Table 3.1 is studied it is seen that, apart from hydrogen, the lighter atoms have similar numbers of neutrons and protons but with increasing atomic number there is an increasing excess of neutrons over protons. This can be shown graphically by plotting the neutron number against the atomic (proton) number for all the stable atoms of the elements (Fig. 3.7). The reason for this gradual change is that as

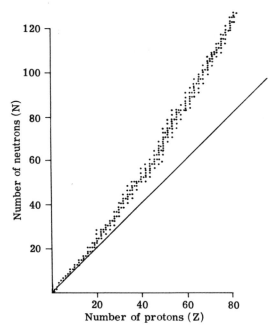

Fig. 3.7 The relationship between the number of proton and number of neutrons for all the stable atoms. The nuclei would all lie on the line at 45 degrees if they had equal numbers of protons and neutrons.

the number of protons increases so does the total electrostatic repulsive force. Although the nuclear force is strong it has a limited range, less than the radius of a large nucleus, and so to keep the nucleus stable extra neutrons are required. These will add to the total nuclear attraction but not affect the electrostatic repulsion.

Nuclear shells

How are the neutrons and protons arranged in the nucleus? A useful but simple model is to think of them arranged in shells, analogous to the arrangement of electrons outside the nucleus. The idea of electrons at certain radii and in motion round the nucleus should not be carried over to the nucleus but rather the concept of energy levels with a certain maximum number of particles in each level. Electron shells are full when they have 2, 8, 18 and 32 in the *K*, *L*, *M*, and *N* shells respectively. Atoms with filled shells are chemically stable and are known as the inert gases—helium, neon, argon and krypton (Ch. 29). In the nucleus the corresponding numbers are 2, 6, 12 and 8; the protons and neutrons have separate shells. When a nucleus has only filled shells an extra nuclear stability is conferred on it, an example is the helium nucleus, with 2 protons and 2 neutrons. It is this special stability of the helium nucleus which explains why it is ejected as a particle in *alpha* decay (Ch. 5) but protons or other elementary nuclei are not expelled from nuclei in radioactive decay events. What is the next especially stable nucleus?

Normally nuclei are in the ground state but can, in special situations exist for a limited time in an excited state. Again an analogy can be drawn with the electronic excitation of atoms where X-radiation is emitted when they de-excite to the ground state. When a nucleus in an excited state falls to the ground state electromagnetic radiation is emitted when they de-excite to the ground state. When a gamma ray is equal to the difference in energy of the two nuclear states.

Figure 3.8 shows some of the nuclear energy levels of an atom of xenon—generally the level schemes are very complex. A nucleus stays in an excited state in most cases for only a very brief period, 10^{-6}–10^{-14} s. However, sometimes nuclei can exist in excited energy states for minutes or hours. These levels, such as the 164 eV level of xenon, are known as metastable states.

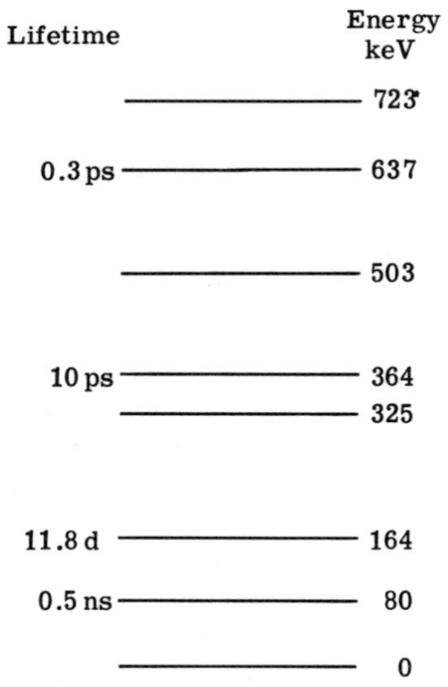

Lifetime	Energy keV
	723
0.3 ps	637
	503
10 ps	364
	325
11.8 d	164
0.5 ns	80
	0

Fig. 3.8 Nuclear energy levels of xenon. The lifetimes of some of the states are indicated (ps = picosecond, 10^{-12}s). The 164 keV level is metastable with a lifetime of 11·8d. Radioactive iodine (^{131}I) decays into xenon.

Nuclide

This is an important term which will be frequently used and denotes a species of atom with a specific atomic number Z, neutron number N and in a defined nuclear state. Normally it is assumed that the nucleus is in the ground state and the same symbolism is used as for an atom, for example, $^{131}_{53}I$ represents an atom of the element iodine with a total mass of 131 and 53 protons. If the nucleus is in a metastable state then this is represented by the superscript m, thus $^{99}_{43}Tc$ is a different nuclide from $^{99}_{43}Tc^m$.

3.6. Isotopes

An isotope is one of a group of nuclides all having the same proton number. This group is therefore made up of different nuclides of the same element. They differ in neutron number and in some cases, nuclear state. Because they only differ in their complement of neutrons they have similar physical properties and the same chemical properties. Three examples will be discussed which illustrate important points:

Hydrogen. There are three isotopes of hydrogen

$$^1_1H \qquad ^2_1H(^2_1D) \qquad \text{and} \qquad ^3_1H$$

Hydrogen   Deuterium   Tritium

These isotopes are unique in that they have separate names and deuterium has the symbol D. The physical properties of compounds made with deuterium differ from their equivalent compounds made with hydrogen due to the factor of two in the mass of the two isotopes. Deuterium oxide, D_2O is known as heavy water and plays an important part in some designs of reactors (Ch. 8). Hydrogen and deuterium are stable but tritium is radioactive.

Chlorine. Natural chlorine is composed of two stable isotopes

$$^{37}_{17}Cl \quad (24 \cdot 5\% \text{ abundance}) \quad \text{and} \quad ^{35}_{17}Cl \quad (75 \cdot 5\% \text{ abundance}).$$

This explains why the relative atomic mass of natural chlorine is $35 \cdot 5$ and not a whole number. There is a further discussion of relative atomic mass in Chapter 30. Isotopes can be, and often are, stable and the term is often misused to imply radioactivity.

Iodine. We will be looking at several isotopes of iodine in the following Chapters. There are 23 isotopes in all, twenty-two are unstable ($^{117}_{53}I \rightarrow ^{139}_{53}I$) and $^{127}_{53}I$ is the only stable one. It will be noticed that about half are lighter and half heavier than the stable isotope. In general the greater the difference in mass between an unstable and stable isotope the greater the instability of the radioactive isotope.

Care should be exercised to use the word radioisotope correctly. It is often mistakenly used in place of the word radionuclide. For example it is correct to say 'there are twenty-two radioisotopes of iodine' but not that 'the radioisotope ^{131}I was used in this investigation'.

4

Radioactivity

4.1. Nuclear instability

Nuclides which do not have a stable combination of neutrons and protons undergo radioactive decay. For a given element, that is a fixed atomic number (Z), there may be several isotopes which are stable. Other isotopes of the element are unstable and the nuclei will at some stage transform to either completely stable or more stable combinations. This transformation, radioactive decay, involves either the expulsion of a charged particle or the capture of an electron by the nucleus. This process will alter the balance of neutrons to protons,

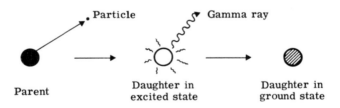

Fig. 4.1 Radioactive decay.

and an atom of a different element is formed. The nucleus may be left in an excited state by the transformation and will in most cases immediately de-excite to the ground state with the emission of one or more gamma rays.

The unstable nuclide is often referred to as the parent and the product as the daughter. The daughter may not always be stable and may itself subsequently decay.

The prefix radioactive is used to denote nuclear instability and hence the potential to undergo spontaneous transformation into another atom. Hence the terms radioactive atom, radioactive isotope and radioactive nuclide—the latter two are usually abbreviated to radioisotope and radionuclide.

A radioactive substance is one which contains radioactive atoms. The atom being transformed in radioactive decay is sometimes said to disintegrate, a rather misleading term as usually only a single particle is involved, either entering or leaving the nucleus.

4.2. Rate of decay and half-life

The rate at which the nuclei of a given radionuclide decay is characteristic of that radionuclide. It is not affected by the chemical environment of the atom—whether the atom is part of a molecule, in a metallic state, or what type of bonding is involved. Neither is it affected by physical conditions, for example temperature, pressure or exposure to light or other radiation.

Radioactive decay is governed by probabilities. For any given radioactive atom there is a constant chance or probability that it will decay in a stated period of time. Each type of nuclide has its own probability. A nucleus of radioactive iodine (^{131}I) has one chance in a million of decaying every second, whilst the probability for the nuclide ^{99}Tc^m is one in thirty thousand per second.

In a collection of radioactive atoms of the same nuclide each nucleus will be completely independent of other atoms as regards when it actually decays. There is no means of predicting when any particular nucleus will decay. However, on average a certain fraction will disintegrate in a stated length of time. In the case of the ^{131}I, if there are one million radioactive atoms, each with a one in a million chance of decay per second, then on average one will decay each second. In some seconds none will decay, in others, two or three or, rarely, more. There is therefore a certain statistical fluctuation in the number of transformations in a time interval. Of an individual nucleus one can say that it has a certain, and known, chance of decay per second. Of all the atoms taken together one can say that on average a known fraction will decay per second.

The period in which half the atoms will, on average, transform is called the half-life ($T_{1/2}$) of the radionuclide. Figure 4.2 shows a plot of the number of radioactive atoms as a function of time. For ^{131}I the half-life is 8·1 days. If there are a million atoms at the start then half, 500 000 will, on average, decay in 8·1 days. It may actually be 501 183 or 499 021 or some other similar value. We will see later with what precision one can predict the actual number in a given situation. At the end of a further 8·1 days only a quarter of a million radioactive atoms will remain.

The number of atoms remaining decreases in an exponential, not linear, fashion (Fig. 4.2). An exponential decrease always occurs when the rate is proportional to the quantity present. After successive half-

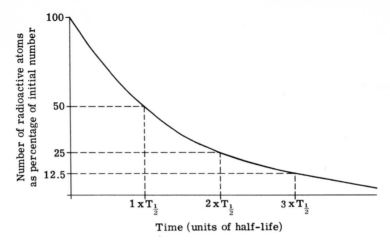

Fig. 4.2 The number of radioactive atoms plotted against time in units of half-life.

lives the fraction remaining is $\frac{1}{2}$, $\frac{1}{4}$, $\frac{1}{8}$, $\frac{1}{16}$ etc. $= 1/2^n$ where n is the number of half-lives which have elapsed and is the exponent of 2 (Appendix 1). The next section describes radioactive decay in a more mathematical form.

4.3. Transformation constant and the decay equation

The chance that a radioactive atom will decay in a stated time is called the transformation constant and will have units of s^{-1}, h^{-1}, d^{-1} or other inverse time interval.

If there are N radioactive atoms and the transformation constant is λ then:

$$\text{Total number decaying per second} = N\lambda.$$

Consider a short period of time t; in this period ΔN atoms will decay:

$$\Delta N = -N\lambda\Delta t. \qquad (4.1)$$

The negative sign is inserted because there is a reduction in the number of radioactive atoms.

This equation can be rewritten:

$$\frac{\Delta N/N}{\Delta t} = -\lambda.$$

This states that the fraction $(\Delta N/N)$ decaying per unit time (Δt) is a constant λ.

A simple equation which is derived in Appendix 2 relates the number of atoms at time t with the initial number N_0 at $t = 0$ and the transformation constant λ

$$N = N_0 e^{-\lambda t}. \tag{4.2}$$

This equation states that the number (N) of radioactive atoms at time t, is equal to the initial number, N_0, multiplied by a factor, $e^{-\lambda t}$. It is a most important equation and can be stated in several ways:

Take $\log_e$ of equation 4.2

$$\log_e N = \log_e (N_0 e^{-\lambda t})$$
$$= \log_e N_0 + \log_e e^{-\lambda t}$$
$$= \log_e N_0 - \lambda t \log_e e$$
$$= \log_e N_0 - \lambda t \qquad (\log_e e = 1)$$

$$\therefore \quad \log_e \left(\frac{N}{N_0}\right) = -\lambda t \quad \text{or} \quad \log_e \left(\frac{N_0}{N}\right) = \lambda t \tag{4.3}$$

now
$$\log_e N = 2 \cdot 303 \log_{10} N \quad \text{(Appendix 1)}$$

$$\therefore \quad \lambda t = 2 \cdot 303 \log_{10} \left(\frac{N_0}{N}\right). \tag{4.4}$$

Half-life

The half-life ($T_{1/2}$) is the period in which half the atoms will decay, that is $N = N_0/2$.

Substituting $t = T_{1/2}$ and $N = N_0/2$ into equation 4.4

$$\lambda T_{1/2} = 2 \cdot 303 \log_{10} 2 = 0 \cdot 693$$

$$\therefore \quad T_{1/2} = \frac{0 \cdot 693}{\lambda} \quad \text{and conversely} \quad \lambda = \frac{0 \cdot 693}{T_{1/2}}. \tag{4.5}$$

In section 4.2 the number of radioactive atoms present was plotted as a function of time and a curve obtained. One property of this curve is that it never actually reaches zero—it is said to tend towards zero. The reason for this is that with every passage of a half-life the number of atoms remaining is halved, so however many half-lives are allowed to elapse the number never reaches zero—a half of something is never zero!

If the number of atoms is plotted on a logarithmic scale then a straight line is obtained. The reason for the straight line can be clearly seen by rearranging equation 4.4

$$\log_{10} N = \frac{-\lambda}{2 \cdot 303} t + \log_{10} N_0$$

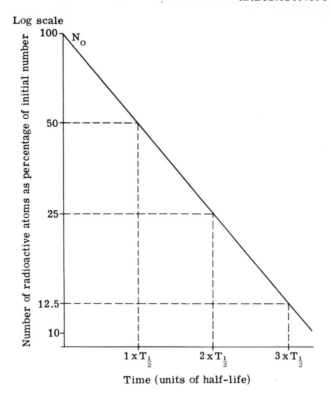

Fig. 4.3 Plot of radioactive atoms versus time. Note the log scale for the number of radioactive atoms and that the time is measured in units of half-life. Compare with Figure 4.2.

now $y = mx + c$ — equation for a straight line (Appendix 1)

so $y \equiv \log_{10}N$

and

$$m \equiv \text{slope} = \frac{-\lambda}{2 \cdot 303}$$

and

$$c = \text{constant} = \log_{10}N_0.$$

The log graph of decay can be plotted either using log-linear graph paper or by taking the log of the activity (using tables or an electronic calculator) and plotting on linear-linear paper (Appendix 1).

Mean life
The average time a radioactive nucleus survives is called the mean life, $\bar{T}$. This is longer than the half-life because, although half the atoms decay in the first half-life, the remainder do not all decay in the second half. The mean life ($\bar{T}$) is related to the half-life by the factor 1·44

$$\bar{T} = 1\cdot44\, T_{1/2}.$$

This relationship can be easily derived. If there are N radioactive atoms and λ is the transformation constant then

number decaying per second, $\Delta N = N\lambda$

$$\therefore \quad \frac{N}{\Delta N} = \frac{1}{\lambda}$$

$$= \frac{T_{1/2}}{0\cdot693} = 1\cdot44\, T_{1/2} \qquad \left(\lambda = \frac{0\cdot693}{T_{1/2}}\right)$$

now

$$\frac{N}{\Delta N} = \bar{T}$$

$$\therefore \quad \bar{T} = 1\cdot44\, T_{1/2}.$$

The mean life is used in dosimetry calculations (see Ch. 9).

4.4. Measurement of activity
The amount of radioactivity is measured in terms of the transformation rate—the number of decays which occur in unit time. The becquerel is the unit of activity and it is equal to one transformation per second and has the symbol Bq. This is an extremely small unit and normally the multiples megabecquerel or gigabecquerels are used (Appendix 3).

> 1 becquerel   (1 Bq) = 1   transformation per second
> 1 megabecquerel (1 MBq) = 10^6 transformations per second
> 1 gigabecquerel   (1 GBq) = 10^9 transformations per second

Until recently, and still widely used in some countries, the unit of activity was the curie, symbol Ci. An amount of radioactive material in which there are $3\cdot7 \times 10^{10}$ transformations per second is said to have an activity of 1 curie. The number $3\cdot7 \times 10^{10}$ was chosen for historical reasons as this is the number of transformations occurring per second in one gram of radium. The millicurie (mCi) and microcurie (μCi) were commonly used.

$$1\,\text{mCi} = 3 \cdot 7 \times 10^7 \text{ transformations per second}$$
$$= 37\,\text{MBq}$$
$$1\,\mu\text{Ci} = 3 \cdot 7 \times 10^4 \text{ transformations per second}$$
$$= 37\,\text{kBq} \text{ or } 0 \cdot 037\,\text{MBq}$$

Specific activity

The specific activity is the activity per unit mass of an element or compound containing a radioactive nuclide. It should always be carefully noted when dealing with compounds whether the mass refers to the element or the whole compound. Thus a solution of radioactive sodium iodide ($Na^{131}I$) might be described as having a specific activity $500\,\text{MBq}/\mu\text{g}$ of Iodine whilst a solution of sodium o-hippurate labelled with ^{131}I might have a specific activity of $5\,\text{MBq}/\text{mg}$ sodium o-iodohippurate. The specific activity is also expressed in terms of activity per mol, for example a solution ^{14}C-thymidine might be $2\,\text{GBq}/\text{mmol}$.

Radioactive concentration

This is the activity per unit volume and has units of Bq per litre ($\text{Bq}\,1^{-1}$) or suitable multiples or fractions of these units such as $\text{MBq}\,\text{dl}^{-1}$.

4.5. Radioactive decay calculations

The basic equation has been stated in terms of number of atoms

$$N = N_0 e^{-\lambda t}.$$

However, the N and N_0 can be replaced by any suitable unit, such as activity, radioactive concentration or percentage of initial activity. Hence:

$A = A_0 e^{-\lambda t}$ A_0 = initial activity

$\qquad\qquad\qquad A$ = activity at time t

or

$C = C_0 e^{-\lambda t}$ C_0 = initial radioactive concentration

$\qquad\qquad\qquad C$ = radioactive concentration at time t.

There are several ways of carrying out this type of calculation:
1. Evaluation of $e^{-\lambda t}$. λ must be a dimensionless quantity and compatible units must be used—if λ is in s^{-1} then t must be in s. Once λt has been calculated then $e^{-\lambda t}$ can be looked up in e^{-x} tables.

2. If exponential tables are not available then the decay equation can be evaluated using equation 4.3 or 4.4 and log tables.

3. It is sometimes convenient to draw a straight line plot of the decay, as in Figure 4.3, and read off the percentage remaining at time t. The plot is conveniently constructed using log-linear graph paper and only the value of the half-life is required.

4. When repeat calculations are done on a particular radionuclide a table of the fraction remaining against time is often constructed.

Time	Fraction remaining
0	1·0
$\frac{1}{2}$ hour	0·94
1 hour	0·89
2 hours	0·79

The fraction remaining after $1\frac{1}{2}$ h will be $0·89 \times 0·94$.

5. If $T_{1/2}$ is given either λ can be calculated using equation 4.5 or $t/T_{1/2}$ is calculated, checking t and $T_{1/2}$ are expressed in the same units, and tables of $e^{-t/T_{1/2}}$ (generalised half-life tables) are used.

The following worked examples should help to clarify some of these points. It is essential that basic radioactive decay problems can be easily handled by the student and practice is essential.

Q. A bottle of ^{131}I is delivered on the 3rd November from the manufacturers and it states on the label that the activity will be 400 MBq at 1200 hours on the 11th November.
What is the activity at 1200 hours on the delivery day and on the 27th?
(Assume half-life of ^{131}I is 8 days).

A. Always check whether a problem can be solved simply using the half-life, as in this case. There are eight days, one half-life, between the delivery and calibration date. The activity will therefore be a factor of two greater, that is 800 MBq. On the 27th November, two half-lives (16 days) have elapsed after the calibration date and therefore the activity will have decayed to a quarter. The bottle will then contain 100 MBq.

Q. A bottle contains 600 MBq of ^{18}F in 5 ml at 0900 hours. What volumes of solution must be withdrawn to make up the following patient doses?

90 MBq at 1050 h
60 MBq at 1050 h
90 MBq at 1240 h

(Half-life of ^{18}F is 110 minutes).

A. This problem can also be solved using half-lives. It is usually easiest in this type of calculation to work in terms of radioactive concentration.

At 0900 h radioactive concentration will be $\dfrac{600}{5} = 120\,\text{MBq ml}^{-1}$

At 1050 h radioactive concentration will be $120 \times \tfrac{1}{2} = 60\,\text{MBq ml}^{-1}$

At 1240 h radioactive concentration will be $60 \times \tfrac{1}{2} = 30\,\text{MBq ml}^{-1}$

Thus:

Volume required for 90 MBq at 1050 h $= \dfrac{90}{60}\left(\dfrac{\text{MBq}}{\text{MBq ml}^{-1}}\right) = 1{\cdot}5\,\text{ml}$

Volume required for 60 MBq at 1050 h $= \dfrac{60}{60}\left(\dfrac{\text{MBq}}{\text{MBq ml}^{-1}}\right) = 1{\cdot}0\,\text{ml}$

Volume required for 90 MBq at 1240 h $= \dfrac{90}{30}\left(\dfrac{\text{MBq}}{\text{MBq ml}^{-1}}\right) = 3{\cdot}0\,\text{ml}$

The reader will note that there is not enough activity to supply all the requests—always check that the total volume to be dispensed is not greater than the original volume.

Q. A dose of ^{131}I for a patient has to have an activity of 40 MBq at 1500 h on the 22nd November. The stock bottle states the activity is 120 MBq at 0900 h on the 21st November and that the activity is in 5 ml of solution. What volume of solution must be withdrawn from the bottle to give the correct activity for administration to the patient?
(Transformation constant, $\lambda = 0{\cdot}0866\,\text{d}^{-1}$).

A. Always check what units λ is quoted in—s^{-1}, h^{-1} or d^{-1}. The radioactive concentration at 0900 h on the 21st November $= 22\,\text{MBq ml}^{-1}$. The decay factor can be calculated several ways:

1. Using e^{-x} tables

   $\lambda t = 0{\cdot}087 \times 1{\cdot}25 = 0{\cdot}11$

   From tables $e^{-0{\cdot}11} = 0{\cdot}90$

   $\therefore$ concentration at 1500 h on 22nd November $= 0{\cdot}90 \times 22$

   $$= 19{\cdot}8\,\text{MBq ml}^{-1}$$

   $\therefore$ for 40 MBq withdraw $\dfrac{40}{19{\cdot}8} = 2{\cdot}02\,\text{ml}.$

2. Using $e^{-\lambda t}$ tables for ^{131}I

From tables

t	$e^{-\lambda t}$
6 hours	0·92
24 hours	0·98

∴   Decay factor $= 0·92 \times 0·98 = 0·90$

3. Using equation 4.4

$$\frac{\lambda t}{2·303} = \log_{10}\left(\frac{A_0}{A}\right)$$

Now

$$\frac{0·11}{2·303} = 0·047 \text{ and antilog of } 0·047 \text{ is } 1·11$$

$$\therefore \quad A = \frac{A_0}{1·11} = 0·90\, A_0$$

4.6. Summary

Half-life $T_{1/2}$: Time taken for the radioactivity to decay to half its initial value.

Transformation Constant λ: The probability that an atom will decay in unit time.

Radioactive Decay:

$$A = A_0 e^{-\lambda t} \qquad A_0 = \text{initial activity}$$
$$A = \text{activity at time } t.$$

Activity: Rate of Decay: measured in units of the becquerel (Bq—one transformation per second).

5

Mechanisms of radioactive decay

5.1. Radioactive decay

The non-radioactive isotopes of the 81 elements with at least one stable isotope make up a total of 274 nuclides. For reasons of nuclear stability (Ch. 3) the heavier nuclides have rather more neutrons than protons and therefore a plot of neutron number against atomic number deviates from a straight line (Fig. 3.7).

There are many more unstable nuclides than stable ones, over a thousand are known. A few of these occur naturally but most are produced using either a nuclear reactor or an accelerator (Ch. 36). When plotted on a neutron-proton chart these radionuclides lie either side of the stable nuclides or are grouped at the high atomic number extremity (Fig. 5.1). The latter have too many nucleons for stability

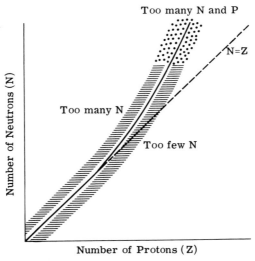

Fig. 5.1 Schematic diagram showing relative position of stable and unstable nuclides. The radionuclides are classified into three groups, those with excess neutrons, those deficient in neutrons and those with an excess of protons and neutrons.

whilst the former have either too few or too many neutrons, depending on which side of the 'line of stability' they occur.

Unstable nuclides achieve stability by radioactive decay, during which they either lose mass by ejection of an alpha particle (helium nucleus) if they have too many nucleons or by changing their ratio of neutrons to protons. This second process is achieved by emitting an electron (beta minus particle) from the nucleus if they have an excess of neutrons or by either emitting a positron (beta plus particle) or capturing an electron if they are neutron deficient (Table 5.1). The new nuclide formed in the decay may be left in an excited nuclear state by the decay process and lose this excess energy by emission of gamma radiation (Fig. 4.1).

Table 5.1 Decay mechanisms

Nuclear instability due to	Mode of decay
Excess neutrons	Beta minus (β^-)
Deficiency in neutrons	Positron (beta plus, β^+)
	or
	Electron capture (EC)
Excess neutrons and protons	Alpha (α)

The decay product (the daughter nuclide) may itself be radioactive and decay (Fig. 5.2). This sequence can be repeated as in the naturally occurring uranium series (Ch. 36).

Figure 5.3 shows an extract from a chart of the nuclides, showing the stable and unstable nuclides, their half-lives and decay mechanisms. The nuclides are arranged according to their proton and neutron number. Apart from showing that the mode of decay is dependent on their position, which is related to the cause of instability, it also shows that, in general, the further a nuclide is from the 'line of stability' the shorter its half-life, reflecting its decreased nuclear stability.

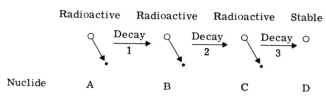

Fig. 5.2 Illustrations of a series of radioactive decays. The final member of the series will be stable.

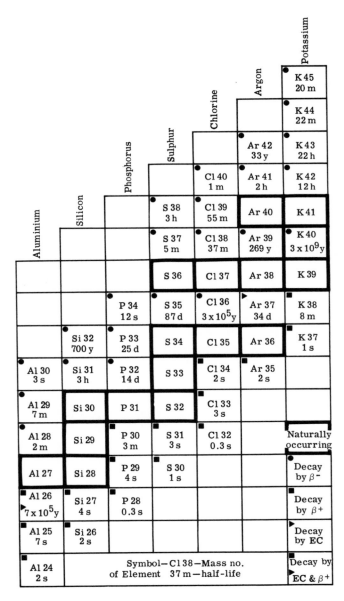

Fig. 5.3 A section from a chart of the nuclides.

The various decay mechanisms (Table 5.1) will be considered in turn, together with the emission of gamma radiation and other processes, such as internal conversion, which can occur during radioactive decay.

5.2.   Nuclides with too many neutrons

Beta decay

Those radioactive nuclides to the left of the stable elements (Figure 5.1) achieve stability by the transformation of a neutron into a proton and electron

$$n \rightarrow p^+ + e^-.$$

The proton stays in the nucleus but the electron (negatron) is emitted from the atom and is called, for historical reasons, a beta particle (β^-). The nucleus as a result has one less neutron and one additional proton (Fig. 5.4).

An example is phosphorus-32 which decays by beta decay into stable sulphur-32

$$^{32}_{15}P \rightarrow ^{32}_{16}S + \beta^-. \hspace{2cm} (5.1)$$

This can be illustrated schematically by the energy level—atomic number diagram shown in Figure 5.5. The energy is that of the total atom, including the rest mass energy. The various states of the parent and daughter are indicated by horizontal lines and atoms of equal

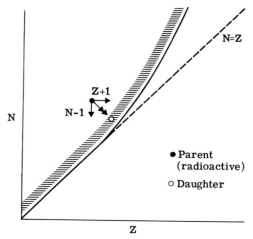

Fig. 5.4 Beta minus decay. The effect on the position of the nuclide of changing a neutron into a proton.

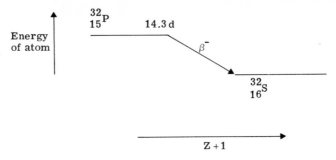

Fig. 5.5 The decay of ^{32}P. Energy of the atom is plotted on the x axis and the atomic number on the y axis.

number are in the same column. Where the daughter nuclide is of higher atomic number than the parent it is displaced to the right; where it is of lower atomic number, to the left. Diagonal lines between two nuclides represent a decay process and vertical lines the emission of gamma radiation. The half-life is usually indicated for radioactive nuclides (14·3 d for ^{32}P) and the energy above the ground state of involved excited nuclear states shown. In this case ^{32}P decays directly to the ground state of ^{32}S by beta decay with the emission of a beta minus particle. Energies shown are relative to the ground state of the nuclide.

The beta particle (an electron) emitted can have a kinetic energy of any value up to a definite maximum energy, which is characteristic of the decay process (Fig. 5.6). The general shape of the spectrum of beta particle energies is similar for many nuclides. Where more complex spectra are observed these are found to be composed of several simple

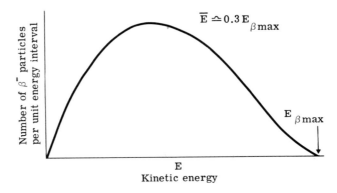

Fig. 5.6 Energy spectrum of beta minus particles.

spectra superimposed. A useful fact to remember is that the average energy is approximately one third the maximum energy.

Beta decay was first fully investigated in the 1920's and 1930's by physicists and the experimental evidence that beta particles had a spectrum of energies rather than a definite discrete value was a major problem. What happened to the difference in energy between the actual energy of the beta particle and the maximum energy? The difference in energy between the parent and daughter nuclides was accounted for when the maximum energy of the beta particle plus any photons emitted was taken into account but not in other situations. There seemed a conflict with the law of conservation of energy. The physicist Wolfgang Pauli suggested in 1931 that an additional particle, called a neutrino, was emitted. This particle would be very hard to detect as it would be electrically neutral and have a very small mass compared with that of the electron. It was not until 1956 that direct evidence of the neutrino was obtained. There are two types, the neutrino (v) and the anti-neutrino (v*) and it is the anti-neutrino which carries off the difference in energy between the beta particle energy and the maximum energy in beta minus decay. Equation 5.1 should be written:

$$^{32}_{15}P \rightarrow ^{32}_{16}S + \beta^- + v*$$

but as the neutrino plays no part in nuclear medicine it is usually omitted from decay equations.

5.3. Gamma radiation

After beta or other decay processes the daughter nucleus is often in an excited state and by emitting electromagnetic radiation (γ-rays) changes to the ground state (Fig. 5.7). This usually happens virtually instantaneously, in less than a millionth of a second, but in certain cases the daughter nuclide can remain in the excited state for a

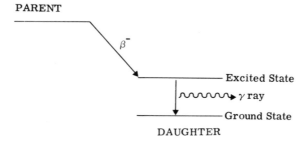

Fig. 5.7 Emission of gamma radiation after beta minus decay.

considerable time (see Section 5.9). This de-excitation is analogous to the situation when an atom in an excited atomic state, caused for example by heating it or bombarding it with electrons, returns to the ground state by emission of electromagnetic radiation (light or X-ray photons). Gamma radiation is a form of electromagnetic radiation and is differentiated from X-rays only by origin; gamma rays coming from the nucleus and X-rays due to changes in the energy of electrons. It is not possible to tell from the energy of a photon whether it is an X-ray or a gamma ray. The gamma rays emitted have discrete (single value) energies, characteristic of the daughter, as they correspond to the energy difference between the two nuclear energy states of the daughter after the primary decay process has taken place.

In many cases the decay schemes of nuclides are more complicated, involving several alternative modes of decay and the emission of gamma rays of different energies. Figure 5.8 shows the decay scheme of cobalt-60. Ninety-nine point eight per cent of ^{60}Co atoms decay by emitting a beta particle (the beta spectrum has a maximum energy of 0·3 MeV) followed by two gamma rays emitted by the daughter nucleus, ^{60}Ni. These two gamma rays, of energies 1·2 and 1·3 MeV, are due to the daughter de-exciting from the 2·5 to 1·3 MeV nuclear state (2·5–1·3 = 1·2) and then from the 1·3 MeV to the ground state. However, 0·2 per cent atoms decay by emitting a beta particle (maximum energy 1·2 + 0·3 = 1·5 MeV) and one gamma ray (1·3 MeV). The overall beta spectrum will be a complex one made up of two simple spectra in the correct intensity ratio (99·8 to 0·2).

5.4. Nuclides with too few neutrons

Nuclides lying to the right of the stable nuclides in Figure 5.1 need to increase their neutron to proton ratio. They can do this by one of two mechanisms, positron emission or electron capture.

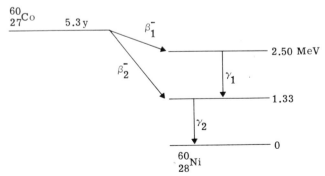

Fig. 5.8 The decay of ^{60}Co.

Positron emission
This is analogous to beta decay but in this case a proton in the nucleus changes into a neutron and a positively charged electron (positron or beta plus particle)

$$p^+ \rightarrow n + \beta^+.$$

The neutron stays in the nucleus but the positron (β^+) is emitted. The resultant nucleus has one less proton and one more neutron and is more stable (Fig. 5.9).

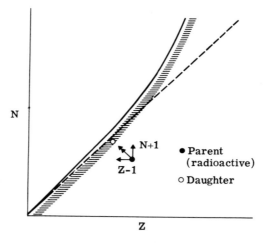

Fig. 5.9 Positron decay and electron capture. The effect on the position of the nuclide of changing a proton into a neutron.

As in the case of electrons emitted during beta minus decay the positrons have a spectrum of energies with a definite maximum energy, characteristic of the decay process. The difference in energy between the maximum energy and the energy of a particular positron is carried away by a neutrino.

An example of positron emission is the decay of fluorine-18 to oxygen-18:

$$^{18}_{9}F \rightarrow ^{18}_{8}O + \beta + \nu.$$

The maximum kinetic energy of the positron is 0·63 MeV. Often the neutrino is omitted from the equation. The decay is shown schematically in Figure 5.10; 97 per cent of ^{18}F atoms decay by this method, the remainder by electron capture.

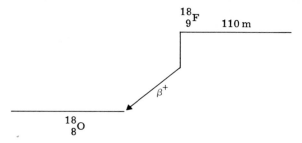

Fig. 5.10 The decay of ^{18}F.

Annihilation radiation

When the positron leaves the nucleus it loses its kinetic energy by interacting with surrounding atoms; when it has lost its kinetic energy it is annihilated by combining with an electron from one of the surrounding atoms, to form two photons, referred to as the annihilation radiation

$$\beta^+ - e^- \rightarrow \gamma + \gamma.$$

The mass of the particles is converted into electromagnetic radiations according to Einstein's equation, $E = mc^2$ (Section 2.3). The two photons each have an energy of 0·51 MeV and they travel in opposite directions so that their net momentum is zero (see Fig. 5.11).

Annihilation radiation is often referred to as a gamma radiation as it results from a nuclear decay process. The special property that the two photons are emitted at 180° to each other can be used in scanning (see Section 26.5).

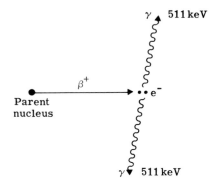

Fig. 5.11 The annihilation of a positron, after being ejected from the atom, with an electron to form two photons of 0·51 MeV.

The term beta decay is sometimes used to cover both decay with the emission of a positron as well as decay with the emission of an electron (negatron) and differentiation between the two is achieved by the use of the terms beta plus and beta minus decay.

Electron capture (K-capture)
This is rather a different mechanism from beta (plus or minus) decay in that no particle (apart from a neutrino) is emitted from the nucleus but an electron is captured from one of the orbitals, most often the *K*-shell, and combines with a proton in the nucleus with the formation of a neutron (and a neutrino)

$$p + e^- \rightarrow n\,(+v).$$

The overall change in the nucleus is exactly the same as in positron decay, one less proton and one more neutron.

An example is the decay of chromium-51 to vanadium-51. Ninety-one per cent of ^{51}Cr atoms decay directly to the ground state of ^{51}V (Fig. 5.12). This is why only nine per cent of the transformations of ^{51}Cr result in a 320 keV gamma ray. The *K*-shell electrons are involved in 90 per cent of captures, the remainder coming from the *L*-shell.

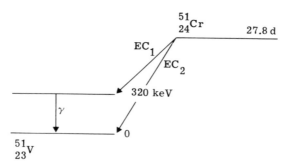

Fig. 5.12 The decay of ^{51}Cr.

Electron capture or positron emission?
Nuclides with too few neutrons can decay by either electron capture (EC) or positron emission, the daughter nucleus being the same in both cases. The probability of which mechanism occurs depends on:

1. *Z* number. The higher the *Z* of the nucleus the closer the *K*-shell is to the nucleus and the greater is the probability of *K*-shell electrons interacting with the nucleus.

2. The difference in energy between the parent and daughter must be at least 1·02 MeV for positron decay to occur. If the energy

difference is less then only electron capture can occur. This is because a positron is ejected from the atom (0·51 MeV) and an orbital electron (0·51 MeV) lost due to the decrease in atomic number of the atom by one. The 1·02 MeV is indicated in the decay diagram by a vertical component in the arrow indicating the transition from the parent to the daughter (Fig. 5.10).

In many cases both mechanisms occur, as we have noted for fluorine-18 where three per cent of transformations occur by electron capture. In the case of chromium-51 the energy difference is only 0·75 MeV, so no positron decay can occur. In general when there is enough energy for positron decay to occur this will predominate, except at higher Z numbers.

5.5.   Internal conversion (IC)

When a daughter nucleus in an excited state makes the transition to the ground state the energy is given off as gamma radiation. However, the situation is rather more complex and the energy may instead be transferred to one of the bound electrons which is ejected from the atom (Fig. 5.13). The process is called internal conversion and can be thought of as analogous to the photo-electric effect, where an external photon interacts with a bound electron and transfers all its energy to

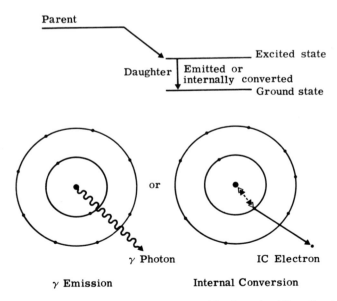

Fig. 5.13 Internal conversion. Gamma rays can either be emitted from the atom or internally converted (IC).

that electron; here the photon can be regarded as emanating from the nucleus—an 'internal photo-electric effect'.

The emitted electron is called the internal conversion (IC) electron and all the energy of the transition is transferred to the electron and used to overcome the binding energy and give it kinetic energy. It should be emphasised that a photon actually never leaves the nucleus when internal conversion takes place.

$$\text{Energy of transition} \rightarrow \text{BE} + \text{KE of electron.}$$

For any given nuclear transition there is a certain probability or chance that the energy will be emitted as IC electrons. The probability increases

1. The higher the Z of the atom.
2. The lower the energy of the transition.
3. The longer the lifetime of the excited state.

The reason for the increased probability with higher Z nuclides is that the K-shell will be physically closer to the nucleus, and thus there will be a greater chance of interaction between the electrons and the nucleus. In general the lower the energy of the transition, the more comparable its energy is with the binding energies of the electrons, and the longer the lifetime the more time there is for the interaction to take place.

Decay of iodine-131

^{131}I decays by beta decay to xenon-131 (Fig. 5.14). Two per cent of ^{131}I atoms decay to the 723 keV excited level of ^{131}Xe, seven per cent to the 637 keV level and 90 per cent to the 364 keV level (Table 5.2). All the nuclei in the 637 and 723 keV levels decay direct to the ground state whilst seven per cent of the nuclei in the 364 keV level decay via the 80 keV level and the remainder (93 per cent) go direct to the ground state. Thus approximately six per cent (seven per cent of 90) of ^{131}I atoms decay via the 80 keV level of ^{131}Xe.

Not all transitions lead to gamma rays and internal conversion occurs. Whilst less than one per cent of the higher transitions are converted the figure for the 80 keV transitions is 61 per cent. The lifetimes of all the states involved are less than 10^{-9} s and this example illustrates that the lower the energy of the transition the greater the probability of internal conversion.

5.6. Auger electrons

Electron capture and internal conversion both leave the daughter atom with an electron vacancy in one of its shells; the vacancy is most

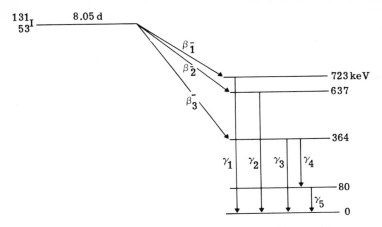

Fig. 5.14 Decay of ^{131}I. Transitions and energy levels involving $<1\%$ disintegrations have been omitted.

likely to occur in the K-shell, with diminishing probability for the other shells. It is filled by electrons transferring from shells of lower energy. In about 90 per cent of times a K-shell vacancy will be filled by an electron from the L-shell, directly from the M-shell in about 10 per cent and very occasionally from shells further out. These transfers will be accompanied by the emission of characteristic radiation

Table 5.2 Decay of ^{131}I. Transitions involving less than 1% of the transformations have been omitted

Beta radiation

	Mean number/ transformation	Maximum energy (MeV)
β_1	0·02	0·25
β_2	0·07	0·33
β_3	0·90	0·61

Gamma radiation

	Transition energy (keV)	Mean number/ transformation	%IC	Mean number/ transformation emitted	Mean number/ transformation IC
γ_1	723	0·02	0	0·02	0
γ_2	637	0·07	0	0·07	0
γ_3	364	0·84	2	0·82	0·02
γ_4	284	0·06	5	0·06	$<0·01$
γ_5	80	0·06	61	0·03	0·03

corresponding to the difference in the energy between the two shells involved.

Iodine-125 decays by electron capture to tellurium-125 (Fig. 5.15) and the binding energies, to the nearest keV, are:

$$K \quad 33$$
$$L \quad 5$$
$$M \quad 1.$$

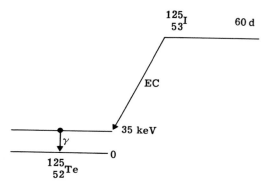

Fig. 5.15 Decay of ^{125}I.

Therefore a transition of an electron from the L to the K-shell will result in an X-ray (K_α) of $(33 - 5) = 28$ keV; similarly a vacancy in the L-shell filled by an electron from the M-shell will lead to an X-ray (L_α) of 4 keV being emitted. It is important to note that the X-rays emitted are discrete and characteristic of the daughter nucleus. The X-rays emitted during the decay of ^{125}I are characteristic X-rays of the daughter nucleus ^{125}Te not ^{125}I.

Not all the X-rays are emitted but some, in an analogous process to internal conversion, are converted and the energy transferred to an outer electron, thereby ejecting it from the atom as an 'Auger' electron (after the French physicist who studied this effect) (Fig. 5.16). The kinetic energy of Auger electrons is low as their energy is the difference between the transition energy of the internal rearrangement of the electrons and the binding energy of the electron ejected.

^{125}I decay

The processes of electron capture, internal conversion and the emission of Auger electrons can be illustrated by the decay of ^{125}I (Fig. 5.15). This, as noted above, decays by electron capture, resulting in vacancies in the various shells, the majority (81 per cent) occurring

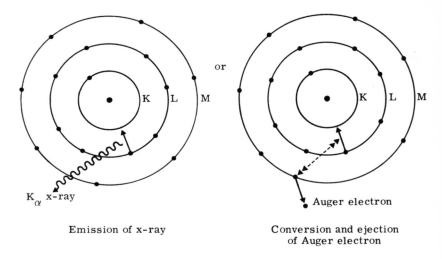

or

K$_\alpha$ x-ray

Auger electron

Emission of x-ray

Conversion and ejection
of Auger electron

Fig. 5.16 Auger effect. The conversion of characteristic X-rays and the production of Auger electrons.

in the K-shell. The transition from the excited nuclear state of [125]Te to the ground state results in a gamma ray of 35·5 keV; this is largely (in 93 per cent of transformations) internally converted giving rise to vacancies (75 per cent in K-shell, 11 per cent L, and eight per cent in M-shell): vacancies are created in the L-shell not only directly from the electron capture process and from internal conversion but also from filling vacancies in the K-shell. This results in there being created, on average, 1·7 vacancies on the L-shell per transformation. Similar processes result in an average of nearly four vacancies in the M-shell per disintegration. There is therefore a complex chain of events finally resulting in the emission of large numbers of X-rays, internal conversion and Auger electrons as detailed in Table 5.3. It should be noted that on average 1·4 photons (X- and γ-rays of more than 20 keV) are emitted per transformation. It is never safe to assume that on average one photon is emitted per transformation; we have already seen with ^{51}Cr that considerably less than one (0·09) may be emitted.

5.7. Alpha decay

In alpha decay the nucleus emits a helium nucleus which consists of two neutrons and two protons. The emitted particle thus carries away a total mass of four and reduces the atomic number by two (Fig. 5.17).

Table 5.3 Decay of ^{125}I. Transition energy is 0·149 MeV

Radiation	Mean number/ transformation emitted	Energy (keV)
Gamma	0·07	35
X-rays		
K_α	1·12 ⎫	27*
K_β	0·24 ⎬ 1·57	31*
L	0·21 ⎭	4
IC electrons		
From K-shell	0·75	4*
From L-shell	0·11	31*
From M-shell	0·08	35*
Auger electrons		
Due to vacancy in K-shell being filled	0·20	24*
Due to vacancy in L-shell being filled	1·49	3*
Due to vacancy in M-shell being filled	3·59	1*

* Mean energy.

It occurs normally in very heavy nuclei, the most well known example being the decay of radium-226:

$$^{226}_{88}\text{Ra} \rightarrow {}^{222}_{86}\text{Rn} + \alpha.$$

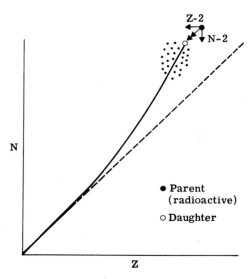

Fig. 5.17 Alpha decay. The effect of a loss of 2 neutrons and 2 protons from a nucleus.

Alpha particles are usually emitted with energies between 3 and 7 MeV and have a very short range due to their mass and their double charge. For this reason they have no use in nuclear medicine and due to their high toxicity (Ch. 10) are only encountered as sealed sources emitting γ- or X-rays. An example is americium-241, where the principal γ-emission of 60 keV is convenient for calibration and for certain other purposes.

5.8. Fission
A very few high mass radioactive nuclides undergo spontaneous fission with the emission of neutrons (Ch. 8). One example is californium-252, this has a half-life of 2·6 years and decays by alpha decay in 97 per cent of transformations and by spontaneous fission in 3 per cent. Encapsulated ^{252}Cf sources have been investigated as mixed neutron and gamma sources for brachytherapy.

5.9.   Isomeric transitions
In Section 5.3 we stated that after radioactive decay the daughter nuclide is often left in an excited state and emits gamma radiation in order to reach the ground state. In most cases this happens virtually instantaneously but in a number of cases the nuclide has an excited level with a relatively long half-life, minutes or hours. These long-lived excited states are called 'metastable levels' and are designated by use of the suffix or superscript m. Thus there is a long lived excited level of technetium-99, designated technetium-99m (^{99}Tc^m) which has a half-life of six hours. When metastable levels decay they emit gamma radiation only—being just an excited state of the decay product. Particulate radiation is only emitted in the form of electrons as the result of internal conversion of the gamma radiation.

Metastable isotopes play a very large part in nuclear medicine because of:

1. The low radiation dose per MBq administered to the patient, due to the absence of beta radiation or IC resulting from EC.

2. In certain cases they can easily be obtained in the laboratory by separating them from their parent isotope by ion exchange processes (Ch. 37).

Two particularly important radionuclides are indium-113m and technetium-99m. Their decay schemes and data on them and their parents tin-113 and molybdenum-99 are shown in Figures 5.18 and 5.19 and Tables 5.4–5.6.

Tin-113 decays by electron capture either to the 647 keV or the 392 keV level of ^{113}In. In the former case a 255 keV photon is emitted and the nucleus de-excites to the 392 keV, resulting in all the decaying

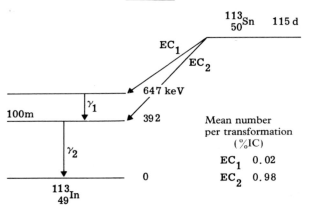

Tin - 113

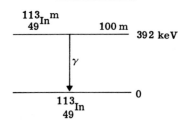

Indium - 113 m

Fig. 5.18 Decay of ^{113}Sn and its metastable daughter ^{113}In^m.

Table 5.4 Decay of ^{113}In^m

Radiation emitted	Mean number/ transformation	Energy (keV)
Gamma	0·62	392
IC electrons	0·38	37*
X-rays: K_α	0·19	24
K_β	0·04	27
L	0·03	3*
Auger electrons	0·99	1–23

* Mean energy.

nuclei of ^{113}Sn going through the 392 keV level of ^{113}In. The 392 keV level is metastable with a half-life of 100 m and has a single direct transition to the ground state. Due in part to the long half-life of the metastable level 38 per cent of the gamma rays are internally converted, with the consequent emission of characteristic X-rays, *IC* and Auger electrons.

The decay of ^{99}Mo is more complex. In this case 86 per cent of the nuclei decay via the metastable (6h) 142·7 keV level. It might be expected that due to the long life of the metastable state and its lower energy compared with ^{113}In^m, there would be nearly 100 per cent internal conversion: this is so (γ_1 is 98 per cent converted) but only 1·4

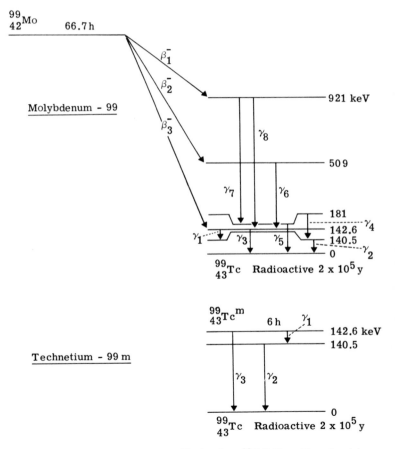

Fig. 5.19 Decay of Mo and its metastable daughter ^{99}Tc^m. Transitions involving less than 1 % of the transformations have been omitted.

per cent of nuclei go direct to the ground state; the remainder go via the 140·5 keV level which has a very short half-life ($< 10^{-9}$ s). It is the transition from this level which is the famous 140 keV transition of ^{99}Tc^m. The 2 keV transition, 142·7 to 140·5 keV is 100 per cent converted as would be expected from the lifetime of the 142·7 keV level and the low energy of the transition. The 140·5 keV transition is 10·4 per cent converted.

Table 5.5 Decay of ^{99}Mo including decay of daughter ^{99}Tc^m. Transitions involving less than one percent of ^{99}Mo atoms have been omitted

Radiation	Mean number/ transformation (%IC)		Transition energy* (keV)
Beta particles:			
β_1	0·18		456
β_2	0·01		868
β_3	0·80		1234
Gamma transitions (emitted and converted)			
γ_1	0·85	(100)	2
γ_2	0·91	(11)	140·5
γ_3	0·01	(98)	142·6
γ_4	0·06	(71)	40·5
γ_5	0·08	(14)	181
γ_6	0·01	(0)	366
γ_7	0·14	(0)	740
γ_8	0·05	(0)	778

* Maximum energy of beta particles.

Table 5.6 Decay of ^{99}Tc^m

Radiation	Mean number/ transformation		Energy (keV)
Gamma transitions (emitted and converted)			
γ_1	0·99	(100%IC)	2·1
γ_2	0·99	(11%IC)	140·5
γ_3	0·01	(100%IC)	142·6
X-rays (emitted)			
K_α	0·07		18*
K_β	0·01		21*
IC electrons			
K	0·10		120*
L	0·01		139*
M	0·99		2*
Auger electrons	1·37		1*

* Mean values.

5.10   Summary

Radioactive decay mechanisms appear more and more complex the deeper one goes into the subject, not an unusual feature in science. However, as long as the basic features and patterns are understood then the reader should be able to understand more than enough for most purposes in nuclear medicine. The basic decay mechanisms are illustrated and summarised below in Figures 5.20 and 5.21.

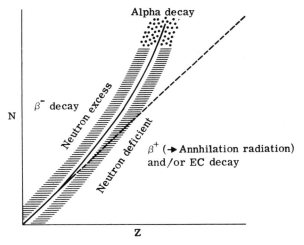

Fig. 5.20 Summary of the basic decay mechanisms.

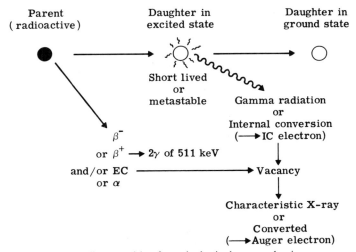

Fig. 5.21 Secondary effects resulting from the basic decay mechanisms.

6

Interaction of electrons with matter

The electrons encountered in nuclear medicine—Auger, internal conversion and beta particles—travel only a short distance in tissue, varying from a few microns to several millimetres. Many thousands of interactions and collisions are needed to stop an electron and three mechanisms are involved, ionization, excitation and the production of X-radiation (*bremsstrahlung*). The first two usually predominate whilst the latter is only of practical importance for activities of at least a hundred megabecquerels of a high energy beta emitting radionuclide.

6.1. Excitation and ionization

The electrostatic interaction between the energetic electron and the atomic electrons causes ionization along the track of the particle (Fig. 6.1), each event contributing to the slowing down of the particle. In tissue the energy expended by an electron in collision processes is roughly equally divided between ionization and excitation. The average energy required to form an ion pair is about 34 eV. When an

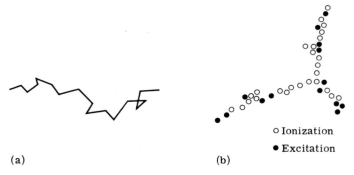

○ Ionization
● Excitation

(a)   (b)

Fig. 6.1 Schematic illustration of track of electron
(a) overall zig-zag path;
(b) one section of path showing ionization and excitation events. One of the atomic electrons has sufficient energy transferred to it to form a short separate track.

atom is ionized the electron produced may have sufficient energy to cause one or more further ionizations and excitations. In a few cases a distinct separate track can be formed. The electron will be scattered not only by interactions with the atomic electrons, but also by elastic collisions with the nuclei. The result is that the electron follows a very tortuous path and so, although the actual track lengths of monoenergetic electrons are similar, the actual penetration in a given direction varies enormously.

Electron range

The absorption of monoenergetic electrons by water is shown in Figure 6.2. The intercept of the line formed by extrapolating the steepest part of the curve to the range axis is often taken as measure of the maximum range. For beta particles this maximum range would refer only to those particles with the endpoint energy. The average penetration is much less, normally about a fifth of the maximum range.

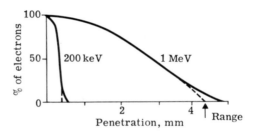

Fig. 6.2 Absorption of monoenergetic electrons by water. The percentage of particles transmitted is plotted as a function of penetration.

The range of an electron depends on the number of electrons with which it collides per unit length of its path. This will be proportional to the density of the material and vary only slightly with atomic number. Hydrogen is an exception as the number of electrons per gram is higher since the proton to neutron ratio is not approximately one as in atoms of other elements.

Point sources

Often the important parameter required is not the fraction of particles which penetrate to a certain distance but the distance within which a certain percentage of the emitted energy is absorbed. This has been calculated for point sources and is called the percentile distance. It is defined as the radius of the sphere around the point source within which a stated fraction of the emitted energy is absorbed. Figure 6.3 is a plot of percentile distance in water for 1 MeV monoenergetic photons and for beta particles emitted by two radionuclides.

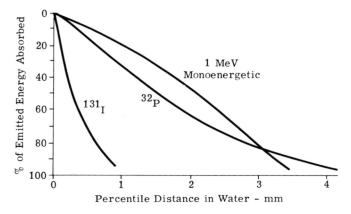

Fig. 6.3. Percentile distance. The percentage of energy emitted from a point source which is absorbed within a sphere around that source. The radius of the sphere is the percentile distance.

Linear energy transfer (LET)

This is the energy deposited per unit length of track and is related to the amount of biological damage caused (Ch. 10). A 1 MeV electron will create about 7000 ions per millimetre (the ionization density) at the start of its track and its LET will be $0.25\,keV\,\mu m^{-1}$. The comparable figures for a 100 keV electron are 12 000 and 0.4. It should be realised that although the ionization density is expressed in ions per millimetre the actual range may well be less than a millimetre; an analogy would be walking at three miles an hour for a hundred yards.

6.2. Bremsstrahlung

When an electron is de-accelerated (slowed down) by interacting with the electric field of a nucleus or the atomic electrons some of its energy is transformed into X-radiation. This radiation appears as a continuous spectrum and is called bremsstrahlung (from the German word meaning braking radiation). The maximum energy of the X-rays produced will be equal to the maximum energy of the particle and corresponds to the electron losing all its kinetic energy in one interaction (Fig. 6.4).

The amount of energy lost by bremsstrahlung production is usually only a few per cent but it is proportional to the energy of the particle

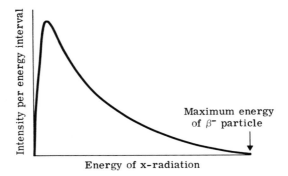

Fig. 6.4 Bremsstrahlung radiation from a pure beta emitter. The decrease in intensity at low energies is due to absorption in the sample and the window material of the detector.

and the atomic number of the material. The dependence of bremsstrahlung production on Z means that a light shielding material, for example plastic, is more suitable material for protection against pure beta-emitters than high atomic number materials.

The bremsstrahlung radiation can be used to determine the *in-vivo* distribution of radionuclides such as ^{32}P. However, imaging by this method is not efficient and therapeutic amounts of the radionuclide are required.

6.3.   Other particles

Alpha particles
These have a very high ionization density and LET due to their large mass and double charge. Their maximum range is less than a tenth of a millimetre. There is no application of alpha particles in nuclear medicine, although alpha emitters may be encountered, either due to the use of other radiation emitted or because of a particular property of a daughter nuclide.

Positrons
The interaction of energetic positrons with matter is similar to that of the electrons and the range is equivalent to that of an electron with the same energy. At the end of their path they annihilate with an electron and two 511 keV photons are created (Ch. 7).

Photons
These are not particles of matter but have some particle-like properties (Ch. 2). They do not cause ionization and excitation tracks

directly, but some or all of their energy can be transferred to electrons, by mechanisms discussed in the next chapter, and these electrons can cause further ionization. Photons are therefore often referred to as indirectly ionizing particles.

6.4. Summary

Electrons have a maximum range in tissue and this is of the order of millimetres for beta particles and microns for Auger and internal conversion electrons.

Electrons lose energy by:

> ionization
> excitation
> production of X-radiation (bremsstrahlung).

Photons are indirectly ionizing particles.

7

Interaction of X and gamma radiation with matter

7.1. Attenuation of X and gamma radiation

There is a major difference between the interaction of charged particles and photons with matter. Charged particles have a definite range but this is not the case with photons. The distance an individual photon will travel before interacting cannot be predicted; however for a beam of photons *the average fraction* which will have interacted within a certain distance can be stated.

If the intensity (I) of a narrow beam of monoenergetic photons is measured firstly without an absorber present (I_0) and then after passing through different thicknesses (x) of an attenuator the characteristic curve shown in Figure 7.1 results when the intensity is plotted against thickness (x). If the results are replotted using a logarithmic scale for I a straight line is obtained. The beam of photons is said to be exponentially attenuated and obeys the equation

$$I = I_0 e^{-\mu x}. \tag{7.1}$$

Here μ is the linear attenuation coefficient; it is the fractional reduction per unit thickness of material. The equation is identical in mathematical form to the one governing radioactive decay ($A = A_0 e^{-\lambda t}$, Ch. 4) and the derivation is given in Appendix 2.2. The linear attenuation coefficient is characteristic of a given material and density when attenuating photons of a specified energy.

In an exactly analogous way to that used to derive equation 4.4 in Chapter 4 equation 7.1 can be written

$$\mu x = 2 \cdot 303 \log_{10} \left(\frac{I_0}{I} \right).$$

Half-value thickness ($D_{1/2}$)

This is the thickness of material which will reduce the intensity of a beam to half its original value. The relationship between $D_{1/2}$ and μ is

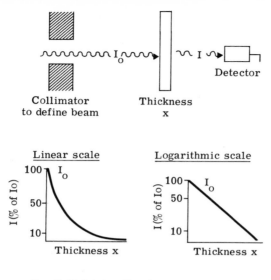

I_0 = Initial intensity of photon beam
I = Intensity after passing through
       material of thickness x

Fig. 7.1 Attenuation of radiation by matter.

identical to that between half-life ($T_{1/2}$) and transformation constant
(λ) and is obtained by substituting $x = D_{1/2}$ and $I = I_0/2$ into 7.1:

$$\mu = \frac{0 \cdot 693}{D_{1/2}}$$

A beam of photons is never completely attenuated by an absorber;
with every half-value thickness of attenuator added the beam
intensity is reduced by one half. Table 7.1 gives the half-value
thickness of water and lead for photons of several energies and for
various radionuclides. In the case of ^{131}I the figure given is only valid
for the first half-value thickness as a number of gamma rays of
different energies are emitted and those of lower energy will be more
rapidly attenuated with depth.

Attenuation, absorption and scatter
The attenuation of a beam is made up of two components, absorption
and scatter. Absorption is when the photon is entirely eliminated
from the beam and scatter is when the photon is deflected out of the
beam (Fig. 7.2).

Table 7.1 The half-value thickness for water and lead of 25–500 keV photons and for photons emitted from four radionuclides. Narrow beam conditions.

Photon energy	Half-value thickness (cm)	
	Water	Lead
25 keV	1·5	0·002
50 keV	3·2	0·008
100 keV	4·1	0·01
250 keV	5·5	0·08
500 keV	7·1	0·40
Radionuclides		
^{125}I	1·7	0·002
^{99}Tc^m	4·5	0·04
^{131}I	6·3	0·24
^{18}F	7·2	0·40

With a narrow beam most of the scattered radiation will not enter the detector whilst with a wide beam photons may be deflected into the detector. Thus the attenuation coefficient will be different whether a narrow or wide beam is being measured (Fig. 7.3). In most situations in nuclear medicine when dealing with photons from a radioactive substance the attenuation coefficients for a wide beam are the most appropriate.

Mass attenuation coefficient
Attenuation depends on the nature of the atom and not on its chemical or physical form. Therefore the linear attenuation coefficient will always be proportional to the density of the material as well as being related to the atomic number of the nuclide. It is therefore

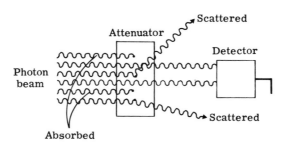

ATTENUATION = ABSORPTION + SCATTER

Fig. 7.2 Absorption and scattering of photons by an attenuator.

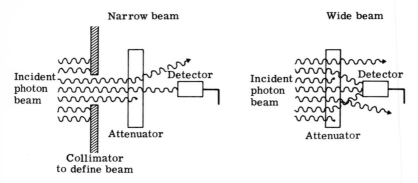

Fig. 7.3 The effect of scattered radiation on the attenuation of a beam of photons.

convenient to define a mass attenuation coefficient, μ_m, given by the linear attenuation coefficient divided by the density ρ.

$$\mu_m = \frac{\mu}{\rho}$$

If μ is in cm^{-1} and ρ is in units of g cm^{-3} then

$$\mu_m = \frac{\text{cm}^{-1}}{\text{g cm}^{-3}} = \frac{\text{cm}^2}{\text{g}} = \text{cm}^2 \, \text{g}^{-1}$$

The SI unit is m^2 kg^{-1} but most tables at present are in cm^2 g^{-1}. The mass attenuation coefficient μ_m therefore eliminates the effect of density. For example, the linear attenuation coefficient for photons of a certain energy will be different for ice, water and steam, but the mass attenuation coefficients will be the same.

Table 7.2 gives some values for the mass attenuation coefficient for photons ranging from 10 keV to 10 MeV. It can be seen that there is a

Table 7.2 Mass attenuation coefficients in cm^2 g^{-1} for photons of various energies in different materials

Photon energy	Water	Air	Aluminium	Lead
10 keV	4·89	4·66	26·5	84·6
100 keV	0·025	0·023	0·16	5·47
1 MeV	0·031	0·028	0·061	0·070
10 MeV	0·015	0·014	0·017	0·053

large variation even for the same material. The later sections of this chapter will explain why this large variation occurs and the mechanisms involved.

Calculations

As the same basic mathematical equation is applicable to both attenuation and radioactive decay the guidance given in Chapter 4 is applicable in evaluating equation 7.1.

Equation 7.1 can be expressed in terms of photons per second per cm^2, coulombs per kilogram per hour ($C\,kg^{-1}\,h^{-1}$), percentage of initial intensity or other suitable unit. $C\,kg^{-1}$ is the SI unit of exposure, however the special unit of the exposure, Röntgen (R), may be used temporarily, and $1\,R = 2\cdot58 \times 10^{-4}\,C\,kg^{-1}$ exactly).

When calculating attenuation it is often sufficiently accurate to approximate to the nearest number of half-value thicknesses. If the attenuation coefficient is used always check whether the mass or linear coefficient is given—only the linear coefficient can be used in equation 7.1.

Q. Calculate the exposure rate of a beam of gamma rays of 360 keV after passing through 1 cm of lead. The initial exposure rate is $0\cdot32\,C\,kg^{-1}\,h^{-1}$. Mass attenuation coefficient of lead $= 0\cdot25\,cm^2\,g^{-1}$. Density of lead, $\rho = 11\cdot3\,g\,cm^{-3}$.

A. Calculate the linear attenuation and then the half-value thickness.
Linear attenuation coefficient, $\mu = \mu_m \times \rho$

$$= 2\cdot8\,cm^{-1}$$

Now the half value thickness, $D_{1/2} = \dfrac{0\cdot693}{\mu} = 0\cdot25\,cm$

$\therefore$ Thickness of lead in terms of $D_{1/2} = \dfrac{1}{0\cdot25} = 4$ half-value thicknesses

The beam will therefore be attenuated by a factor $(\frac{1}{2})^4 = \frac{1}{16}$. Thus the exposure rate of attenuated beam

$$= \frac{0\cdot32}{16} = 0\cdot02\,C\,kg^{-1}\,h^{-1}.$$

If the thickness of the lead had not been an exact number of half-value thicknesses then an accurate result could be calculated using equation 7.1.

7.2. Mechanisms of attenuation

There are four ways by which a photon can interact with atoms

1. Scattering—elastic.

2. Scattering—inelastic (Compton effect).

3. Absorption—Photoelectric effect.

4. Absorption—Pair production.

All four mechanisms contribute to attenuation and the total attenuation coefficient is the sum of the four separate attenuation coefficients. The symbol μ_m with an appropriate superscript, for example c for Compton, is used to denote the separate attenuation coefficients.

As illustrated in Figure 7.3, in scattering the photon is deflected—it may or may not lose energy in the process. When absorption occurs the photon disappears in a single interaction.

Elastic scattering

In this process the photon is deflected from its path but suffers no loss in energy. It contributes to attenuation but is not important in nuclear medicine as it only contributes significantly to the attenuation at very low energies. A great deal of information can be gained about the structure of crystals by studying how they scatter an X-ray beam, a subject called X-ray crystallography. Using this technique the structure of DNA (deoxyribonucleic acid), the material from which genes and chromosomes are made, was discovered by Crick and Watson in 1952.

Bound and free electrons

An electron is said to be 'free' if the energy of the interacting photon is considerably greater than its binding energy. Therefore for a photon of 50 keV, only the outer electrons of an atom of lead can be considered free—the K-shell electrons are 'bound'. For photon energies of several hundred keV or more all the electrons in a solid are 'free'. The terms 'bound' and 'free' are therefore used relative to the energy of the photon.

7.3. Compton scattering

In this process the incident photon interacts with a 'free' electron, transfers some of its energy to the electron (recoil electron) and is scattered. The scattered photon will therefore have a lower energy than the incident photon (Fig. 7.4).

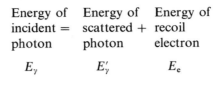

$$E_\gamma \qquad\qquad E_\gamma' \qquad\qquad E_e$$

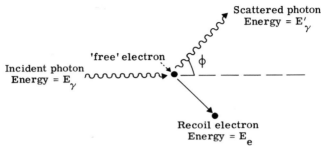

Fig. 7.4 Compton scattering of a photon by a 'free' electron.

Mass attenuation coefficient, μ_m^C
Compton scattering occurs with free electrons and except for hydrogen all elements contain approximately the same number of electrons per gram (about 3×10^{23}). This is because the ratio of neutrons to protons is similar, only slowly increasing with Z. Hydrogen is an exception as it has no neutron and hence the number of electrons per gram is approximately twice that of other elements. Therefore in general and for energies greater than the binding energies of the atoms, the mass attenuation coefficient is independent of Z. This means that, gram for gram and for photons of the same energy, all materials will cause a similar amount of Compton scattering.

The attenuation coefficient decreases with increasing energy (Fig. 7.5a)—high energy photons are scattered less than low energy ones.

The scattered photon
The proportion of photons scattered in different directions varies with the energy of the incident photon. Very low energy photons are scattered nearly equally in all directions but as the energy increases a greater percentage is scattered in a forward direction (Fig. 7.5b). The fraction of the incident photon energy which is transferred to a recoil

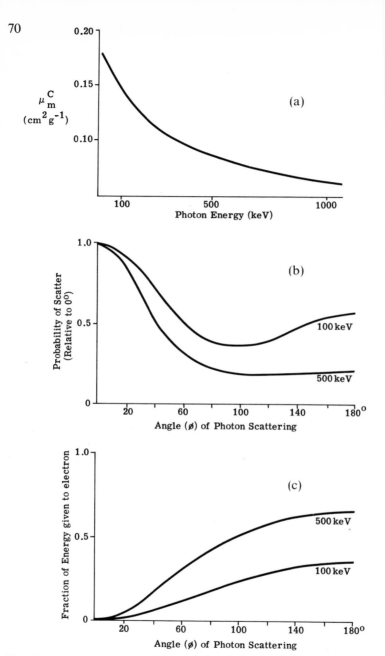

Fig. 7.5 Compton scattering. (a) The variation of the mass attenuation coefficient μ_m^C, with photon energy. (b) The variation, with angle of scatter, ϕ, of the probability of scatter, expressed as a fraction of the probability of 0° scatter. Graphs are given for 100 and 500 keV photons. (c) The fraction of the incident photon energy transferred to the recoil electron as a function of scattering angle, ϕ. Graphs are given for two photon energies, 100 and 500 keV.

electron depends on both the energy of the photon and on the angle of scatter, ϕ (Fig. 7.5c). The change in energy of a photon which is deflected by a few degrees is slight whilst one which is deflected through 180° and its path reversed transfers the maximum amount of energy to the recoil electron.

Scattered radiation is important as it affects the resolution of imaging systems and is a major factor when selecting the energy analyser settings of scanners and cameras. In Figure 7.6 both the relative amounts of $^{99}Tc^m$ radiation which is scattered in various directions and the energy of the scattered photons are shown.

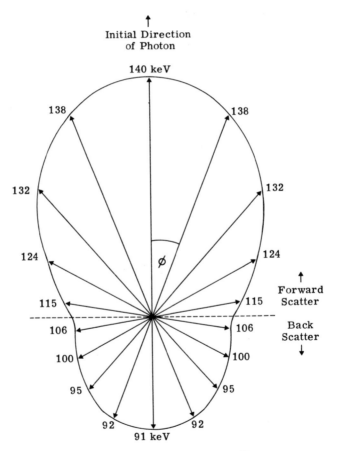

Fig. 7.6 Compton scattering of the 140 keV photons from $^{99}Tc^m$. The magnitude for various directions is indicated by the length of the arrows and the energy of the scattered photons is shown numerically.

Recoil electron

The recoil electron will be slowed down, principally by causing ionisation and excitation, and therefore its energy will be absorbed locally.

7.4. Photoelectric effect

In this process the photon completely disappears in one interaction and a bound electron is ejected, resulting in an ionized atom. The energy of the photon goes into overcoming the binding energy of the electron and any remaining energy is transformed into kinetic energy (KE) of the electron (Fig. 7.7).

Energy of = Binding energy + Kinetic Energy
photon   of electron   of electron

$$E_\gamma \quad = \quad BE \quad + \quad E_{pe}$$

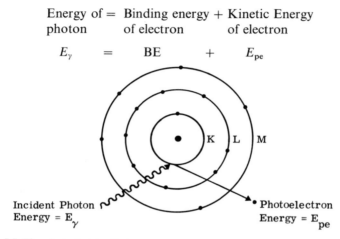

Fig. 7.7 The photoelectric effect.

Consider a 100 keV photon interacting with an atom of lead.

If photon ejects *K*-electron, BE 88 keV,   then KE = 12 keV
                     L-electron, BE 15 keV,   then KE = 85 keV

The photoelectron tends to travel in a forward direction, especially at high photon energies.

Characteristic X-radiation

The ejection of an electron from a shell will leave a vacancy. This will be filled by an electron from another shell with the emission of an X-ray with an energy corresponding to the difference in the binding energy of the two shells. The resulting vacancy will itself be filled and the sequence repeated until an electron from outside the atom is trapped (Fig. 7.8). The X-rays are emitted in random directions.

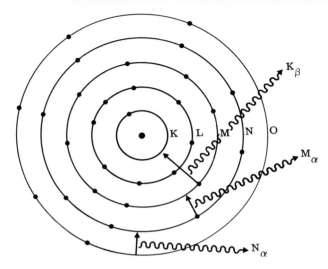

Fig. 7.8 One possible sequence of events after a vacancy has been created in the K-shell of an atom by a photoelectric event.

Mass attenuation coefficient, μ_m^{PE}
The attenuation coefficient falls rapidly with increasing energy and obeys a cube law over the important part of the energy range.

$$\mu_m^{PE} \propto \frac{1}{E_\gamma^3}$$

The variation with atomic number also, in general, obeys a cube law

$$\mu_m^{PE} \propto Z^3$$

Absorption edges
The photon must have at least the binding energy of the electron for a photoelectric interaction to take place. This results in a sharp increase in the attenuation coefficient just above the binding energy of each shell. Photons with energies just less than the binding energy of a shell are unable to eject electrons from it but those with the energies just greater are able to do so. The effect is superimposed on the fall in attenuation coefficient as the cube of energy (Fig. 7.9).

Photoelectron
The photoelectron will cause ionisation and excitation as it slows down and therefore its kinetic energy will be absorbed locally.

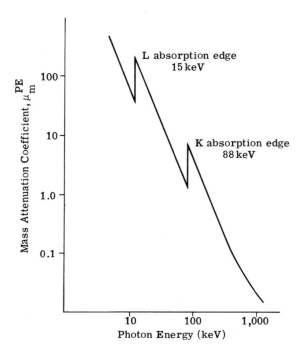

Fig. 7.9 The change in the mass attenuation coefficient for lead as a function of energy.

7.5.   Pair production

Photons with energy greater than $1 \cdot 02$ MeV when passing close to a nucleus can create an electron-positron pair. The difference between the photon energy and $1 \cdot 02$ MeV, the total rest mass energy of an electron and a positron, is given to the electron and positron as kinetic energy. The photon disappears and the process is an example of creation of mass from energy (Ch. 2).

The electron and positron lose their kinetic energy by ionisation and excitation. The positron then interacts with an electron and annihilation occurs with the creation of two $0 \cdot 51$ MeV photons travelling at 180° to each other. An identical process occurs after the ejection of a positron from an atom in beta plus decay. The overall result is that two $0 \cdot 51$ photons are created and some energy $(E_\gamma - 1 \cdot 02 \text{ MeV})$ is deposited locally by the ionisation and excitation caused by the electron and positron when slowing down.

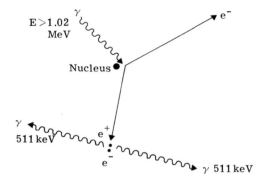

Fig. 7.10 Pair production. The creation of an electron-positron pair and subsequent annihilation of the positron with an electron to form two 511 keV photons.

Mass attenuation coefficient μ_m^{PP}

For photon energies greater than 1·02 MeV the coefficient is approximately proportional to the energy

$$\mu_m^{PP} \propto (E_\gamma - 1·02)\, \text{MeV}$$

The electron-positron pair are created in the nuclear field and the coefficient is proportional to Z.

$$\mu_m^{PP} \propto Z.$$

7.6. Attenuation coefficients

The total mass attenuation coefficients is the sum of the coefficients of the three important processes involved:

$$\mu_m = \quad \mu_m^{PE} \quad + \quad \mu_m^{C} \; + \mu_m^{PP} \;(+\text{elastic scattering})$$

Total   Photoelectric   Compton   Pair

Both the total coefficient and the relative contributions of the individual coefficients are important, and Figures 7.11 and 7.12 illustrate these coefficients for water and lead. The relative contributions to the total coefficient are plotted as percentages of the total coefficient. For example for the photoelectric effect the relative contribution will be

$$\frac{\mu_m^{PE}}{\mu_m} \times 100 \text{ per cent.}$$

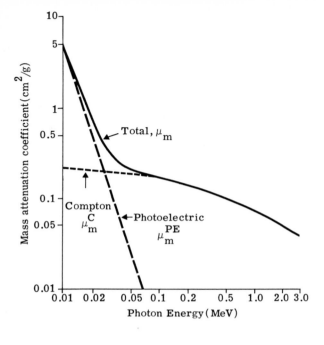

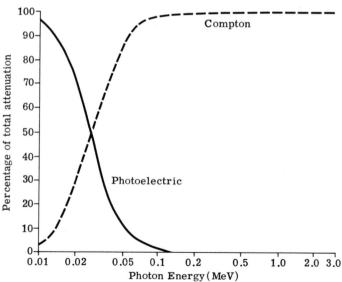

Fig. 7.11 Photoelectric, Compton and pair production. Mass attenuation coefficients and their relative contribution to the total attenuation coefficient, μ_m, for water.

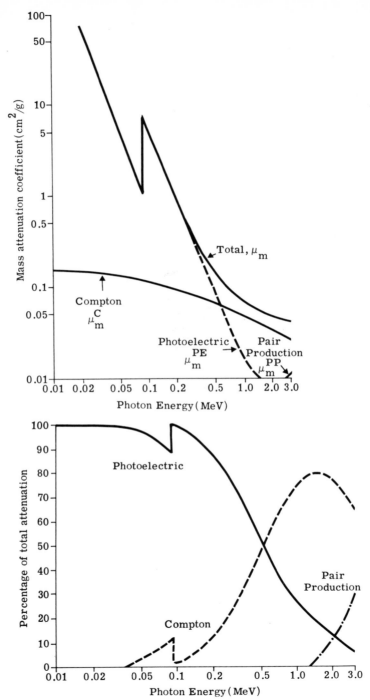

Fig. 7.12 Mass attenuation coefficients (Compton and photoelectric) and their relative contributions to the total attenuation coefficient, μ_m, for lead.

There is an enormous range in the attenuation coefficients as was noted in 7.1. This is primarily due to the cubic dependence of the photoelectric effect on atomic number and energy.

In low Z materials such as tissue, the Compton effect is the most important form of interaction for photons from 50 keV up to several MeV—the range of energies normally encountered in nuclear medicine. After one or more Compton interactions the photon will be sufficiently degraded in energy that it comes in the region where a photoelectric interaction is most probable. The effect of scattered radiation on the gamma ray energy spectrum is discussed in Chapter 17.

In materials with a high atomic number, such as lead, the photoelectric effect is important up to 500 keV. It is the combination of the high density and high atomic number which makes lead such an excellent material for protection. The cubic dependence of the photoelectric effect explains why the lead half-value thicknesses for $^{99}Tc^m$ and ^{131}I are so different although their main gamma ray energies differ by only a factor of two and a half. Lead is also widely used as a collimator material for the same reasons that it is used in protection. Other high Z materials can be used, such as tungsten, gold and uranium, but they have disadvantages such as cost or difficulties in fabrication.

When imaging the radionuclide distribution in a patient, the photons interact with a scintillation crystal, usually sodium iodide. The atomic number of iodine is 53 and to absorb entirely all the energy requires a certain thickness of crystal which depends on the energy. This will influence the design of detectors, the choice of instruments and also of radionuclides used in nuclear medicine. All these aspects of the interaction of radiation will be dealt with in more detail at the appropriate stages in this book.

7.7.   Summary

1. *Attenuation of radiation*

$$I = I_0 e^{-\mu x}$$

I_0 = initial intensity

I = intensity after traversing distance x

μ = linear attenuation coefficient

2. *Half-value thickness* $(D_{1/2})$

This is the thickness of material which will reduce the intensity of a beam to half its original value

$$\mu = \frac{0 \cdot 693}{D_{1/2}}$$

3. *Mass attenuation coefficient* μ_m

$$\mu_m = \frac{\mu}{\rho} \qquad \rho = \text{density}$$

4. *Attenuation = absorption + scatter*

5. *Mechanisms*

Mechanism of attenuation	Symbol for mass attenuation coefficient	Dependence of μ_m on atomic number	Dependence of μ_m on energy
Photoelectric effect	μ_m^{PE}	Z^3	$1/E^3$
Compton scatter	μ_m^C	Independent	$1/E$
Pair production	μ_m^{PP}	Z	$(E - 1 \cdot 02)$

$$\mu_m = \mu_m^{PE} + \mu_m^C + \mu_m^{PP}$$

6. *Relative importance of different mechanisms of attenuation*

Photon energy	Water	Lead
10–50 keV	{ Photoelectric / Compton	Photoelectric
50–500 keV	Compton	Photoelectric
500 keV–2 MeV	Compton	Compton

8

The nuclear reactor and the cyclotron

It was only after the availability of nuclear reactors, during the late 1940's, that the widespread application of radionuclides to medicine became possible. From the discovery of radioactivity in 1896 by Henri Bequerel until 1919 when Lord Rutherford showed that radioactivity could be induced in stable nuclei by bombarding them with fast alpha particles, only naturally occurring radionuclides were available for clinical investigation and treatment. The development of high voltage equipment for accelerating particles, such as protons and deuterons, by Cockcroft and Walton (1932) allowed the production of a wider range of radionuclides; however they were available only in limited quantities. The machine now most widely used for accelerating charged particles for radionuclide production is the cyclotron. Although cyclotron-produced radionuclides play an important part in nuclear medicine the main bulk of radionuclides used are created by neutron bombardment in nuclear reactors. It is helpful to understand the basic principles of the nuclear reactor and cyclotron in order to appreciate the various methods of production discussed in Chapter 36. Two concepts and their units which will be used both in this and later chapters are that of flux and cross-section.

8.1. Radiation flux and cross-section

If we have a steady beam of particles or photons then the number of particles per unit time passing through a unit area perpendicular to the beam is known as the flux of the beam. Thus a neutron beam might have a flux of 10^{18} neutrons per second per square metre ($10^{18} \, \text{n m}^{-2} \text{s}^{-1}$). If the beam is composed of charged particles then this is equivalent to a current of electricity, the total current being given by

$$\text{Current} = \text{Flux} \times \text{Charge per particle} \times \text{Area of beam}$$

The concept of flux can be used even when we are not dealing with a beam and the particles are moving in all directions, for example the neutrons in a nuclear reactor. The flux in this situation is defined as:

Number of particles or photons per unit volume × average speed

i.e. Density × average speed

The two definitions of flux are equivalent and the units are the same, as can be seen by substituting the appropriate component units in the above formula.

The concept of cross-section is used in discussing the strength of the interaction of particles or photons with nuclei. If a beam of particles or photons is interacting with a target then the cross-section is the average area perpendicular to the direction of the radiation which has to be assigned to each nucleus in order to account geometrically for the total number of interactions. The unit of cross-section is therefore in terms of area and is called the barn.

$$1 \text{ barn} = 10^{-28} \text{ m}^2$$

The cross-section can be thought of as the 'area of influence or interaction' and is completely separate from its physical dimensions. Its size depends not only on the type of nucleus but also on the type and energy of the particles. Like the concept of flux, cross-section is not limited to beams—in general:

$$\text{Cross section} = \frac{\text{Number of interactions per unit time}}{\text{Radiation Flux} \times \text{Number of Nuclei}}$$

8.2.   Nuclear energy

Mass defect
The fundamental basis of nuclear energy is the conversion of matter into energy according to Einstein's formula, discussed in Chapter 2.

$$E = mc^2 \qquad \begin{aligned} E &= \text{energy} \\ m &= \text{mass} \\ c &= \text{velocity of light} \end{aligned}$$

Only by knowing that mass and energy are interchangeable under certain circumstances can the surprising fact that the mass of a nucleus is less than the sum of the masses of the constituent protons and neutrons be understood. The difference in mass, called the mass defect, is given off as energy during the formation of the nucleus. To illustrate this consider the stable carbon nucleus, composed of six neutrons and six protons. The masses of individual protons and neutrons are similar but not, as has been assumed till now, identical. They are 1.6725×10^{-27} kg and 1.6748×10^{-27} kg respectively.

The mass of a ^{12}C nucleus would be expected to be

$$1\cdot6725 \times 10^{-27} \times 6 = 10\cdot035 \times 10^{-27}\,\text{kg}$$
$$1\cdot6748 \times 10^{-27} \times 6 = \frac{10\cdot049 \times 10^{-27}\,\text{kg}}{20\cdot084 \times 10^{-27}\,\text{kg}}$$

However, in fact the mass of a ^{12}C nucleus is only $19\cdot920 \times 10^{-27}$ kg.

$$\therefore \quad \text{Mass defect} = (20\cdot084 - 19\cdot920) \times 10^{-27}\,\text{kg}$$
$$= 0\cdot164 \times 10^{-27}\,\text{kg}$$

Converting to energy using Einstein's equation:

$$E = 0\cdot164 \times 10^{-27} \times (3 \times 10^8)^2 \text{ joules}$$
$$= 1\cdot476 \times 10^{-11}\,\text{J}$$

Now $1\,\text{MeV} \simeq 1\cdot6 \times 10^{-13}\,\text{J}$

$$\therefore \quad E = \frac{1\cdot476 \times 10^{-11}}{1\cdot6 \times 10^{-13}}\,\text{MeV}$$
$$= 92\,\text{MeV}.$$

The mass defect *per nucleon*, which for ^{12}C $= \frac{92}{12}$ or $7\cdot7$ MeV, varies with the mass of the nuclide, being greatest for medium mass nuclides (Fig. 8.1). We cannot take individual protons and neutrons and construct nuclei but we can take either two very light nuclei and combine them to form a medium mass nucleus, or take a heavy nucleus and split it into two medium mass nuclides. The two processes are known as fusion and fission respectively. In both cases the mass defects per nucleon of the nuclei after the process, being of medium mass, are less than those of the initial nuclei. The difference in mass defect is given off as energy.

Fusion
An example of a fusion reaction is the combination of two deuterium nuclei

$$^2_1\text{H} + ^2_1\text{H} \rightarrow ^3_1\text{H} + ^1_1\text{H} + 4\,\text{MeV}$$

Fusion reactions, or thermonuclear reactions as they are sometimes called, are responsible for the energy in the sun and stars and very high temperatures, many millions of degrees, are required to initiate the reactions. The hydrogen bomb is an example of an uncontrolled thermonuclear reaction. Major efforts are being made to produce a controlled reaction so that the energy released can be used to create electricity but the problems are formidable and it is likely to take a number of years before this is achieved.

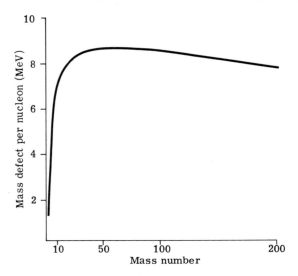

Fig. 8.1 Mass defect per nucleon as a function of mass number. Data have been smoothed.

Fission

Fission can take place spontaneously but is normally induced by a neutron. The most frequently used reaction in nuclear reactors is the induced fission of uranium-235; this may split into a variety of pairs of nuclides but an example is

$$^{235}_{92}U + {}^{1}_{0}n \xrightarrow{\text{fission}} {}^{137}_{55}Cs + {}^{97}_{37}Rb + {}^{1}_{0}n + {}^{1}_{0}n + \text{Energy (about 200 MeV)}$$

The sum of the masses of the product nuclei must be 234, whilst the sum of the atomic numbers of the products must equal the atomic number of uranium ($55 + 37 = 92$) for the equation to balance.

Figure 8.2 shows the relative amounts of the products of ^{235}U fission (note the log scale used for the relative amounts). One product comes from each of the peaks. Over 60 primary products have been detected; as most of these are radioactive and decay into other nuclides, the total number of nuclides present is very large.

On average 2·5 neutrons are produced for each fission, leading to the possibility of an uncontrolled reaction. If a nucleus in a mass of ^{235}U undergoes fission, the two neutrons released are able to cause two further fissions, hence releasing four neutrons and so on in a chain reaction. This is the basis of the atomic bomb. The controlled release of energy requires that, on average, only one of the neutrons created per fission causes further fission.

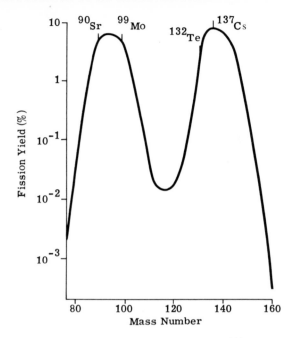

Fig. 8.2 Distribution of the yield of fission products from ^{235}U as a function of mass number.

Natural uranium is composed mainly of ^{238}U (99·3 per cent) and ^{235}U makes up only 0·7 per cent. Unfortunately ^{238}U is not a suitable nuclide for controlled fission as other nuclear processes occur, the most important one being neutron capture forming plutonium-239, and a controlled chain reaction cannot be maintained. To separate ^{235}U from ^{238}U is extremely expensive as, being isotopes, one can only use their difference in mass which is about one per cent. However, if one can slow down the high energy neutrons emitted by the fission of ^{235}U the resulting slow neutrons do not interact with the ^{238}U to the same extent and the probability of causing a fission reaction in ^{235}U is greatly increased. This can be restated in terms of cross-sections (Table 8.1). The cross-section for fission of ^{235}U is low for fast neutrons, as given out in fission. The non-fission cross-section for fast neutrons for ^{238}U is high but low for slow neutrons. The cross-section for fission of ^{235}U by slow neutrons is high.

To slow down or 'moderate' the fast neutrons a low atomic mass material which does not capture neutrons is incorporated into the reactor. Heavy water, D_2O (D is the isotope ^2_1H) and graphite (a form

Table 8.1 Cross-sections for fission and non-fission capture of neutrons by ^{235}U and ^{238}U

		^{235}U	^{238}U
Slow neutrons	Fission	High	Low
	Non-fission	Very low	Low
Fast neutrons	Fission	Low	Very low
	Non-fission	Very low	High

of carbon) are suitable. Low atomic mass materials are used as a fast neutron will transfer most of its energy to a light nucleus during an inelastic collision, whilst a similar collision with a heavy nucleus leads to only a small transfer of energy.

8.3. The nuclear reactor

There are many different types of reactor, although most are based on the fission of ^{235}U. The one described here is a type which has been operating for many years; in fact the first reactor, built in 1942 in Chicago, operated in a similar fashion. The moderator is graphite and the fuel natural uranium which is contained in cylindrical rods (fuel rods) with diameters of a few centimetres. These rods are inserted, in a lattice arrangement, into blocks of the graphite moderator. To control the rate of the reaction, and hence output of heat, control rods which have the property of absorbing neutrons and thereby reducing the number of neutrons available to cause fission are also incorporated. Steel enriched with boron or cadmium is a suitable material for these rods which are inserted or removed according to whether the reaction requires to be slowed down or speeded up. It is also normally necessary to have a coolant, either a suitable gas (for example, carbon dioxide) or a liquid. In reactors used for producing electrical power this coolant is used to produce steam for the steam turbines which in turn drive the generators.

Around the core, described above, a reflector is incorporated; this is usually the same material as the moderator and its role is to reduce the 'waste' of neutrons leaving the core by reflecting some of them back into the reactor. Surrounding the reflector is massive radiation shielding of special high density concrete. Access has to be provided to the core through the shielding for the insertion and removal of both the fuel and control rods, the coolant pipes, and also for the insertion of material (referred to as targets) to be irradiated by the neutrons. Figure 8.3 shows a cutaway drawing of the core of a typical reactor.

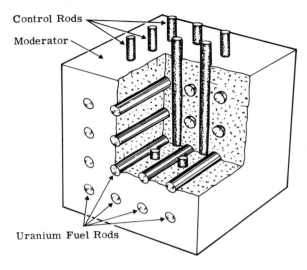

Fig. 8.3 Cut-away diagram showing the core of a nuclear reactor. Cooling system not shown.

The basic components of a reactor are therefore

uranium fuel rods ⎫
control rods   ⎬ The core
moderator   ⎪
coolant   ⎭
reflector
shielding

The major use of nuclear reactors is as a source of heat for the production of electricity by the method outlined above. Other uses include the production of fissile material for making nuclear weapons and the use we are interested in—as an intense source of low and high energy neutrons for the production of radionuclides for medical and other peaceful purposes.

8.4. The cyclotron

Charged particles need to have considerable kinetic energy, a minimum of a few MeV, before they can overcome the electrostatic repulsive force of the nucleus and cause a nuclear reaction. There are various ways in which this can be achieved but the most common machine used in the production of radionuclides is the cyclotron. We need not go into details of this type of machine but the basic principles should be understood.

The charged particle is accelerated by an electric field created by a voltage across two electrodes (Fig. 8.4). The particle is made to move in a circle by a magnetic field. Any charged particle moving in a magnetic field will have a force exerted on it in a direction perpendicular to the magnetic field and to the direction of motion (Fig. 8.5).

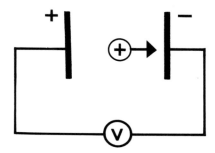

Fig. 8.4 A positive ion being accelerated towards a negative electrode.

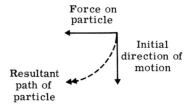

Fig. 8.5 Motion of a charged particle in a magnetic field results in a force on the particle perpendicular to the initial movement of the particle. The resultant path is circular.

A cyclotron consists of two hollow metal boxes, the electrodes, known as 'dees' or 'D's because of their shape. There is a slight gap between the two dees as shown in Figure 8.6. The charged particle is introduced between the dees and when a potential is applied it is accelerated towards the appropriate electrode. The dees are hollow and when the ion reaches the electrode it goes between the upper and lower surfaces (a region of zero electric field). The dees are placed between the two pole pieces of a large electromagnet and due to the magnetic field the particle will move in a circle. Whilst it is circulating in the dee the voltage between the two dees is reversed and on emerging the particle is attracted to the other dee. This process continues and the voltage polarity is switched so that the particle is

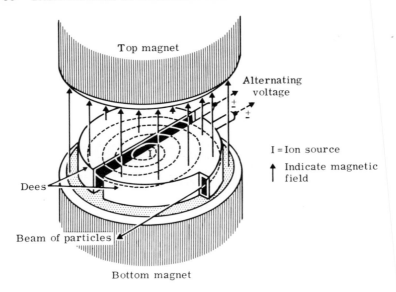

Fig. 8.6 Schematic diagram of a cyclotron showing the dees located between the pole pieces of an electromagnet and the spiral path followed by the charged particles.

accelerated twice per circuit. Since its speed steadily increases with each successive acceleration whilst the magnetic field stays constant, the particle will follow a spiral rather than circular path.

The source of charged particles can be a simple discharge tube in which ions are extracted from the tube by an electrode system and fed to the centre of the dees. The target is placed either inside the cyclotron or the ions are extracted and directed by a set of electric fields onto an external target. The volume in which the ions move must be a vacuum and the alternating voltage applied to the dees has a frequency of several MHz. In a typical cyclotron for production of radionuclides, as illustrated in Figure 8.7, the radius of the dees is about 40 cm. The most massive part of the cyclotron is the electromagnet.

Set out in Table 8.2 is the performance of one commercially available cyclotron. It can be seen that the internal current is much higher than the external current. The disadvantage of using the internal beam is the difficulty in changing the target; the external beam can be easily switched from one target to another.

There are now available some ultra-compact cyclotrons specifically designed for the production of ^{11}C, ^{13}N, ^{15}O and ^{18}F. The energy of

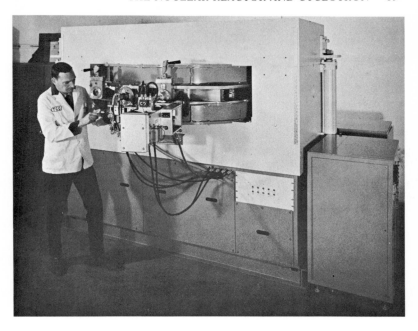

Fig. 8.7 A commercial cyclotron designed for the production of radionuclides. (*Courtesy of The Cyclotron Corporation, U.S.A.*).

the deuterons is typically 7 MeV whilst the current for protons and deutrons is in the range 50–100 μA. They are suitable for the production of the above nuclides but are limited in other respects. A cyclotron for a hospital often has a dual role and is used as a neutron source for radiotherapy as well as for the production of radionuclides. Protons of at least 15 MeV, preferably 30 MeV, are required for neutron therapy.

Table 8.2 Performance ratings of a variable energy cyclotron designed for the production of radionuclides

Particle	Energy	External current	Internal current
Protons	2–24 MeV	70 μA	500 μA
Deuterons	3–14 MeV	100 μA	500 μA
Helium -3^{++}	5–36 MeV	70 μA	150 μA
Helium -4^{++}	6–28 MeV	50 μA	100 μA

Radiation and biology

9

Dosimetry

The absorption of radiation, particulate or electromagnetic, involves the transfer of energy from the radiation to matter. In the case of particles the energy transferred, by ionisation and excitation, is their kinetic energy. Photons are indirectly ionizing particles and can be scattered or absorbed by matter (Ch. 7). The ionisation and excitation caused by both types of radiation give rise to biological effects which are discussed in Chapter 10.

The absorbed dose is the energy deposited per unit mass by ionizing radiation and in this Chapter the method of calculating the dose to the whole body and to various organs will be described. This is important in evaluating the radiation risks to a patient from a diagnostic procedure involving the administration of a radionuclide, as the value of the information to be obtained from the test must be balanced against the risk from the radiation. There is no completely safe limit and all absorbed radiation doses should be kept to a minimum consistent with carrying out the test satisfactorily and in a reasonable time. In most current nuclear medicine procedures the risks are small and the doses received are less than the maximum allowed per year for occupationally exposed radiation workers. If a radionuclide is being administered therapeutically the radiation dose to the whole body or an organ which is not the target may be the limiting factor. It is therefore vital that the radiation dose be assessed not only for the target organ or volume but also for other parts of the body.

9.1. Absorbed dose
This is the energy deposited at a point per unit mass of a material by ionizing radiation. The unit of absorbed dose is the gray (Gy), defined as 1 joule per kilogram. Until recently, and still widely used in some countries, was the rad, defined as 0.01 J per kilogram (originally 100 ergs per gram).

The absorbed dose is essentially the concentration of energy deposited — energy per unit mass. For example, a liver weighing two kilograms which has uniformly absorbed five joules of radiation energy will have received a dose of $5/2 = 2\cdot5$ joules per kilogram, that is $2\cdot5$ Gy or 250 rad. In the case of a whole body irradiation of 1 Gy (100 rad) every part of the body has absorbed one joule per kilogram (1 Gy).

Table 9.1   Units of absorbed dose

Name	Symbol	Definition
gray	Gy	1 J per kg
rad	rad	$0\cdot01\,\mathrm{J\,kg^{-1}}\,(100\,\mathrm{erg\,g^{-1}})$

1 gray = 100 rad

9.2.   Calculation of absorbed dose

Although the basic principles of dosimetry are simple, the subject can easily become very confusing due to different approaches and terminologies. In this Chapter the approach and terminology is based on that used by the International Commission on Radiation Units and Measurements (ICRU Report 32, *see* Appendix 8) who, of course, use SI Units. Other authors and bodies have adopted a similar approach and only changes in formalism and units is required to transfer from one system to another. In particular, the Committee on Medical Internal Radiation Dose (MIRD) of the American Society of Nuclear Medicine have issued a series of valuable reports and compilations of data. Unfortunately they are not based on SI units but microcuries and rads. However as the 'MIRD System' is widely used a separate section (9.10) is devoted to it at the end of this Chapter.

The hardest part in a dosimetry calculation is usually assembling and evaluating the all-too-often sparse biological data rather than the mathematics or obtaining the physical data required. Having understood the basic concepts and ideas of dosimetry, it is essential to carry out calculations so as to clarify the formalism used.

Basic principles
The radiation energy given out by radionuclides in an organ will be wholly or partially absorbed in that organ. If the total energy given out and the fraction absorbed by the organ are known then the total energy absorbed is the product of the two: by dividing by the mass of the organ the absorbed dose is obtained. For a pure beta emitter it can be assumed (as the range of the beta particles is small) that all the energy emitted is absorbed in the organ and therefore the absorbed

fraction is unity. In the case of γ-emitting nuclides, the fraction of the energy emitted from the radioactivity in one organ (the source organ) which is absorbed by a second organ (the target organ) must be known. Then, given the mass of the target organ, the absorbed dose to the target organ can also be calculated.

In carrying out the calculation, it is easiest to work in terms of the dose rate per unit activity in the source, as only physical data are required to calculate this quantity and all the other information needed, such as activity administered, percentage uptake in the organ, retention and excretion, is contained in a quantity called the time integral activity, $\tilde{A}$ (sometimes called the cumulated activity).

Absorbed dose = dose rate per unit activity × time integral activity:

$$\bar{D} = \frac{\Delta \times \phi}{m_v} \times \tilde{A} \qquad (9.1)$$

where

$\bar{D}$ = absorbed dose (in grays).

Δ = mean energy of radiation emitted per nuclear transformation (in joules).

ϕ = the fraction of the energy emitted which is absorbed by the target organ (no units of course!).

$\tilde{A}$ = The time integral activity. This gives the total number of transformations which occur (becquerels × seconds).

m_v = mass (in kilograms) of the organ whose absorbed dose is being calculated.

The basic concepts and the fundamental methods of calculating the absorbed dose to an organ will be illustrated by two easy examples before we discuss each of the factors in equation 9.1 in more detail. We will then be in a position to consider the full equation for the calculation of absorbed dose (equation 9.1 is a simplified form of the full equation).

Example 1. Absorbed dose to thyroid from ^{131}I. Radioactive (^{131}I) sodium iodide is used both in diagnosis and treatment of thyroid disease. Over 90 per cent of the dose to the thyroid is due to the beta particles emitted and so we will only consider these particles in this example; they have an *average* energy of thirty femtojoules ($\Delta = 30 \times 10^{-15}$ J — Table A.5.1 in Appendix 5) per nuclear transformation. Virtually no particles escape from the thyroid due to their short range and so all their energy is deposited in the thyroid ($\phi = 1$). If we divide by the mass of the thyroid ($m_v = 0.02$ kg — Table

9.5) we obtain the absorbed dose per nuclear transformation in the thyroid:

$$\frac{30 \times 10^{-15}}{0 \cdot 02} = 1 \cdot 5 \times 10^{-12} \, \text{gray} \qquad \left(\text{this is } \frac{\Delta \times \phi}{m_v} \right)$$

Typically, in a euthyroid person, about 30 per cent of the administered activity is taken up by the thyroid. If we make the assumption that none of the radioiodine leaves the thyroid then we can make use of the relationship

Mean life $= 1 \cdot 44 \times$ Half-life   (section 4.3)

to calculate the total number of transformations which occur as the ^{131}I decays away to a negligible activity. The half-life of ^{131}I is $8 \cdot 1$ days ($8 \cdot 1 \times 24 \times 60 \times 60 \simeq 7 \times 10^5$ s). Thus if 1 MBq is administered to a patient the total number of transformations in the thyroid will be:

$$1 \times 10^6 \times 0 \cdot 3 \times 1 \cdot 44 \times 7 \times 10^5$$

| Injected | % | |
| activity | taken-up | Mean life |

$$\simeq 3 \times 10^{11} \qquad \text{(this is } \tilde{A})$$

The absorbed dose per megabecquerel administered is:

$$1 \cdot 5 \times 10^{-12} \times 3 \times 10^{11}$$

$$= 0 \cdot 45 \, \text{Gy per MBq administered.}$$

Example 2. Liver scan with ^{99}Tc^m—sulphur colloid. Approximately, 85 per cent of an intravenous injection of ^{99}Tc^m labelled sulphur colloid is taken up by the liver and there is no evidence that any ^{99}Tc^m leaves the liver. If we consider the 140 keV gamma rays we need first to calculate the average energy emitted per nuclear transformation. A 140 keV gamma ray is given out in $0 \cdot 88$ of transformations (*see* Table 5.6) and remembering to convert from electronvolts to joules (1 eV $\simeq 1 \cdot 6 \times 10^{-19}$ J)

$$\Delta(140 \, \text{keV gamma rays}) = 0 \cdot 88 \times 140 \times 10^3 \times 1 \cdot 6 \times 10^{-19}$$
$$= 19 \cdot 7 \times 10^{-15} \, \text{J}$$

Not all the gamma rays will be absorbed by the liver itself—the figure is about 16 per cent ($\phi = 0 \cdot 16$). The mass (m_v) of the liver is

1·8 kg (Table 9.5) and therefore the energy absorbed per unit mass (the absorbed dose) per nuclear transformation is:

$$\frac{19·7 \times 10^{-15} \times 0·16}{1·8} \simeq 1·8 \times 10^{-15} \, J$$

A typical activity administered for a liver scan is 80 MBq and, using the same relation ($\overline{T} = 1·44 \, T_{\frac{1}{2}}$) as in Example 1 above, to calculate the time integral activity ($\tilde{A}$), we obtain

$$\tilde{A} = 80 \times 10^{6} \times 0·85 \times 1·44 \times 6 \times 60 \times 60$$
$$= 2·1 \times 10^{12}$$

Hence the absorbed dose to the liver due to 140 keV gamma rays from $^{99}Tc^{m}$ is the liver arising from an injection of 80 MBq is:

$$1·8 \times 10^{-15} \times 2·1 \times 10^{12}$$
$$= 3·8 \times 10^{-3} \, Gy$$

Dosimetry results are often quoted as mGy per MBq, this would give a value of $3·8/80 = 0·047$ mGy per MBq. A more sophisticated calculation which takes into account the Auger and K electrons emitted by $^{99}Tc^{m}$ (*see* Table 5.6) and the contribution to the absorbed dose from activity elsewhere in the body gives total dose to the liver about twice the above value (Table 9.2).

Source and target organs
In the above examples we only dealt with absorbed dose to an organ from activity within that organ. In most cases we need to consider other organs as well and the first step when presented with a dosimetric problem is to separate the various organs and radioactive distributions involved. In the case of a radioactive colloid injected intravenously this will be initially in the blood and will then accumulate in the liver, spleen and bone marrow. The absorbed dose to the liver will comprise the sum of the doses:

1. Due to activity in the liver

2. Due to activity in the blood
    Due to activity in the spleen   } all radiation from outside the organ
    Due to activity in the bone marrow

The adsorbed dose to another organ which does not take up the activity, such as the pancreas, will arise only from activity outside that organ.

In practice many of the contributions to the absorbed dose of an organ are small and can, depending on the accuracy of the estimate

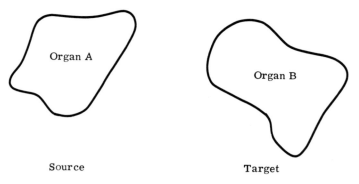

Fig. 9.1 All dosimetry problems are built up from calculations involving two organs, the source and target. The activity is assumed to be uniformly distributed in Organ A, the source.

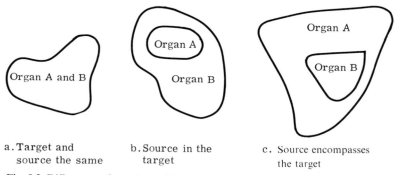

a. Target and   b. Source in the   c. Source encompasses
   source the same   target   the target

Fig. 9.2 Different configurations of the source and target organs.

required and the biological data available, be ignored. In the above example the contribution from the blood to the liver dose is very small, less than one per cent.

In general two organs are involved, the one containing the radioactivity, referred to as the source organ (Organ A in Fig. 9.1), and the organ being irradiated for which the absorbed dose is required, the target organ (Organ B). In the case of the liver dose from activity in the liver, the source and target organs are one and the same (Fig. 9.2a). Organ B can also encompass A (for example where A is the liver and B the blood — Fig. 9.2b) or be within it (for example where A is the whole body and B the liver — Fig. 9.2c). No change in the method of calculation is required.

Penetrating and non-penetrating radiations
Having resolved the problem into irradiation of Organ B by activity
in Organ A the next step is to consider the different types of radiation
involved. All particulate radiation, electrons (beta minus particles,
internal conversion electrons and Auger electrons) and positrons can
be considered non-penetrating as their range is, at the most, a few
millimetres. The same applies to low energy and gamma radiation,
usually taken as less than 11 keV since 95 per cent of the radiation of
this energy is absorbed within 1·0 cm of a point source in tissue.
Electromagnetic radiation above this energy is sufficiently penetrating for a significant amount to escape from the source organ. Each
gamma or X-ray, or groups of rays with similar energies, must be
treated separately. When the target organ is physically separated
from the source only penetrating radiation will be involved. The dose
to the target organ will be the sum of the individual doses due to the
non-penetrating and the separate penetrating radiations. An example
is given in Table 9.2.

9.3. Physical and biological data

Mean energy per nuclear transformation, Δ
Each type of radiation from a radionuclide has a value of Δ_i, the mean
energy of radiation of the *i*th type per nuclear transformation.
Consider a radionuclide which gives out a beta particle of average
energy $\bar{E}_i$ joules in a certain fraction, n_i, of disintegrations. Then the
energy emitted in the *i*th form per transformation is simply $n_i\bar{E}_i$.

$$\Delta_i = n_i\bar{E}_i$$

If the energy is given in MeV, as often occurs, then

$$\Delta_i = 1\cdot6 \times 10^{-13} n_i\bar{E}_i$$

(See Table A3.6 in Appendix 3 for conversion factor)
where Δ_i is in J and $\bar{E}_i$ is in MeV

Table 9.2 Absorbed dose to the liver from $^{99}Tc^m$ activity uniformly distributed in the
liver. Contributions to the dose from activity in other organs is less than 0·003 mGy. (It
is assumed 85 per cent of the activity is taken up into the liver).

Dose due to:		Dose per MBq administered
Non-penetrating radiation	=	0·040 mGy
Penetrating radiations		
	K X-rays =	0·003 mGy
	140 keV γ-rays =	0·047 mGy
Total dose	=	0.090 mGy

In the specific case of phosphorous-32, the only radiation emitted is a single beta particle of mean energy 0·6948 MeV. In the case n_i will equal 1, and

$$\Delta_i = 1\cdot6 \times 10^{-13} \times 1 \times 0\cdot6948$$
$$= 1\cdot111 \times 10^{-13} \text{ joules}$$

The units of Δ have been stated as joules. However it will have been noted that $\Delta \times \phi/m_v$ (equation 9.1) is the dose rate per unit activity. As ϕ has no units and m_v that of kg, it would be expected that Δ should be a rate (it is) and for this to be reflected in its unit. The explanation of this apparent anomaly is that the unit of joule for Δ is derived from $J\,Bq^{-1}s^{-1}$ and as $Bq \equiv s^{-1}$ we get $Bq^{-1}s^{-1} \equiv 1$. Generally the full expression is used $(J\,Bq^{-1}s^{-1})$, usually with the prefix $f(10^{-15})$ or $p(10^{-12})$ as very small numbers are involved. Thus Δ_i for P-32, in the example above, might be stated as $11\cdot1\,pJ\,Bq^{-1}s^{-1}$.

In the case of most radionuclides, it is not necessary to calculate Δ_i for each type of radiation as they are available in tables. Table 9.3 shows radionuclide data for $^{99}Tc^m$. The input data show what happens in the nucleus and the output data then takes into account the effect of internal conversion and the Auger effect. It is the output table which is important as regards the dosimetry and it can be greatly simplified by dividing it into penetrating and non-penetrating radiation. All the Δ_i for non-penetrating radiation can be summed and the information required for dosimetry presented as in Table 9.4. Data for other common radionuclides are given in Appendix 5.

Absorbed fraction

The absorbed fraction, ϕ, is the energy absorbed in the target organ divided by the total energy emitted by the radioactivity in the source organ:

$$\phi = \frac{\text{energy absorbed by target}}{\text{energy emitted by the source}}$$

For non-penetrating radiation the absorbed fraction will be unity when the source organ is also the target organ and zero for all other cases.

In the case of penetrating radiation the absorbed fraction will depend on the energy of the photons, the mass and shape of the two organs, their separation and the absorption and scatter of the photons by the tissue of the body. Therefore the calculation of absorbed fractions is very complex and many simplifications need to be introduced. Calculations have been carried out, with the help of computers, on phantoms which approximate the body shape and

Table 9.3 Nuclear data and decay scheme for $^{99}Tc^m$. See Section 5.9 for a discussion of the decay scheme. (Adapted from MIRD pamphlet 10, 1975, with permission from the publisher)

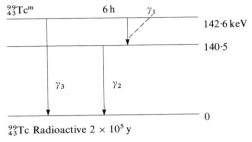

$^{99}_{43}Tc$ Radioactive 2×10^5 y

		INPUT DATA	
$^{99}_{43}Tc^m$		Decay: Isomeric Transition	$T_{\frac{1}{2}} = 6.03$ h
Transition		Mean Number/ Transformation	Transition Energy (MeV)
Gamma 1		0.986	0.002
Gamma 2		0.986	0.140
Gamma 3		0.014	0.143

		OUTPUT DATA		
$^{99}_{43}Tc^m$		Decay: Isomeric Transition $= 6.03$ h		
Radiation			Mean Number/ Transformation n_i	Mean Energy/ Particle $\bar{E}_i$ (MeV)	Δ_i fJ Bq^{-1} s^{-1}
		Gamma 1	0.000	0.002	0.00
M	IC	Electron	0.986	0.002	0.26
		Gamma 2	0.879	0.141	19.74
K	IC	Electron	0.091	0.119	1.74
L	IC	Electron	0.012	0.138	0.25
M	IC	Electron	0.004	0.140	0.08
		Gamma 3	0.000	0.143	0.01
K	IC	Electron	0.009	0.121	0.16
L	IC	Electron	0.004	0.140	0.07
M	IC	Electron	0.001	0.142	0.02
K	Alpha-1 X-Ray		0.044	0.018	0.12
K	Alpha-2 X-Ray		0.022	0.018	0.06
K	Beta-1 X-Ray		0.010	0.021	0.03
KLL	Auger	Electron	0.015	0.015	0.03
KLX	Auger	Electron	0.005	0.018	0.01
LMM	Auger	Electron	0.109	0.002	0.03
MXY	Auger	Electron	1.236	0.000	0.08

Table 9.4 Summary of essential nuclear data for $^{99}Tc^m$. Data from Table 9.3

Element	Nuclide	Mean number per trans-formation (n_i)	Mean energy (MeV) (E_i)	Δ_i (fJ Bq^{-1} s^{-1})
Technetium	$^{99}Tc^m$ $T_{\frac{1}{2}}$ 6 h Decay IT			
	Non-penetrating			2·8
	Penetrating	0·08	0·019*	0·2
	Penetrating	0·88	0·140	19·8

* Weighted mean of K X-rays

dimensions — the organs are represented by simple geometric forms. The various parameters are normally based on 'Reference Man', a mythical homosapiens made up from mean values for the various organs of men, or women where appropriate, of 20–30 years of age and weighing 70 kg.

Data are given in MIRD pamphlet 5 (revised) for one set of calculations. In the phantom used 22 internal organs are included, the mass of the principal ones being listed in Table 9.5. Absorbed fractions for photons ranging from 10 keV to 4 MeV were calculated and a simplified example of the results is given in Table 9.6. Further results are given in Appendix 5.

Table 9.5 Mass of organs. Based on MIRD pamphlet 5 (revised) with permission of the publisher

Organ	Mass (kg)
Bladder*	0·24
Red bone marrow	1·50
Brain	1·45
Kidneys	0·28
Liver	1·81
Lungs†	1·00
Ovaries	0·01
Pancreas	0·06
Total skeleton	7·47
Spleen	0·17
Testicles	0·04
Thyroid	0·02
Total body	69·88

* Model used in study consisted of organ plus average contents.
† Density of lungs is approximately 0.3 g cm^{-3}.

Table 9.6 Absorbed fractions, ϕ, for a source uniformly distributed in the liver. Adapted from MIRD pamphlet 5, with permission of the publisher.

Target organ	Photon Energy, E, (MeV)					
	0·020	0·030	0·050	0·100	0·500	1·00
	Source organ — Liver					
Kidneys	0·001	0·004	0·006	0·004	0·004	0·003
Liver	0·784	0·543	0·278	0·165	0·157	0·144
Lung	0·009	0·016	0·015	0·010	0·008	0·008
Marrow	0·008	0·023	0·032	0·021	0·010	0·009

It will be noticed from Table 9.6 that above 100 keV there is little variation in the absorbed fraction (Fig. 9.3). It is usually acceptable to combine all the gamma rays above 100 keV from a radionuclide into a mean value. This has been done for the nuclear data presented in Appendix 5 and Table 9.7 shows the derivation of data for ^{131}I. Each gamma ray below 100 keV should be treated separately, except for those very close together. For accurate work the absorbed fraction for energies not given can be obtained by interpolation.

The absorbed fraction relates to the whole target organ. If the absorbed fraction is divided by the mass of the target organ then the absorbed fraction per unit mass of target organ is obtained, called the specific absorbed fraction.

$$\Phi = \frac{\phi}{m_v}$$

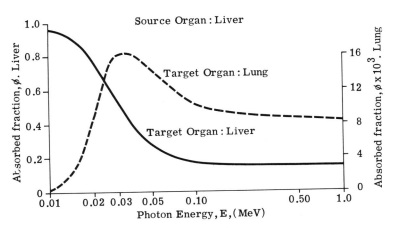

Fig. 9.3 The absorbed fractions of the liver and bone marrow as a function of energy for a source uniformly distributed in the liver.

Table 9.7 Nuclear data for dosimetric purposes for [131]I. (*See also* Table 5.2)

Radiation	Mean number per transformation n_i	Energy (MeV) E_i	Weighted Mean Energy (MeV) $\bar{E}_i$	Δ (fJ Bq^{-1} s^{-1}) Δ_i or Δ_s
Non-penetrating				30·6
Penetrating				
(a) Below 0·1 MeV				
K α-1 X-ray	0·025	0·030 ⎫		
K α-2 X-ray	0·013	0·030 ⎬ 0·031		0·2
K β-1 X-ray	0·007	0·034 ⎬		
K β-2 X-ray	0·001	0·034 ⎭		
Gamma 1	0·026	0·080		0·3
(b) Above 0·1 MeV				
Gamma 3	0·058	0·284 ⎫		
Gamma 4	0·820	0·364 ⎬		59.8
Gamma 5	0·065	0·637 ⎬		
Gamma 6	0·017	0·723 ⎭		

Gamma rays with n_i less than 0·01 have been omitted.
Δ = Mean energy emitted per nuclear transformation.
$\Delta_s = \sum \Delta_i$ Used for non-penetrating radiation and where several X or γ-rays have been summed.

Time integral of the activity (cumulated activity), $\tilde{A}$
This gives a value for the total number of transformations which occur in the source organ and has units of Bq s. It is the product of the rate of transformation (Bq) and the time (s). The activity in an organ is continuously changing with time due to various factors — uptake of the radiopharmaceutical excretion from the organ and physical decay. To calculate the time integral of the activity two main methods are available.

Graphical integration. The total activity in the organ is plotted as a function of the time (Fig. 9.4). The area under the curve will be the product of the Bq and the time — the time integral of the activity. Data to plot this curve can be obtained by several techniques. If the organ is the thyroid the percentage uptake can be measured at regular time intervals with a scintillation probe detector, and, knowing the administered activity, the absolute activity in the organ can be calculated. For other organs quantitative scanning can be used. Activity in the blood can be measured by taking samples and measuring the radioactive concentration. The area under the curve can be evaluated by using a 'planimeter', a simple device which, when used to trace the perimeter, indicates the total area directly on a dial. Another method is counting squares.

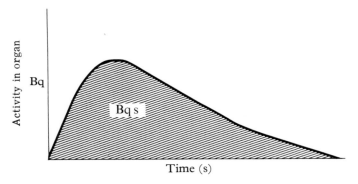

Fig. 9.4 Plot of activity in an organ as a function of time.

Effective half-life. It is often found that the amount of activity in an organ decreases in an exponential manner or that an exponential decrease is a reasonable approximation. This is obviously the case if the decrease is entirely due to physical decay, for example, in liver scanning with technetium sulphur colloid. However, many biological processes also result in exponential decreases as the rate of clearance is often proportional to the amount of material present. The clearance of $^{99}Tc^m$–DTPA from the blood is exponential, after an initial period, due to glomerular filtration by the kidneys.

If two processes are operating, each on its own involving an exponential clearance, then the result of the two processes is also exponential. If one is physical decay and the other a biological process then the resultant rate is known as the effective rate, or if described in terms of the half-life, the effective half-life.

$$\lambda_E = \lambda_P + \lambda_B$$

Now $\lambda = \dfrac{0.693}{T_{\frac{1}{2}}}$

$$\frac{0.693}{T_E} = \frac{0.693}{T_P} \frac{0.693}{T_B}$$

λ: transformation constants

T: half-lives

$$\frac{1}{T_E} = \frac{1}{T_P} + \frac{1}{T_B}$$

subscripts:

E effective
P physical
B biological

or $\quad T_E = \dfrac{T_P T_B}{T_P + T_B}$

The effective half-life is determined from plotting, on log-linear graph paper, the results of measurements on the uptake in the organ or measurements on blood samples. The clearance of activity from the blood can often be analysed in terms of only two or three separate exponential clearances. The technique of separating several exponentials — known as curve stripping — is described in Chapter 13.

The cumulated activity is given by the product of the total initial activity and the mean life (*see* Section 4.3).

$$\tilde{A} = A \times 1.44 \times T_E \text{ Bq s}$$

9.4.   Formula for calculation of absorbed dose

In equation 9.1 a simplified formula was given for calculation of an absorbed dose. The full equation is:

$$\bar{D} = \frac{\tilde{A}}{m_v} \sum \Delta_i \phi_i \tag{9.2}$$

Each separate Δ_i (or summed value where appropriate) must be multiplied by the appropriate absorbed fraction, ϕ, and all the products ($\Delta_i \phi_i$) then summed. This result is then multiplied by the time integral of activity, $\tilde{A}$, and divided by the mass of the target organ, m_v. To summarise and clarify the sources of the data:

$\bar{D}$ = total average dose to target organ in grays.

$\tilde{A}$ = time integral of activity (also known as cumulated activity) in source organ, in Bq s.
(From biological data and administered activity [*see* Section 9.3])

m_v = mass of target organ. (From Table 9.5 or MIRD pamphlet 5).

Δ_i = mean energy of radiation of the ith type per nuclear transformation.
(From Appendix 5 or ICRU Report 32).

ϕ_i = absorbed fraction for ith type radiation from the source organ and absorbed by the target organ.
(From Appendix 5 or MIRD pamphlet 5).

Pure beta emitters represent a special case as only non-penetrating radiation is involved. Only the source organ will be irradiated and ϕ will be unity.

9.5.   Reciprocity relations

In certain situations reciprocal relationships exist between pairs of organs. The specific absorbed fraction is independent of which organ is the target and which is the source. Therefore if the absorbed fraction of the spleen for activity in the liver is known then the absorbed fraction of the liver for activity in the spleen can be calculated. Thus:

$$\frac{\phi_s}{m_s} = \frac{\phi_l}{m_l}$$

where ϕ_s = absorbed fraction by spleen from activity in liver

ϕ_l = absorbed fraction by liver from activity in spleen

m_s = mass of spleen

and m_l = mass of liver

In general it is valid to use the reciprocity relationship in most practical situations.

9.6. Worked example

Problem. Four megabecquerels of ^{51}Cr-EDTA are injected intravenously to measure glomerular filtration rate. Calculate the total absorbed dose to the kidneys and total body.

Assume that the ^{51}Cr-EDTA rapidly diffuses into the extravascular space and clearance is with a half-time of 100 minutes. Also assume that 5 per cent of the total activity is in the kidneys.

Answer: Break down the problem into component parts.

Source Organ	Target Organ	Comments
Total body	Total body	Calculation 1 below
Total body	Kidneys	Similar to total body dose
Kidneys	Kidneys	Calculation 2 below
Kidneys	Other organs	Small compared with dose from whole body

N.B. There will be a significant dose to the bladder wall and other organs from activity in the bladder. Not dealt with here.

1. *Dose to total body from activity in total body.*

Physical Data:

From Appendix 5 and Table 9.5

	Δ_i $(fJ\ Bq^{-1}\ s^{-1})$	ϕ_i
Non-penetrating	0·83	1
Penetrating (320 keV)	4·58	0·34

Mass (total body) = 70 kg

Time integral activity:

$$\tilde{A} = \text{Activity} \times 1\cdot44 \times T_E$$
$$= 4 \times 10^6 \times 1\cdot44 \times 100 \times 60$$
$$= 3\cdot46 \times 10^{10} \text{ Bq s}$$

Apply equation 9.2:

$$\bar{D} = \frac{3\cdot46 \times 10^{10}}{70}(0\cdot83 \times 1 + 4\cdot58 \times 0\cdot34) \times 10^{-15}$$
$$= 0\cdot118 \times 10^{-5} \text{ Gy}$$
$$= 0\cdot0012 \text{ mGy}$$

2. *Dose to kidney from activity in kidney.*

Physical data: Δ_i as for calculation 1 above

	Δ_i
Non-penetrating	1
Penetrating	0·07
Mass kidneys = 0·284 kg	

Time   activity in kidneys

$$A = \frac{5}{100} \times 4 \times 10^6 \times 1\cdot44 \times 100 \times 60$$
$$= 17\cdot28 \times 10^8 \text{ Bq s}$$

Apply equation 9.2:

$$\bar{D} = \frac{17\cdot28 \times 10^8}{0\cdot284}(0\cdot83 \times 1 + 4\cdot58 \times 0\cdot07) \times 10^{-15}$$
$$= 70 \times 10^{-7} \text{ Gy}$$
$$= 0\cdot007 \text{ mGy}$$

The total dose to the kidneys will be that from the kidneys (0·007 mGy) and from the total body (0·0012 mGy) giving a value of 0·008 mGy. The dose to the bone marrow and gonads will be similar to the total body dose (0·001 mGy). The only organ, apart from the kidneys, to receive a dose significantly greater than the total body dose is the bladder.

9.7. Dosimetry of individuals

Adults
Very few individuals will be adequately represented by 'Reference Man'; for diagnostic applications this is not usually very important

but if therapy applications are being considered then calculations for the individual are necessary. In normal persons the weight of organs is nearly proportional to body weight and so the activity administered can be scaled accordingly.

$$\frac{M}{70} \times A \qquad (9.5)$$

M = weight of individual in kg
A = activity administered to 'Reference Man'.

The approximation ignores changes in the absorbed fraction which will alter with mass and shape of the organ. However, if therapy level doses are being administered then most of the absorbed dose will arise from the non-penetrating radiation and so any changes in absorbed fraction will have a small effect on the total absorbed dose.

In ill patients the weight of organs may be very different from that expected from considering the individual's body weight. If the absorbed dose is to be accurately calculated then the weights of the relevant organs must be determined. This is not easy but, depending on the organ, various imaging methods such as radionuclide imaging, ultrasound and computerised tomography may be used.

Children
The discussion in the previous section is generally relevant to children but although the weights of most organs are proportional to the weight of the child the brain is an exception. A further important consideration is the percentage uptake in the organ — for example the thyroid uptake of iodine in euthyroid infants during the first two weeks is very high. Bearing these considerations in mind, and also the need to keep the radiation dose to a minimum, the formula given above (equation 9.5) can be used.

An alternative approach is based on the child's age. A formula which will give a reasonably correct proportion of the adult dose is:

$$\frac{(x + 1)}{(x + 7)} \times A \qquad \text{x is the child's age in years}$$
A is activity used in the adult

A reference to more detailed considerations of radiopharmaceutical dosimetry in paediatrics is given in Appendix 8.

9.8. Special situations

Absorbed dose to wall of cavity containing radioactivity
The dose to the wall of a container filled with a radioactive solution is

often of importance. The situations where this occurs are the walls of the bladder, the surface of peritoneal and pleural cavities with ^{198}Au-gold therapy and the dura mater in cisternography.

For non-penetrating radiation the dose to the surface is half the dose in the centre of the container. At the centre a point is subjected to radiation from all directions whilst the surface receives radiation only from the liquid (Fig. 9.5).

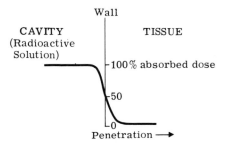

Fig. 9.5 Absorbed dose to surface of a cavity containing a solution of a beta emitting radionuclide. The rate of fall-off of dose with depth in tissue is approximately exponential (Ch. 6).

Blood
Absorbed fractions for blood or for organs arising from activity in the blood are not listed in MIRD pamphlet 5. However, it is reasonable to use the values for the distributed activity in the total body when calculating the absorbed fraction to other organs from activity in the blood. The gamma radiation dose to blood, either from activity in the blood itself or from another organ, will be very similar to the total body dose. In this case if the total body absorbed fraction is used then the total body mass must be used also.

Breast
The female breast is one of the most sensitive organs of the body to the induction of cancer by radiation (*see* Table 10.4); however, absorbed fractions are not currently available. An average mass of 720 g can be assigned to the sum of the two breasts. One method of deriving an absorbed fraction is to assume that, where an absorbed fraction is available for 'other tissues' (muscle and adipose), the absorbed fraction is proportional to the mass of the breasts.

$$\phi_{breast} = \frac{m_{breast}}{m_{other\ tissue}} \times \phi_{other\ tissue}$$

9.9. Absorbed dose from diagnostic nuclear medicine procedures

In Table 9.8 are listed some values for absorbed doses for diagnostic procedures. These have all been calculated for 'Reference Man' and are based on the best biological information available. The radiopharmaceutical may concentrate in organs apart from the one required for visualisation and the radiation dose to the other organs must always be borne in mind. Two examples may be cited from Table 9.7, the dose to the stomach wall from $^{99}Tc^m$-pertechnetate and to the kidney from $^{99}Tc^m$-DTPA.

It is difficult to compare absorbed dose in diagnostic X-ray procedures with that received in nuclear medicine procedures. In diagnostic X-ray the dose is almost entirely limited to the area being examined, the whole body radiation dose due to scattered radiation being low, whilst there is usually a significant whole body dose from radionuclides. Another major difference is that an organ is uniformly irradiated in radionuclide procedures but the entrance and exit doses

Table 9.8 Absorbed doses for various radiopharmaceuticals used in diagnosis.

Nuclide	Form	Typical activity administered (MBq)	Absorbed dose per procedure (mGy)			
			Gonads	Marrow	Total body	Other
^{67}Ga	Gallium Citrate	80	6	12	5	Liver 9
^{75}Se	Seleno-methionine	10	27	20	20	Liver 60 Kidney 50
$^{99}Tc^m$	Pertechnetate	400	2	2	2	Stomach wall 25 Thyroid 13
$^{99}Tc^m$	Sulphur Colloid	80	<0·2	0·6	<0·2	Liver 7 Spleen 4
$^{99}Tc^m$	DTPA	200	1	1	1	Bladder wall 27
$^{99}Tc^m$	Macro-aggregated albumin	80	0·4	0·4	0·4	Lung 4
$^{99}Tc^m$	Diphosphonate	400	1	2	1	Bladder 40 Bone 4
^{123}I	Sodium Iodide	8	<0·1	<0·1	<0·1	Thyroid 26 Stomach wall 0·4
^{131}I	Sodium Iodide	0·8	<0·1	<0·1	0·1	Thyroid 260 Stomach wall 0·3

can differ by a factor of 100 in X-ray procedures. Some values are given in Table 9.9.

The ultimate method of comparing different diagnostic procedure is to calculate the actual risk of cancer mortality and of genetic damage. This is discussed in more detail in the next Chapter (10) but Table 9.10 categorises a number of common diagnostic procedures.

9.10. The MIRD system

This system is based on the use of the rad and Curie but the formalism is the same and equation 9.2 is applicable. The terminology is slightly different in places but the method of calculation is the same.

Table 9.9 Representative values of radiation dose from diagnostic X-ray procedures

| Examination | Absorbed dose per examination (mGy) | | | |
	Skin	Bone Marrow (Mean)	Gonad (F = Female)	Other organ (Centre)
Skull (Radiography)	14	0·4	<0·01	Brain 2
Chest (Radiography)	0·25	0·05	<0·02	Lung 0·1
Chest (Fluoroscopy)	20		<0·1	
Angiocardiography (Cardiac Catheterisation)	200	14	0·4(F)	
Abdomen (Radiography)	14	1	2(F)	
Barium Meal (Fluoroscopy)	160	8	3(F)	
Intravenous Pyelography (IVP)	17	6	8	Kidney 3

Table 9.10 The risk of cancer mortality from some common diagnostic procedures.

Risk	NM Procedures	X-Rays
Less than 1 in 10^6		Chest (PA) Dental
10^6–10^4	^{51}Cr Red Cell Volume ^{99}Tc^m Liver scan ^{99}Tc^m Lung scan ^{99}Tc^m Renogram ^{123}I Thyroid scan	Skull X-ray Barium meal Cholecystogram Lumbar spine Head-CT
More than 1 in 10^4	^{75}Se Pancreas Scan ^{131}I Thyroid scan ^{99}Tc^m Dynamic (20 MBq)	Lung-CT (Female) Cardiac catheterisation

Most of the biological data required for the estimation of dose are embodied in the cumulated activity $\tilde{A}$, while the remaining part of equation 9.2 involves physical and anatomical data. This information has been brought together in one unit, S, called the absorbed dose per unit accumulated activity. MIRD pamphlet 11 gives tabulations of S for a wide range of radionuclides and source target configurations.

$$S = \frac{1}{m_v} \sum_i \Delta_i \phi_i = \sum_i \Delta_i \Phi_i \qquad (9.3)$$

The total absorbed dose is therefore given by

$$\bar{D} = \tilde{A}S \text{ rad} \qquad (9.4)$$

To reiterate the meaning of these terms, using the terminology and units used in the MIRD system — sources of data are also given.

$\bar{D}$ = total absorbed dose to target organ in rads

$\tilde{A}$ = the cumulated activity in source organ, in μCi-h. Calculated in identical fashions except for the units used, as described in Section 9.3.

m_v = mass (in grams) of target organ (From Table 9.5 or MIRD pamphlet 5)

Δ_i = equilibrium dose constant for the ith type radiation (g-rad/μCi-h)

ϕ_i = absorbed fraction for the ith type of radiation emitted from the source organ and absorbed by the target organ

Φ_i = specific absorbed fraction = $\dfrac{\phi_i}{m_v}$

S = absorbed dose per unit accumulated activity. Units are rad per μCi-h. (MIRD pamphlet II).

Mean energy per nuclear transformation, Δ

The name used for this quantity in the MIRD system is the 'equilibrium dose constant'. The units are g-rad per μCi-h and a simple derivation will show how this unit is arrived at. Consider a radionuclide which gives a particle of average energy $\bar{E}_i$ Mev in a certain fraction, n_i, of transformations.

Energy emitted *per transformation* in this ith form of radiation

$$= n_i \bar{E}_i \text{ MeV}$$

converting to joules:
(1 eV = 1·6 × 10^{-19} J) $= 1\cdot6 \times 10^{-13} n_i \bar{E}_i$ joules

converting to g-rad:
(1 rad = 10^{-5} J per g) $= 1\cdot6 \times 10^{-13} n_i \bar{E}_i \times 10^5$ g-rad
                                                    $= 1\cdot6 \times 10^{-8} n_i \bar{E}_i$ g-rad

Now

$$1 \mu Ci = 3\cdot7 \times 10^4 \text{ transformations per second}$$
$$= 60 \times 60 \times 3\cdot7 \times 10^4 \text{ transformations per hour}$$
$$= 1\cdot33 \times 10^8 \text{ transformations per hour}$$

Therefore

Energy emitted *per* μCi *per hour* in the ith form of radiation

$$\Delta_i = 1\cdot33 \times 10^8 \times 1\cdot6 \times 10^{-8} n_i \bar{E}_i \text{ g-rad per } \mu\text{Ci-h.}$$

$$= 2\cdot13 \, n_i \bar{E}_i \text{ g-rad}/\mu\text{Ci-h}$$

The use of 'S' removes the need to calculate Δ_i and greatly simplifies the calculation of absorbed dose.

Example 4. Absorbed dose to liver from $^{99}Tc^m$ sulphur colloid. Making the same assumption as example 2 (85 per cent uptake and all the $^{99}Tc^m$ stays in the liver until it has physically decayed) we can easily calculate the dose by looking up 'S' in pamphlet 11;

$$S = 4\cdot6 \times 10^{-5} \text{ rad}/\mu\text{Ci-h} \qquad \begin{array}{l} \text{source organ: liver} \\ \text{target organ: liver} \end{array}$$

$\tilde{A}$ is calculated as before, but remembering to use the correct units

$$\tilde{A} = 1\cdot44 \times 0\cdot85 \times 2 \times 1000 \times 6 \text{—for 2 mCi (74 MBq) injected}$$
$$= 14688 \, \mu\text{Ci-h.}$$

Therefore

$$\text{Absorbed dose, } \bar{D} = 4\cdot6 \times 10^{-5} \times 14688$$
$$= 0\cdot68 \text{ rad}$$

It will be noted that this takes into account all the radiation emitted whilst example 2 only took into account the 140 keV gamma rays.

9.11.   Summary of methods for calculating absorbed dose

Procedure:

1. Breakdown problem into single source-target organ calculations.
2. Calculate the cumulated activity, $\tilde{A}$, either by using the effective half-life or by graphical integration.
3. Look up physical data.
   Mass target organ, m_v (kg)   (Table 9.5)
   Absorbed fractions, ϕ_i (Appendix 5)

Mean energy per nuclear transformation,

Δ_i $(\text{J Bq}^{-1}\text{s}^{-1})$

for penetrating (grouped) and
non-penetrating radiations   (Appendix 5)

4. Calculate absorbed dose for each source-target organ by substituting into

$$\bar{D} = \frac{\tilde{A}}{m_v}\sum \Delta_i\phi_i$$

5. Sum all the contributions to the dose for a particular organ.

MIRD System. Steps 1, 2 and 5 are identical. Either steps 3 and 4 can be carried in a similar manner but using the appropriate units and tables of data stated in Section 9.10 or just 'S', the absorbed dose per unit accumulated activity (rad per μCi-h), may be looked up in MIRD pamphlet 11 and then (stage 4 above) make use of the equation

$$\bar{D} = \tilde{A}S \text{ rad}$$

9.12.   Conclusion
The concept of the absorbed dose has been introduced and the basic principles of dosimetry outlined. The essentials of a method for calculating absorbed dose have been discussed and are summarised in Section 9.11. There are many problems which have not been dealt with in detail but it is hoped that sufficient information has been imparted for the reader to tackle the more extensive works listed in Appendix 8.

10

Biological effects of radiation

10.1. Introduction

The absorption of radiation energy by living cells always produces effects which are potentially harmful to the irradiated organism. The type of injury produced depends on the amount of radiation energy absorbed and may range from acute sickness and death within days or weeks to the induction of cancer twenty or more years after exposure. All radiation injury results primarily from radiation-induced chemical changes in one or more of the complex molecules which are present in living cells.

The induction of biological damage can be considered to occur in four stages, three of which are very rapid and one is slow. The molecular damage occurs during the first three rapid stages and the expression of these molecular changes into functional or structural damage to the cells and to the whole organism occurs during the slow phase. The phases of induction of radiation injury will now be considered in more detail.

10.2. The phases of induction of radiation injury

In all biological systems water is the most abundant molecule and radiation-induced splitting of the water molecule, the *radiolysis of water*, is a primary event in the initiation of biological damage.

The first phase of the induction of radiation injury which may be called the *initial physical phase* is the shortest lasting about 10^{-16} seconds. During this phase energy is deposited in the cell causing ionisation and excitation of ions and molecules. The absorption of energy by a water molecule results in the ejection of an electron (e^-) leaving a positively charged species H_2O^+

$$H_2O \longrightarrow\!\!\!\wedge\!\!\!\wedge\!\!\!\wedge\!\!\!\rightarrow H_2O^+ + e^-$$

In the second, or *physico-chemical phase* which lasts about 10^{-6} seconds the positive ion dissociates to yield a hydrogen ion, H^+, and a *hydroxyl free radical*, $OH^\bullet$.

$$H_2O^+ \longrightarrow H^+ + OH^\bullet.$$

116

The electron reacts with other water molecules which then dissociate to form hydrogen free radicals $H^{\bullet}$, and hydroxyl ions OH^{-}.

$$H_2O + e^- \longrightarrow H_2O^-$$

$$H_2O^- \longrightarrow H^{\bullet} + OH^-.$$

The principal products of these two phases are hydrogen and hydroxyl ions and free radicals. Hydrogen and hydroxyl ions are normally present in living cells and do not contribute to the radiation damage. The free radicals, which contain unpaired electrons, are very reactive species and may undergo many reactions, for example two $OH^{\bullet}$ radicals may combine to form hydrogen peroxide, H_2O_2, which is a powerful oxidising agent.

$$OH^{\bullet} + OH^{\bullet} \longrightarrow H_2O_2$$

Similar types of reaction may occur with other components of cells and tissues producing excited ions, excited molecules and other types of free radicals.

In the third or *chemical phase*, lasting a few seconds, the products of earlier reactions, especially the free radicals react with organic molecules within the cell. Reactions with proteins and the deoxyribonucleic acid (DNA) of the cell nucleus are particularly important. The reaction of these macromolecules with the products of the radiolysis of water may produce changes in the secondary or tertiary structure of proteins (see Ch. 35), as a result of the disruption of hydrogen bonds (see Ch. 30), or inter- or intramolecular cross-linking in the double-stranded DNA molecule. These changes may produce severe alterations in the biological properties of the molecules, for example a protein enzyme may completely lose its enzymatic activity. The breakage or cross-linking of DNA molecules may have particularly serious effects, ranging from loss of the cells' capacity to divide to the production of mutations which may lead to cancer or the birth of genetically damaged offspring.

The last phase of the induction of radiation injury is the *biological phase* during which the chemical changes are transformed into cellular changes. Three main types of cellular changes may be recognised. These are early cell death, prevention or delay of cell division (mitosis) and the production of permanent, inheritable changes which may be passed on to daughter cells at mitosis. These cellular changes may lead to other changes which affect the whole organism, be it plant, mouse or man.

This phase of the development of radiation injury shows the longest and most variable time scale. Some effects may develop within a few hours while others, for example cancer induction, may take many years to become apparent.

10.3.   Classes of radiation injury

Radiation-induced biological effects are divided into two main classes. *Somatic effects*, which arise from damage to the ordinary cells of the body resulting in injuries which affect only the irradiated person or organism, and *hereditary effects* which arise from damage to the germ cells in the ovary or testis and which are reflected only in injury to future generations.

10.4.   Somatic effects of radiation

The somatic effects of radiation arise mainly from the depletion of the numbers of mitotic, dividing, cells or from interference with the processes of cell division. Acute damage is most likely to occur in those cells which are undergoing very rapid cell division, for example the cells of the lymphoid and granulocyte systems and the cells lining the gastrointestinal tract. Because of their higher rate of growth young animals are often more susceptible to irradiation damage than adults.

The somatic effects of radiation also fall into two classes. The *acute effects* which are observed within a few days or weeks of exposure to relatively large doses of radiation, and the *long-term effects* which arise years after exposure to much lower doses.

Acute effects. Following exposure of man, or other mammals, to acute doses of radiation greater than about 0·25 Gy the lymphocyte count in the peripheral blood falls rapidly. If the radiation dose received is fairly small and the subject is going to recover the lymphocyte count begins to rise again after a few days, but full recovery may take some months. The lymphocyte count is a useful indicator of the radiation dose received by a subject over the range of 0·25 to 4 Gy of whole body exposure. At doses greater than 4 Gy, too few cells survive to permit accurate counting. The platelet count and the red blood count in the peripheral blood also fall a few days after exposure and then recover if the radiation dose received is not too large. The monitoring of the red and white blood cell counts provides useful information on the severity of, and pattern of recovery from, radiation exposure. Blood counts are used extensively to monitor patients undergoing radiation therapy, and also in the surveillance of persons occupationally exposed to serious risk of radiation injury.

At higher doses of radiation a number of other symptoms may be observed. The sequence of symptoms which may be expected to occur in human subjects after exposure to radiation doses of 4 to 6 Gy of X- or gamma rays is summarised in Table 10.1. Temporary or permanent sterility may also be produced by exposure to acute irradiation as a result of damage to the germ cells in the gonads. Information on the acute effects of irradiation has been obtained from observations on patients undergoing radiotherapy, atomic bomb casualties and from the victims of the few radiation accidents which have occurred in the past thirty years. More information has been obtained from experimental studies in a variety of animal species.

Table 10.1 Acute effects of exposure to a whole body radiation dose of 4–6 Gy

Time	Symptoms
0–48 hrs	Loss of appetite, nausea, vomiting, fatigue and lethargy.
2 days to 2–3 weeks	Recovery from these symptoms patient appears quite well.
2–3 weeks to 6–8 weeks	Purpura, haemorrhages, diarrhoea, loss of hair, fever, severe lethargy. Some deaths may occur.
6–8 weeks to several months	Recovery stage, surviving patients show general improvement and severe symptoms disappear.

The severity of the symptoms observed following exposure to a large dose of radiation appears to show wide individual variations. With doses of around 1 Gy about 15 per cent of exposed persons would show some of the symptoms listed in Table 10.1. At 2 Gy almost all the exposed individuals would exhibit symptoms and a few deaths would be expected, and the death rate would rise to 50 per cent after exposure to doses of 4·5 to 5 Gy. Studies in experimental animals and the limited experience of human exposure to high doses of radiation suggest that radiation doses in excess of 10 Gy to the whole body are likely to cause death within 3 to 5 days as a result of gross destruction of the cells lining the gastro-intestinal tract. Exposure to doses of between 5 and 10 Gy may result in death after about two weeks due to secondary infections which probably result from severe damage to the immune system.

The severity of the biological effects observed varies with the rate at which the radiation is received, the dose-rate, and the type of radiation to which the organism is exposed. The effects also vary with the proportion of the total body, or the specific organ which is irradiated. For instance while a dose of 5–10 Gy, delivered to the whole human body would almost certainly cause death within a few days the same dose delivered to a small area of the body, for example to a tumour, would produce relatively little systemic effect. The importance of dose-rate in the induction of biological damage is illustrated by the following example. When rats are exposed to whole body doses of 7–9 Gy of X- or gamma rays delivered over a few minutes the animals die within 14 to 21 days, but rats of the same age and strain will live in good health for months when exposed to continuous gamma rays at a dose rate of 0·05 Gy per day. Experimental studies in some systems have shown that the absorption of one Gy from alpha-particle or neutron irradiation may produce far more severe damage than one Gy of X- or gamma rays.

Long-term effects. The biological effects of radiation which arise a long time after the radiation dose is received include the induction of leukaemia and other types of cancer, cataract formation and life-shortening. These effects may be observed after exposure to radiation doses much lower than those which will produce the acute effects discussed earlier.

Cancer induction may require periods ranging from about 7 to 30 years to become apparent, Table 10.2. The relationship between the radiation dose received by an individual and the risk of cancer induction is not yet clearly understood, especially in relation to the risks following exposure to very low doses of radiation. There is considerable uncertainty about whether the risk of cancer induction increases linearly with radiation dose from the lowest dose upwards or whether there is a 'threshold' dose below which cancer induction is not observed.

Cataract formation appears to occur after a latent period of 5 to 10 years, but in this type of injury there appears to be a threshold dose of about 4 Gy below which cataracts are not seen.

10.5.   Hereditary effects of radiation

The hereditary effects of radiation arise from radiation induced mutations which occur in the egg cells, or ova, in the ovary of the female, or in the sperm cells of the testis in the male. Most genetic damage will probably result in embryonic or foetal death; however some may be non-lethal and permit the birth of a viable child suffering from severe abnormalities of one type or another. For this reason in

Table 10.2 Long-term effects of radiation

Effect	Latent period
Cataract formation (eye)	5–10 years
Leukaemia	8–10 years
Lung tumours	10–20 years
Bone tumours	15 years
Thyroid tumours	15–30 years

all medical investigations involving radiation care is taken to avoid any unnecessary irradiation of the gonads of either the patients or the investigators.

10.6.   Effects of radiation on the embryo

Irradiation of the pregnant female may cause serious damage to the developing embryo or foetus. A large number of observations on children born to women who were exposed to diagnostic or therapeutic X-rays during pregnancy have shown that irradiation *in utero* may lead to serious abnormality in the offspring. A variety of defects have been observed in these cases including mongolism, hydrocephalus, microopthalmia and limb malformation.

The human experience combined with the results of studies in experimental animals, suggests that the risks of damage to the embryo are greatest during the first 2 months of pregnancy and gradually decrease at later times. The risks of intra-uterine death or severe malformation are probably greatest during the first 38 days of pregnancy, that is during the pre-implantation stage (up to day 11) and the period of organogenesis.

This high risk of radiation damage to the embryo during the very early stage of pregnancy makes it extremely important to avoid any unnecessary radiation exposure during this time. Since it is possible that a fertile woman may not be aware that she is in the early stages of pregnancy when she attends for a radiographic or radionuclide investigation the so-called *ten-day principle* has been introduced into clinical radiological practice. This recommends that radiographic examinations, particularly of the abdomen and pelvis, in any woman for whom a possibility of pregnancy exists should normally only be carried out during the ten days following the onset of menstruation since during this time pregnancy is highly improbable. The applicability of the ten-day principle to investigations involving radiopharmaceutical administration is, at present, a matter of some controversy. However, all non-essential irradiation of the pregnant female should be avoided. In the unfortunate event that a foetus was exposed to a radiation dose of more than $0 \cdot 2$ Gy many experts would recommend that the pregnancy should be terminated.

10.7.   The concept of dose equivalent

We learned in Section 10.4 that radiation-induced biological injury depends not only on the amount of energy which is deposited in the cell or tissue but also on the type of radiation to which it is exposed. For example alpha particles, which give up their energy over a very short distance, produce more injury than X-rays which dissipate their energy over a long distance. The rate at which radiation energy is transferred to the atoms of the medium through which it passes is known as the Linear Energy Transfer, or LET, and is expressed in $keV \mu m^{-1}$ (see Ch. 6). The shorter the distance over which a given amount of energy is dissipated, the higher the LET. Biological studies in animals exposed to charged particles and radiation of different LET shows that for a given radiation dose the severity of the effects observed is greater for high LET than low LET radiation.

In radiation protection work it is necessary to be able to assess the risk of injury from exposure to different types of radiation and it is desirable to have a unit of radiation dose for which the risk of injury, or the 'detriment to health', can be regarded as similar for all types of radiation exposure. This requirement has led to the concept of *dose equivalent* which has a special unit, the sievert (Sv) where $1\ Sv = 1\ J\,kg^{-1}$. The former unit of dose equivalent, which is still widely used, was the rem which is equivalent to 0.01 Sv.

The dose equivalent (H) at any point in a tissue is given by the expression:

$$H = DQN$$

where D is the absorbed dose in Gy; Q is the *quality factor* for the radiation and N is the product of all other modifying factors which, for example, may take account of absorbed dose rate and fractionation of the radiation exposure. At the present time N is ascribed the value of 1 and Q has a value of 1 for X-rays, gamma rays and beta particles, 10 for neutrons or protons and 20 for alpha particles.

10.8.   Human exposure to radiation

In the preceding sections we have been considering the effects produced by exposure to large doses of radiation. Under normal circumstances none of the acute or long-term effects of irradiation are likely ever to be observed in any worker who is occupationally exposed to radiation or in any patient undergoing diagnostic investigation with radionuclides or radiation.

All radiation exposure is potentially harmful and in the case of the radiation worker, the patient undergoing radionuclide or radiographic investigations and the general public at large it is necessary to prescribe radiation dose levels at which the risk of serious injury to the individual, while never non-existent, is so low that it may be generally regarded as acceptable by both the exposed individual and by society.

Before we go on to consider these dose levels it is important to recognise that throughout his period of life on earth mankind has been exposed to radiation at low dose levels from a number of natural sources. These include radiation by cosmic rays from outer space and the radiations emitted by the naturally occurring radioactive substances in the earth's crust such as uranium and thorium and their decay products. Some of these naturally radioactive elements enter our food chains and become incorporated into bone and other tissues thus, as the atoms decay, irradiating the organs and tissues from within the body. This type of radiation we call *internal* irradiation to distinguish it from the *external* radiation, from cosmic and naturally occurring gamma rays, which impinges upon the body from outside.

The dose rates from natural radiation received by individuals in different parts of the world vary considerably. The dose from cosmic rays increases with increasing latitude, up to about 50°N or S, and with increasing altitude above sea level. In medium latitudes, such as in Great Britain and much of Europe, the mean annual dose rate at sea level is about 300 μSv while at the equator the annual cosmic ray dose is about 250 μSv. At about 10,000 feet, 3100 metres, in the Andes Mountain region of Peru the annual cosmic ray dose is about twice as high as that observed at sea level in the same latitude. The natural gamma ray dose rate from the uranium and thorium in the rocks and soil of the earth varies greatly depending on the type of rock formation found in the particular geographical area. In London, England where the strata are mainly clay and chalk the mean annual dose rate from terrestrial gamma rays is about 300 μSv but in the granite regions around Aberdeen in Scotland the corresponding annual dose rate is about 1500 μSv. Much higher dose rates from terrestrial gamma rays are found in other areas of the world; for example in regions where there are deposits of monazite, a thorium-containing sand, such as in Kerala in India or in parts of Brazil dose rates of between 15 and 120 mSv have been measured.

Another important source of natural radiation comes from radon decay products. The radioactive gas radon-222 is produced by the decay of the radium-226 which is naturally present in rocks and soil; the gas diffuses ifto the atmosphere and is rapidly dispersed in the air. In the open air the dose rates are low, but radon enters dwellings and other buildings through the floor and also from the decay of radium-226 which is often present in very small quantities in the bricks and other building materials; because the air flow in most buildings is much less than in the open air the radon concentration inside builds up. Radon decays to yield solid radioactive daughter products which attach themselves to the walls and ceilings and also to dust particles which may be inhaled and irradiate the lungs. The effective annual dose equivalent from radon daughters in the United Kingdom has been estimated to be 800 μSv on the average, or about 40 per cent of the total natural radiation dose. There are considerable variations in this dose rate, depending on the type of construction and the degree of ventilation of individual buildings and in some instances the dose rate from radon decay products may be more than ten times greater than the average.

Man-made radiation sources also contribute to the general level of radiation received by man; the principal source of man-made radiation is the use of X-rays and other radiation sources in medicine but small contributions are made by fallout from nuclear weapons testing, the disposal of radioactive waste, occupational radiation exposure and miscellaneous sources such as TV sets and luminous watches.

The estimated radiation dose equivalents received annually in the United Kingdom from natural and man-made sources are shown in Table 10.3. Similar dose rates are found in other western countries; in less developed regions the contribution from man-made sources will often be very much lower.

10.9. Dose Equivalent Limits

The recognition of the potentially harmful effects of radiation led to the creation in 1928 of the body which is now known as the International Commission on Radiological Protection (ICRP). This body keeps a watching brief on all aspects of protection against

Table 10.3 Average annual radiation dose equivalents in the United Kingdom from natural and man-made sources. (Data taken from 'Living with Radiation', National Radiological Protection Board, HMSO, London, 1982).

Source	Dose (μSv)
Cosmic radiation	310
Terrestrial gamma rays	380
Radon decay products	800
Potassium-40	170
Carbon-14, Lead-210, Polonium-210 and other internal radiation	200
Total radiation from natural sources	1860
Diagnostic radiology and other medical procedures	500
Fall-out from nuclear weapons	10
Discharge of radioactive waste into the environment	3
Occupational radiation exposure	9
TV, luminous watches and other sources	8
Total radiation from man-made sources	530
Total radiation from all sources	2390

ionizing radiations and makes recommendations concerning basic principles and radiation dose limits. The ICRP makes recommendations only and it is the responsibility of the governments of individual countries to implement those recommendations which they consider appropriate to their own national circumstances.

The latest recommendations of the ICRP, published as ICRP Publication 26 in 1977, define a system of dose limitation based on the following principles:

1. No radiation practice shall be adopted unless its benefits exceed its risks.

2. All exposures shall be kept as low as reasonably achievable, economic and social factors being taken into account — this is now often called the ALARA Principle.

3. The dose equivalent to individuals shall not exceed the limits recommended for the particular circumstances.

In setting the dose equivalent limits the ICRP has recognised two classes of detrimental effects which are defined as follows: *Stochastic* effects are those for which the probability of the specific effect occurring, rather than its severity, is regarded as a function of dose without any threshold. *Non-stochastic* effects are those for which the severity of the effect varies with radiation dose and for which there is a *threshold dose* below which no effect is likely.

Whereas the earlier ICRP recommendations were based on the concept of the 'critical organ' in which the dose equivalent limit to the organ or tissue at greatest risk determined the dose limit for the individual, the ICRP now recommend a procedure which takes account of the total risk attributable to the exposure of all the tissues irradiated. The new dose limits are intended to prevent non-stochastic effects and to limit the occurrence of stochastic effects to an acceptable level. The ICRP believe that these aims may be achieved for stochastic effects by an annual dose equivalent limit for uniform irradiation of the whole body of 50 mSv (5 rem) and for non-stochastic effects by applying a dose equivalent limit of 0·5 Sv (50 rem) for all tissues except the lens of the eye for which the lower limit of 0·15 Sv is recommended (a limit of 0·3 Sv for the lens of the eye was originally recommended in ICRP Publication 26 but this was reduced by the Commission in 1980). These limits apply to radiation workers, for members of the general public lower limits of 5 mSv to the whole body for stochastic effects and 50 mSv to any tissue for non-stochastic effects are recommended.

In order to calculate the effective dose equivalent to the whole body when only a part of the body is irradiated the ICRP have proposed a series of *weighting factors* by which the dose to the individual irradiated organ may be multiplied to give the equivalent whole body dose. The values of these weighting factors are shown in Table 10.4.

The new dose equivalent limits recommended by the ICRP differ markedly in concept from the earlier recommendations which had been in effect for more than twenty years and which had been incorporated into national legislation and codes of practice in many countries. However, in the numerical values of the dose limits the principal difference is that specific dose limits are no longer recommended for particular tissues, except the lens of the eye. The basic limit for whole body irradiation remains unchanged at 50 mSv (5 rems) per year.

Table 10.4 The values of the weighting factors to be used for the calculation of the effective dose equivalent to the whole body (from ICRP Publication 26, 1977).

Tissue	Weighting factor
Gonads	0·25
Breast	0·15
Red bone marrow	0·12
Lung	0·12
Thyroid	0·03
Bone surfaces	0·03
Remainder (excluding the skin, lens of the eye, hands and forearms, feet and ankles)	0·30

In applying these dose limits to practical situations both the stochastic and non-stochastic limits must be considered and either one may prove to be the limiting dose. For example, if a procedure is expected to cause uniform irradiation of the whole body the over-riding dose limit will be given by the stochastic limit, 50 mSv, since this is lower than that for non-stochastic effects, 500 mSv: If only the thyroid gland is likely to be irradiated the over-riding dose limit will be the non-stochastic limit, 500 mSv, since this is smaller than the thyroid dose limit derived from the stochastic limit, 50/0·03 or 1666 mSv.

In nuclear medicine and other fields where radioactive solutions, or other 'unsealed' radionuclide sources, are used radioactive material may enter the human body accidentally by swallowing; inhalation of gases, aerosols or dusts; or through the skin or a wound.

The ultimate fate of radionuclides entering the body depends on their chemical properties and on their interactions with the natural components of cells and tissues. Some materials may be widely distributed throughout the body while others may localise in specific organs or tissues, for example the radionuclides of iodine concentrate in the thyroid gland while those of calcium and radium deposit predominantly in the skeleton. The fate of a radionuclide in the body may be markedly influenced by the chemical form in which it is administered. For instance if ^{131}I is administered as sodium iodide about 30 per cent enters the thyroid gland from which it is released with an average biological half time of about 70 days; in contrast if the same nuclide is administered in the form of ^{131}I-labelled Hippuran essentially all the radioactivity will be eliminated through the kidneys within a few hours. The retention of radionuclides in the body may vary widely from complete elimination within a few hours to retention times of many years, depending on the chemical and physical properties of the deposited material.

For radiation protection purposes it is necessary to limit the intake of radioactive materials into the body to such an amount that the prescribed annual dose equivalent limits are not exceeded. This amount is called the annual limit on intake (ALI). In calculating the ALI the chemical form and biological behaviour of the radioactive material must be taken into consideration together with other factors such as the physical half-life and radiation characteristics of the radionuclide. The values of the ALI vary widely from radionuclide to radionuclide, thus for ^3H_2O in which the critical organ is the whole body the ALI is $9 \cdot 6 \times 10^7$ Bq/yr, while for the long lived alpha emitting nuclide ^{226}Ra which is deposited and retained in bone for many years the ALI for ingested soluble material is only 3×10^3 Bq/yr.

10.10   Concluding remarks

The discussion in this Chapter has been concerned with the short-term and long-term injuries to human health which may result from exposure to relatively large doses of ionizing radiation. It was emphasised, Section 10.8, that under normal circumstances no radiation worker or person undergoing diagnostic investigation by radionuclide or radiographic procedures should ever suffer from any acute or long-term injury.

The dose limits recommended by the ICRP are designed to 'prevent detrimental non-stochastic effects and to limit the probability of stochastic effects to levels deemed to be acceptable'. In recent years much attention has been devoted to the assessment of the risks of radiation injury in numerical terms. The computation of these risk estimates is difficult due to the fact that there is frequently very little direct human data available on which to base our assessment, and most estimates are based on extrapolation of risk at high doses. The present estimate of the risk of fatal cancer induction for protracted whole body irradiation at the annual dose equivalent limit is about 10^{-2} Sv^{-1}. This risk must be considered in relation to the other risks of life such as death from disease, motor vehicle accidents, sporting accidents, smoking or the use of oral contraceptives. In the United Kingdom the average death rate from disease amongst a population ranging in age from 20 to 65 years is about 6000 deaths/10^6 persons/yr for males and 3500 for females. A comparison of various activities which carry a one in a million risk of death is presented in Table 10.5.

Table 10.5 Activities carrying a one in a million risk of causing death. (Compiled from E. E. Pochin — *Community Health* **6**, 2, 1974)

Whole-body exposure to 100 μSv of ionising radiation
Smoking 1·5 cigarettes
Travelling 50 miles (80 Km) by motor car
Travelling 250 miles (400 Km) by passenger aircraft
Rock climbing for 1·5 minutes
Canoeing for 6 minutes
Working in a typical factory for 1 to 2 weeks
Being a woman aged 18 years for 1 day
Being a man aged 30, or a woman aged 35 years, for 9 hours
Being a man aged 42, or a woman aged 47 years, for 3 hours
Being a man aged 53, or a woman aged 59 years, for 53 minutes
Being a man aged 63, or a woman aged 71 years, for 17 minutes

---

In all work with radiation, including clinical investigation the cardinal rule should be to follow the ALARA principle and to reduce the radiation exposure of the individual to the minimum level which is consistent with the satisfactory performance of the investigation.

11

Choice of radiopharmaceutical

Nuclear Medicine embraces a wide range of both diagnostic and therapeutic procedures (Table 11.1). All, except *in vitro* tests, require the administration of a radiopharmaceutical to the patient. The term radiopharmaceutical emphasises the essential characteristics that it contains a radionuclide as an integral part and also that it is a medicinal product and therefore must be suitable for administration

Table 11.1 Nuclear medicine procedures with the requirement of the radiopharmaceutical, especially the radionuclide component, being the principal factor in choosing the categories.

Procedure	Example
Imaging	
Static	Brain scan
Dynamic	Brain perfusion study
Uptake and retention measurements	Thyroid uptake
Tests involving only measurements on specimens	Plasma volume measurements
Therapy procedures	Treatment of thyrotoxicosis with radioiodine
In vitro tests	Assay of blood level of thyroxine

to humans. A wide selection of radiopharmaceuticals is available to meet the very different requirements of the various procedures. Radiopharmaceuticals differ both in their physical and chemical form as well as in the radionuclide involved.

In considering a radiopharmaceutical both its pharmacological behaviour and its nuclear properties must be understood. The radiopharmaceutical must distribute itself in such a manner that the aim of the test is fulfilled and an accurate understanding of its biological behaviour is essential. The properties required of the radionuclide will differ according to the procedure and correct selection of the radionuclide will, in the case of diagnostic procedures, minimise the radiation dose to the staff and patient and maximise the information gained.

There are four basic factors involved in choice of a radiopharmaceutical:

1. *Biological behaviour.* The radiopharmaceutical must achieve a satisfactory distribution in the body or trace a particular metabolic absorptive, excretory or other pathway.

2. *Radionuclide characteristics.* The radionuclide must have suitable properties as regards radiation emitted and half-life.

3. *Availability.* This will depend on the mode of production of the radionuclide (Ch. 36 and 37), the nature of the radiopharmaceutical (Ch. 38) and the cost. This last consideration is not usually a major factor.

4. *Pharmaceutical.* Most agents are injected intravenously and must therefore be of high pharmaceutical quality. This aspect will be discussed in Ch. 38.

11.1.   Biological behaviour

To image an organ it is necessary to localise the radionuclide selectively in that organ. To image a lesion such as a tumour or abscess requires either that the radionuclide concentrates in that lesion to a greater extent than in surrounding tissue or the converse. In the former case a 'hot' lesion is produced — an area of increased radioactivity — whilst in the latter a 'cold' lesion is detected. The term target is used to denote the organ or volume in which it is desired to concentrate the radiopharmaceutical. A very high target to non-target ratio is essential if a therapeutic effect is required.

The achievement of an adequate target to non-target ratio is not the only factor when considering the physiological behaviour of a radiopharmaceutical. It is important that there is not another organ in which the radiopharmaceutical concentrates, even if this does not interfere directly with the test. The radiation dose to the other organ may determine the total activity which can be reasonably administered for a diagnostic procedure. A compound of mercury was once widely used for brain scanning but the high radiation dose to the kidneys per unit administered activity limited its value. There are a variety of mechanisms which are used to obtain the desired distribution of the radiopharmaceutical or affect the way it is handled by the body. The major ones are listed in Table 11.2 and will be discussed in turn. The examples chosen are illustrative.

Metabolic activity

The measurement of uptake of radioiodine by the thyroid gland was one of the earliest nuclear medicine procedures. In the thyroid gland iodine is concentrated from the blood through an almost specific

Table 11.2 Mechanisms used to achieve desired *in vivo* distribution of radionuclides or involved in physiological fate of radiopharmaceuticals

Mechanism	Example Organ	Radiopharmaceutical
Metabolic activity	Thyroid	Iodine
Phagocytosis	Liver	Colloids
Diffusion	Brain	Pertechnetate
Cell sequestration	Spleen	Damaged red cells
Capillary blockade	Lung	Aggregates
Compartmental localisation	Vascular space	Labelled protein
Other	Tumour	Gallium citrate

iodide-trapping mechanism; inside the gland the iodine is stored and converted into the iodine-containing thyroid hormones. The advent of scanners allowed the organ to be imaged. The high uptake of radioiodine results in a very high target to non-target ratio — sufficient even for therapeutic purposes as will be discussed in 11.4. In this case one would expect that only isotopes of iodine could be used and with 22 radioisotopes of iodine a reasonable choice of nuclear decay characteristics is provided. However, the pertechnetate ion, TcO_4^-, has a similar size to that of iodide, I^-, and is taken up by the thyroid gland via the iodide-trapping mechanism; it is not however converted into thyroid hormones and, unlike iodine, it can be relatively easily released from the gland. In a normal person only 1·5–3·0 per cent of an oral dose of $^{99}Tc^m$-pertechnetate is taken up by the thyroid as compared to 15–40 per cent of an oral dose of iodine; however, the uptake of $^{99}Tc^m$ is adequate to give good images of the gland.

Another example of metabolic activity is the use of seleno-methionine for pancreas scanning. This organ has a large requirement for amino acids in order to synthesise the enzyme proteins which it secretes into the duodenum. Methionine has a sulphur atom but unfortunately there is no suitable gamma emitting isotope of sulphur. It was found that if methionine was prepared with the sulphur atom substituted by an atom of selenium, which has a gamma emitting isotope (^{75}Se), then this molecule, selenomethionine is also incorporated into protein. Amino acids labelled with the positron emitting isotope of carbon, ^{11}C, also localise in the pancreas and some, for example ^{11}C-tryptophan, yield good images. However, the very short, 20 min., half life of ^{11}C and the special facilities required for the production of ^{11}C radiopharmaceuticals limit the applicability of these agents.

Phagocytosis

Certain cells in the body, for example Kupfer cells in the liver, have the capacity to ingest small particles, usually those with diameters in the range 10–10 000 nm—this process is called phagocytosis—and a radionuclide in particulate or colloidal form injected intravenously will tend to concentrate exclusively in such cells.

The chemistry of colloids — small particles permanently dispersed in a liquid — will be discussed in Chapter 33. In the liver the Kupfer cells are fairly uniformly distributed throughout the organ, thus the uptake of colloidal particles labelled with an appropriate radionuclide enables an image of the liver to be obtained. The Kupfer cells are part of the reticuloendothelial system, the other major components being the phagocytic cells in the spleen and the bone marrow. Because of the high blood flow to the liver it normally takes up over 80 per cent of the colloid.

Diffusion

Radiopharmaceuticals used for brain scanning are characterised by the fact that normal brain tissue is relatively impermeable to their passage from the blood due to the so-called blood-brain barrier. In contrast, most mass lesions in the brain are more permeable than the normal tissue and so the lesions can be imaged due to diffusion of the radioactivity into the lesion. With some radiopharmaceuticals there are probably other processes also operating.

Cell sequestration

The spleen can be visualised using radiocolloids but this technique is limited by the low uptake and the close proximity of the liver. Erythrocytes can be labelled with a radionuclide and if they are slightly damaged before injection they will be selectively removed by the spleen from the bloodstream.

Capillary blockade

When radioactive particles larger than the size of the blood capillaries (about 8–10 μm diameter) are injected intravenously they will become lodged in the capillaries of the lung. Fewer than a million particles in a size range 20–70 μm are injected and they block less than point one per cent of the capillaries of a normal lung. It is essential that particles are chosen so that they are broken down in a reasonable period of time, hours or days, after being trapped. Particles prepared by aggregation of labelled molecules of the protein human serum albumin are widely used and are known as macroaggregated albumin.

Compartmental localisation
Certain types of cells and molecules are found to be distributed in, effectively, only one particular body compartment. Thus if such cells or molecules are labelled with a suitable radionuclide they may be used as markers to visualize, or to measure the size of, that compartment. For example the volume of red blood cells in the vascular compartment may be measured by injecting intravenously ^{51}Cr- or ^{99}Tc^m-labelled red cells; or the volume of the plasma compartment may be measured by intravenously injecting a labelled plasma protein, for example ^{125}I-labelled Human Serum Albumin. The red blood cells are found virtually exclusively in the vascular compartment, while the diffusion of labelled plasma proteins out of the plasma space is so slow that it is almost negligible when measurements are completed within a few minutes.

Other types of localisation
The method by which a radiopharmaceutical localises in a tissue is not always understood, this is especially true in the case of the radiopharmaceuticals currently used to visualise tumours and inflammatory lesions. Gallium-67 was found empirically to concentrate in various space-occupying lesions and is used for the localisation of both tumours and abscesses. Despite a decade of research it is still not clear how and why ^{67}Ga localises in such lesions; it appears likely that in tumours the iron-transport protein transferrin and a specific transferrin-receptor site on the tumour cell surface play important roles. The mechanisms by which ^{67}Ga, and other similar metallic radionuclides, are taken up by inflamed and normal tissues are still unknown but there is increasing evidence to suggest that they are different from those found in tumours.

One type of mechanism which may permit us to develop sensitive and specific methods for the localisation of tumours, or even of specific cell types, in the body is the antigen-antibody reaction. Most, probably all, cell types in the body have specific molecules on their surface, antigens, which will react only with a specific protein antibody. If these specific antibodies can be isolated in very pure form and labelled with a suitable radionuclide, the labelled antibody may be expected to react only with its own particular antigen on the tumour cell surface thus labelling the tumour but not the normal tissues. This is a potentially very promising and exciting approach to tumour localisation.

Many types of specific antibody can now be produced in pure form in the laboratory by the use of cells or bacteria which have been altered using genetic engineering techniques so that they contain the human or animal gene which makes the desired antibody — such antibody preparations are called monoclonal antibodies. The resulting antibody can be extracted, purified and labelled with a suitable radionuclide, for example ^{123}I. Preliminary studies with such labelled antibodies are yielding encouraging results.

11.2. Choice of radionuclide

The principal factors which need to be considered when selecting a radionuclide are the types of radiation emitted, the energy and abundance of the gamma rays and the half-life. The range of choice for the radionuclide will depend on the physical and chemical form of the radiopharmaceutical. In some cases there may be a choice of element whilst in others only a choice of isotope. In the next three sections when considering the various factors involved only imaging will be considered initially. Any modification for other diagnostic procedures or for therapy will be discussed subsequently in Section 11.4.

Type of radiation emitted. For all diagnostic imaging gamma, or sometimes X radiation, of a suitable energy is required. Particulate radiation is of no value as it is absorbed within the patient. The radiation should be of high abundance; thus ^{198}Au which emits 96 photons of 412 keV per 100 disintegrations is a more suitable radionuclide in this respect than ^{51}Cr which emits only 9 photons of 323 keV per 100 disintegrations. It is also normally an advantage, but not essential, if the gamma rays are monoenergetic rather than spread out over a range of energies as in the case of ^{67}Ga which has principal gamma rays at 92, 182, 300 and 390 keV. In some exceptional cases with radionuclides of high atomic number the characteristic X-rays can be used instead of gamma rays for imaging — the use of the 69 keV ^{198}Au K X-rays in the decay of ^{197}Hg is an example. With therapeutic levels of a pure beta emitter, such as ^{32}P, an image can be obtained using the bremsstrahlung X-radiation.

All radiation emitted contributes to the absorbed dose. It is therefore desirable to minimise the amount of radiation which is not of use in the imaging process. This can be best achieved by using radionuclides which decay by isomeric transition. Even with this type of decay there is some low energy radiation due to internal conversion. With ^{99}Tc^m only 8·5 per cent of the 140 keV gamma rays are converted but in the case of the 390 keV transition of ^{113}In^m the conversion is 33 per cent. Although radionuclides which decay by electron capture emit no particulate radiation from the nucleus, low energy electron and X-radiation are emitted due to the vacancies created by the electron capture and the internal conversion of any gamma radiation. [111]In is an example of a radionuclide which decays by electron capture and can be successfully used for imaging.

In the case of radionuclides which decay by beta, or positron, emission the kinetic energy of the particles is deposited locally. Depending on the energy of the particles their presence can severely restrict the activity that can be safely administered. In the case of ^{131}I for thyroid scanning, over 90 per cent of the radiation dose to the gland arises from the beta particles.

Energy of gamma radiation. The gamma rays to be used for imaging must be of sufficient energy not to be unduly absorbed in the body. One hundred keV is a desirable lower limit; below this the half-value thickness in tissue is less than 4 cm (Table 7.1). Another disadvantage of low energy radiation is that it is more difficult to overcome the problem of the radiation scattered in the body and this reduces the spatial resolution obtainable.

The upper limit is set by the decrease in efficiency of the detectors. This is due to two reasons, the collimator efficiency (Ch. 23) and the NaI(T1) crystal efficiency, especially for gamma cameras which have only a 12·5 mm thick crystal (Ch. 24). Five hundred keV is the upper limit for most purposes. If there is more than one gamma ray emitted the collimator chosen should correspond to the gamma ray with the highest energy, even if it is not being used for the imaging, or else a loss of resolution occurs due to septal penetration. With ^{123}I, although the 159 keV is used for imaging, a medium energy collimator must be used because over 2 per cent of disintegrations result in gamma rays of over 500 keV.

Half-life. The absorbed dose to an organ depends on the effective half-life of the radiopharmaceutical (Ch. 9). If the biological half-life is longer than the physical one then the dominant effect on the effective half-life will be the rate of physical decay. In this situation the physical half-life of the radionuclide should be comparable to the length of the investigation in order to minimise the radiation dose. Many investigations, such as brain scanning, are completed within a matter of hours of injection and therefore a nuclide with a half-life of a few hours is suitable. The lower limit is often set by logistic problems— the supply of the radionuclide and preparation of the radiopharmaceutical.

When the biological half-life is similar to the investigation period and the radionuclide is excreted from the body a long half-life radionuclide may be used. However, problems may arise in this situation. It only requires a small retention, a few per cent, either in the organ of interest or in the whole body, to give a substantial radiation dose which can limit the amount of activity which may be injected.

Handling and protection problems are also increased. In general it is desirable to use as short lived a radionuclide as possible.

The 'ideal' radionuclide

There is no single ideal radionuclide because of the nature of the different investigations. The characteristics required and which have been discussed above are summarised in Table 11.3. For many investigations $^{99}Tc^m$ comes close to fulfilling the ideal requirements — it is readily available in hospitals (Ch. 38); it can be made into a variety of radiopharmaceuticals; it decays by isomeric transition emitting a 140 keV gamma ray in high abundance and its half-life of six hours is a convenient length, long enough that all doses required for a day's investigations can be prepared together but short enough that large activities, up to half a gigabecquerel for some radiopharmaceuticals, can be administered.

Table 11.3 Desirable characteristics of a radionuclide for organ imaging

1. Gamma Emitting:
   Single gamma ray
   Energy 100–500 keV range
   High abundance
   Low internal conversion
   No high energy gamma rays.

2. Decay mechanism. Order of preference:
   Isomeric transition
   Electron capture
   Positron
   Beta minus

3. Half-life:
   Similar to length of investigation.

Uptake and retention measurements

Most of these procedures involve measuring uptake by the whole body after an oral dose or the retention by an organ after an intravenous dose. The radiopharmaceuticals are measuring physiological function and therefore it is essential that labelling the compound does not interfere with or alter the characteristics of the compound. When a direct substitution occurs, radioactive ^{57}Co for stable ^{59}Co in Vitamin B-12, for example, there is no problem but if a labelled analogue is used caution must be exercised.

The properties required of the radionuclide are similar to those for imaging as external detectors are used. However, the requirements are often less stringent as lower activities are generally used — only about

0·1 MBq of ^{131}I are required for an uptake test whilst about 1·0 are needed to produce an adequate image. The half life of the radionuclide must be adequate for the length of the test, which for whole body retention tests may be a period of weeks or months.

Tests involving only measurement on specimens
These tests involve the administration of a radiopharmaceutical to the patient and then taking samples, for example, of blood. Collection of urine, and sometimes faeces, may be required and tissue samples from operation or biopsy specimens can be measured. Other fluids which may be sampled are saliva and nasal secretions.

There is a greater range of radionuclides available as a gamma emitting nuclide is not essential, though convenient due to the easier counting of samples. The activity required to be injected is usually low — a few kilobecquerels — as the sensitivity of sample counting is very high. The radioactivity of beta emitting samples can be measured using liquid scintillation counting.

11.3.   Types of radiopharmaceutical
Table 11.4 summarises the main categories, together with an indication as to whether there is a choice of element or only of isotope for the radionuclide component.

11.4.   Therapy procedures (unsealed sources)
Phosphorus-32 was the first radionuclide to be administered to a patient for treatment purposes. This took place in 1938 and the aim was to treat leukaemia. Like diagnostic applications the widespread use of radionuclides for therapy did not occur until the 1940's and a number of procedures quickly established their value. Until the late 1950's therapy treatments were as numerous as diagnostic tests; since then there has been an enormous growth in diagnostic uses, but the role of radionuclides in therapy has remained fairly static — a valuable but limited form of treatment.

The essential aim of radionuclide therapy is the same as with any radiotherapy, to maximise the radiation dose to the treatment volume and to minimise the dose outside this volume.

Beta emitting radionuclides are almost always used for therapy, for exactly the same reason that they are not very satisfactory for diagnostic applications. The beta particles are absorbed locally and therefore the absorbed dose pattern is the same as the radionuclide concentration pattern. It is therefore essential to have a high target (the treatment volume) to non-target ratio. It is the difficulty of achieving this which limits the number of useful therapy procedures.

Table 11.4 Major categories of radiopharmaceuticals, with examples and comments on choice of radionuclide

Type of radiopharmaceutical	Examples	Comments
Simple Inorganic	$Na^{131}I$ $Na^{99}Tc^mO_4$	Only choice of isotope for any given compound
Colloid	$^{99}Tc^m$-sulphur colloid ^{198}Au-colloid	Virtually all radionuclides can be made in colloidal form but some pharmacological restrictions as to which forms can be administered to humans.
Aggregates Microspheres	^{131}I-albumin macroagregates $^{99}Tc^m$-albumin microspheres	As for colloids
Organic molecules labelled analogues	^{131}I-albumin	Limited number of elements, e.g. I and F, can be used.
Organic molecules substitution	^{57}Co-Vitamin B-12	Choice of isotope only
Complexes	$^{99}Tc^m$-DTPA $^{99}Tc^m$-HIDA	Many elements can be complexed
Labelled cells	^{51}Cr-red blood cells ^{111}In or $^{99}Tc^m$-neutrophils, platelets or lymphocytes	Limited number of elements can be used
Gases	^{133}Xe $^{81}Kr^m$	Restricted number of elements

Method of localisation

There are only two methods which have been widely used, metabolic incorporation and compartmental localisation. Other methods, such as the use of phagocytosis in the treatment of liver disease, have been tried but none have been widely adopted.

The most important and widespread form of radionuclide therapy is in the treatment of the thyroid (Table 11.5), either for the non-malignant condition of thyrotoxicosis or in carcinoma of the thyroid. The method of localisation is metabolic incorporation. Orally administered radioactive sodium iodide is absorbed by the body and selectively concentrated in the thyroid. With an euthyroid patient 15–40 per cent of the administered dose is taken up but this rises to 60 per cent or higher in hyperthyroid patients. In a certain number of patients with carcinoma of thyroid the malignant cells are sufficiently differentiated to concentrate iodine and therefore secondary deposits, wherever they are located in the body, can be treated. The use of radioiodine to treat patients with advanced cancer was the first

Table 11.5 The main radionuclides used for therapy with examples

| Radionuclide | $T_{1/2}$ | Decay | Principal radiation | | Chemical form | Example of use | | Typical dose (GBq) |
			Gamma (MeV)	Beta (max.MeV)		Method of localisation	Condition	
P-32	14·3d	β^-	—	1·7(100%)	Sodium Phosphate	Active transport	Polycythemia rubra vera	0·2
Y-90	2·7d	β^-	—	2·3(100%)	Colloid	Compartmental localisation	Intrapleural –effusions	0·4–1
							Intraperitoneal –ascites	1–1·8
							Intraarticular –joints	0·2
I-131	8d	β^-	0·36(80%) 0·64(9%) 0.72(3%)	0·33(9%) 0·61(87%)	Sodium Iodide	Active transport	Thyrotoxicosis Carcinoma thyroid	0·1–0·4 3–7
Au-198	2·7d	β^-	0·41(96%)	0·96(99%)	Colloid	Compartmental localisation	Intrapleural –effusions	3
							Intraperitoneal –ascites	4–5

successful method of treating disseminated disease. The uptake in secondary deposits is lower than in normal thyroid tissue but enough radioiodine can be concentrated to be therapeutic.

Phosphorus-32 is incorporated into dividing cells and has been used to treat a variety of diseases of the bone marrow. With the advent of chemotherapy its use is now usually limited to polycythaemia rubra vera.

Compartmental localisation is used to treat pleural and peritoneal neoplastic effusions. A radioactive colloid solution is injected into the cavity where it is physically trapped. The fluid in the cavity is irradiated and over a matter of hours the colloid deposits out on the surface, thereby giving a high local dose to the wall of the cavity.

Choice of radionuclide

Beta emitting radionuclides are used almost universally. There are advantages and disadvantages to having gamma radiation also emitted. Gamma radiation allows external monitoring and can improve homogeneity of the absorbed dose distribution. The disadvantages are the whole body absorbed dose, which is not usually a limiting factor, and increased protection problems.

The choice of the energies of the beta particles is normally not critical; in general a reasonably high energy is desirable to give a significant penetration, for example, when treating pleural and peritoneal microscopic deposits.

A half-life of several days is usually satisfactory. With a short lived isotope very large activities have to be administered, whilst if the half-life is too long protection problems arise and small variations in distribution and retention can significantly affect the dosimetry.

11.5. *In vitro* tests

There are now available and widely used a large number of *in vitro* tests and assays which involve the use of radioactive compounds. These compounds are not radiopharmaceuticals as they are not administered to the patient but it is convenient to discuss them in this chapter.

Radioimmunoassay and saturation analysis are techniques involving the use of labelled compounds to measure the concentration of a hormone or other compound in plasma or other fluid. These techniques are discussed in Chapter 14.

The amount of radioactivity involved per test is about a kilobecquerel and either pure beta or gamma emitting radionuclides may be used. Iodine-125 is widely used as many compounds can be labelled with iodine, it can be detected conveniently in a gamma counter using its 28–35 keV X- and gamma radiation and its half-life of 60 days provides a conveniently long shelf life for labelled compounds. As with any labelled compound used as a tracer it is essential that it behaves in an identical fashion after labelling to that before.

12

Basic principles of tracer techniques I — Static studies

12.1. Introduction

During the past forty years radioactive tracer techniques have led to many important fundamental advances in our understanding of biochemistry and physiology. Similar methods now permit the measurement of many physiological and biochemical parameters which are important to our understanding of human disease and in its investigation and management. Physiological quantities such as blood volume, blood flow, lymphocyte and neutrophil circulation, absorption from the gastrointestinal tract, kidney function and the rates of secretion of some hormones may now be measured *in vivo* using radionuclide tracer techniques. Modern developments of the simple organ visualization techniques mentioned in Chapter 1 using computer-coupled gamma cameras, or tomographic or positron scanners, now offer exciting possibilities for the quantitative measurement of metabolic activity in different areas of the brain and heart; the range and scope of such measurements must be expected to grow as new radiopharmaceuticals based on normal metabolic substrates, or substrate analogues, are developed.

In the next two chapters we shall be discussing some of the simple static and dynamic tracer techniques and the basic principles upon which they are based.

12.2. The isotope dilution principle

This concept forms the basis for very many tracer tests and permits the study of masses and volumes; rates of transfer and excretion of substances; and of biochemical pathways.

The basic principle of dilution analysis is very simple. It depends on the fact that if a radioactively labelled substance is mixed with a quantity of the same unlabelled substance the amount of radioactivity per unit mass of the substance will be less than that of the original radioactive substance. In other words the radioactive material has been *diluted* with the inactive substance. Thus if we can measure the reduction in radioactivity per unit mass of substance we can calculate the amount of the diluting substance.

If we consider a tracer compound C^* with a radioactivity A_0 and a mass W_0, the specific activity S_0 of the compound will be:

$$S_0 = \frac{A_0}{W_0} \tag{12.1}$$

The inactive form of the same compound (C) has no radioactivity but it has a mass W_u. If we mix C and C^* the radioactivity is still A_0 but the mass is now $W_u + W_0$. The specific activity S_1 of the compound is therefore:

$$S_1 = \frac{A_0}{W_u + W_0} \tag{12.2}$$

Provided that we know A_0 and W_0 and that we can measure S_1, we can calculate W_u from the expression:

$$W_u = \frac{A_0}{S_1} - W_0 \tag{12.3}$$

The great advantage of this method is that it is not necessary to separate the whole of $W_u + W_0$ in order to measure S_1. Provided that the labelled and inactive substances are in the same chemical form and have been thoroughly mixed, the specific activity S_1 will be independent of the amount of material used to measure it. Thus as long as some of the substance can be separated in a pure state, and the radioactivity and mass of the sample can be measured, then we can calculate the amount of inactive material, W_u, in the whole system.

If the specific activity of the radioactive tracer compound is very high the mass, W_0, of tracer compound added may be very small compared with W_u and may be neglected, thus equation (3) may be simplified to:

$$W_u = \frac{A_0}{S_1} \tag{12.4}$$

This is a general statement of the isotope dilution principle in which we have considered the determination of an unknown mass. The same procedure can be applied to the estimation of volumes or spaces. As an example let us consider a water tank with a volume V. If we introduce into this tank a tracer amount of tritiated water, ^3H_2O, having an activity A and a volume t and mix the contents thoroughly before removing a sample of volume y and if this sample has a radioactivity of S then the volume of water in the tank will be:

$$V = \frac{A.y}{S} - t \qquad (12.5)$$

or if t is very small compared with V then

$$V = \frac{A.y}{S} \qquad (12.6)$$

12.3.   Measurement of volumes and spaces

Some of the applications of the isotope dilution principle to clinical investigation are given in Table 12.1.

A typical procedure for the measurement of plasma volume is as follows: 350 kBq of ^{125}I-labelled human serum albumin (^{125}IHSA) is injected into a vein in 10 cm^3 solution. A known volume of the same ^{125}IHSA solution, say 1 cm^3 is placed in a volumetric flask and diluted to 100 cm^3 to enable the total injected activity to be determined, this is called the 'standard'.

Table 12.1 Some applications of the isotope dilution principle to clinical investigation

Measurement	Radioactive indicator
Plasma volume	^{125}I-human serum albumin
Red cell mass	^{51}Cr-labelled red cells
Total body water	^3H_2O
'Chloride' space	^{82}Br
Total exchangeable sodium	^{24}Na
Total exchangeable potassium	^{42}K

Following injection three blood samples are collected, from another vein, at say 15, 30 and 45 minutes and placed in heparinised tubes. The plasma is separated by centrifugation and 2 cm^3 of plasma are pipetted into counting tubes. A 2 cm^3 aliquot of the diluted ^{125}IHSA is placed in another counting tube. All the samples are then counted in a scintillation counter (see Ch. 21) and the background counting rate is subtracted from the observed counting rate of each sample.

Three blood samples are taken in order to correct for any loss of ^{125}IHSA from the circulating plasma during the initial mixing period. In normal patients this loss is only about 6 to 10 per cent per hour but in patients with burns it may rise to about 18 per cent per hour. The observed net counting rates of the plasma samples are plotted against time on semilogarithmic paper and the resulting straight line is extrapolated to zero time, Figure 12.1. If only one blood sample can be obtained this should be taken at about 15 minutes and the counting rate of this sample used in the calculation of plasma volume instead of the extrapolated value; in these circumstances the error of the estimation is larger than that obtained by the extrapolation method.

The calculation of the plasma volume is illustrated by the following example. A, y and S refer to equation 12.6.

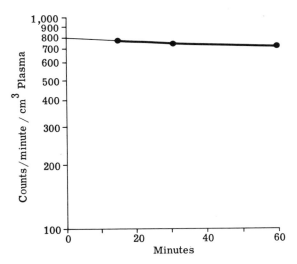

Fig. 12.1 Plasma clearance of [125]IHSA.

Volume of [125]IHSA solution injected = $10\,cm^3$ ($=y$)

Standard = $1\,cm^3$ of [125]IHSA in $100\,cm^3$

Counting rate of standard = $25\,500$ counts/minute/$2\,cm^3$

Hence

$$A = \frac{25\,500 \times 100}{2}$$

Counting rates of samples

15 minutes = 7973 counts/minute/$2\,cm^3$

30 minutes = 7852 counts/minute/$2\,cm^3$

45 minutes = 7810 counts/minute/2 cm^3

Plasma counting rate at zero time (Figure 12.1)

$$= 8095 \text{ counts/minute/2 cm}^3 \quad \left(\text{hence } S = \frac{8095}{2}\right)$$

Applying equation 12.6

$$\text{Plasma Volume} = \frac{25\,500 \times 10 \times 100}{2} \times \frac{2}{8095}$$

$$= 3150 \text{ cm}^3$$

An essentially similar technique is used for the determination of red cell volume using ^{51}Cr-labelled red blood cells as a tracer.

A slightly more complicated example of the use of the isotope dilution principle in clinical investigation is the measurement of 'total exchangeable sodium' using ^{24}Na. A known volume of a solution of ^{24}NaCl, containing about 900 kBq ^{24}Na, is injected intravenously, or given orally, and all urine passed during the next 24 hours is collected and pooled. At the end of the 24 hour period a single blood sample is collected and the plasma is separated rapidly. Part of the plasma sample is set aside for the determination of the total sodium concentration by flame photometry, and the other part is used to determine the ^{24}Na activity by scintillation counting. A 'standard' is prepared by diluting the same volume of the ^{24}Na solution as was administered to the patient to 1 litre with saline and aliquots of this solution and of the patients urine are assayed for ^{24}Na.

During the 24 hour observation period the ^{24}Na becomes uniformly mixed with the total mass of exchangeable sodium in the body and the specific activity of the ^{24}Na in the plasma will be the same as that in the tissues. Thus if we know the total amount of ^{24}Na remaining in the body at 24 hours we can calculate the total mass of exchangeable sodium.

The method of calculation is illustrated in the following example.

Volume of ^{24}Na solution administered = 5 cm^3

'Standard' = 5 cm^3 of ^{24}Na solution in 1000 cm^3

Volume of urine passed = 1420 cm^3

Plasma sodium concentration = 135 mmol/dm^3

Plasma ^{24}Na = 928 cpm/cm^3

Urinary ^{24}Na = 433 cpm/cm^3

Standard ^{24}Na $= 16\,550\,\text{cpm/cm}^3$

^{24}Na remaining in the body after 24 hours is:

(The total activity administered — activity excreted in the urine)

$= (16\,550 \times 1000) - (433 \times 1420)$

$= 16\,550\,000 - 614\,860 = 15\,935\,140\,\text{cpm}$

Total exchangeable sodium

$$= \frac{^{24}\text{Na remaining in the body} \times \text{plasma sodium}}{\text{Plasma } ^{24}\text{Na}}$$

$$= \frac{15\,935\,140 \times 135}{928 \times 1000}\,\text{mmol Na}$$

$= 2318\,\text{mmol}$

or if the patient weighed 62 kg

$$\frac{2318}{62} \quad \text{or} \quad 37{\cdot}4\,\text{mmol/kg}.$$

An essentially similar method using ^{42}K as the tracer may be used to determine the total exchangeable potassium. The 'chloride space' of the body may also be determined by this type of technique but in this case, since no convenient chlorine radionuclide is available we use its analogue ^{82}Br as the tracer.

13

Basic principles of tracer techniques II —Kinetic studies

The type of measurement discussed in Chapter 12 yields information on mass or volume at the time of measurement. Frequently we need information on the rates at which a substance moves in and out of the plasma or some other body compartment. The isotope dilution principle can be applied also to this type of measurement. In order to understand the basis of these techniques we must learn some simple elements of kinetic theory.

Let us consider an open tank from which water is lost through a hole in the bottom, Figure 13.1. The rate at which water runs out of the tank depends on the height (h) of the water in the tank, or in other words on the volume of water in the tank. If the volume of water in the tank is $V_0 \, cm^3$ and the rate of flow is $F \, cm^3 \, s^{-1}$ then at any time

$$F \propto V_0$$

or

$$\frac{F}{V_0} = \text{constant } (k) \tag{13.1}$$

The constant k represents the fraction of the total volume which is lost per unit of time, and is called the 'rate constant'.

At any time t the volume, V, remaining in the tank can be shown to follow a simple exponential function (Appendix 1)

$$V = V_0 e^{-kt} \tag{13.2}$$

or

$$V/V_0 = e^{-kt}. \tag{13.3}$$

If the volumes of water remaining in the tank at various times are measured and the logarithm, to the base e, of the ratio V/V_0 is plotted against the time t the values will lie on a straight line since

$$\log_e V/V_0 = -kt \tag{13.4}$$

and k is a constant, Figure 13.2. (See Appendix 2).

148

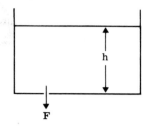

Fig. 13.1

The slope of this line is defined by the constant k. Instead of calculating the value of k from the slope of the curve we may derive it from the 'half-time', $t_{\frac{1}{2}}$, which is the time taken for the value of V/V_0 to decrease to half its original value. From equation 13.4 and Figure 13.2 we see that after one half-time V/V_0 is equal to 0·5 and therefore:

$$\log_e V/V_0 = -kt_{\frac{1}{2}} = \log_e 0·5$$

and

$$kt_{\frac{1}{2}} = -(\log_e 0·5) = \log_e 2 = 0·693$$

thus

$$t_{\frac{1}{2}} = \frac{0·693}{k} \qquad (13.5)$$

This process is analogous to that of radioactive decay (Ch. 4).

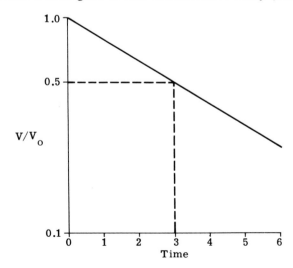

Fig. 13.2

If the water from the tank empties into another tank from which a proportion is pumped back into the first tank we have a slightly more complicated situation in which equation 13.2 becomes

$$V = V_0(a_1 e^{-k_1 t} + a_2 e^{-k_2 t}) \qquad (13.6)$$

where k_1 and k_2 are the rate constants for the outflow and inflow and a_1 and a_2 are the fractions of the total volume lost and returned.

In this situation a plot of $\log_e V/V_0$ against t yields a curve rather than a straight line, Figure 13.3a and b. These curves comprise the sum of the individual exponential components and the individual half-times, and hence the rate constants, for each exponential can be derived from the graph by the use of the technique known as 'curve stripping'. This technique in its simplest form may be illustrated by analysis of the data shown in Fig. 13.3a which shows a two component exponential curve. Inspection of the data for the time points between 25 and 65 minutes shows that these lie on a straight line with a half-time of 45 minutes and rate constant. k_2, of $0.693/45$ or 0.0154. If this line is extrapolated back to zero time it is possible to read off from this line the values of V/V_0 corresponding to this longer term component at each of the time intervals measured between 0 and 25 minutes, at $t = 0$ this value is 0.05. If we subtract this value from the observed value for each time point and plot the net values against time

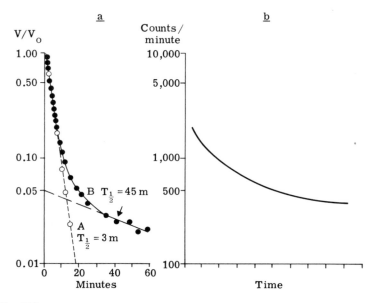

Fig. 13.3

we obtain the straight line, marked A on Figure 13.3a, which represents the first exponential term of the curve. This term has a half-time of 3 minutes or a rate constant, k_1, of $0.693/3$ or 0.231 and intercepts the axis at $V/V_0 = 0.95$. Thus the equation to this curve is:

$$V = V_0(0.95e^{-0.231t} + 0.05e^{-0.0154t})$$

Let us now consider a slightly different situation in which our tank is closed and remains completely full because water flows into it at the same rate as it flows out, Figure 13.4.

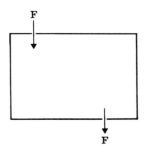

Fig. 13.4

In this case the volume V remains constant, but water molecules are continually entering and leaving the tank. If we disperse a radioactive marker into the tank the concentration of the marker will decrease as the labelled fluid leaks out and is replaced by unlabelled fluid. In this case the rate at which the radioactive marker leaves the tank will depend on the concentration of the marker in the tank, and equation 13.2 can be re-written as:

$$C = C_0e^{-kt} \qquad (13.7)$$

Where C_0 is the initial concentration and C is the concentration at any time 't'. If instead of one tank we have two interconnected tanks, equation 13.7 will be similar to equation 13.6 but with concentration 'C' replacing volume 'V'. In the much more complex situation where we have a larger number 'n' of interconnecting tanks or compartments, equation 13.7 must be expanded to become:

$$C = C_0(a_1e^{-k_1t} + a_2e^{-k_2t} + \cdots a_ne^{-k_nt}) \qquad (13.8)$$

This type of system in which the volume or mass of substance does not change, but there is a continual inflow and outflow, is called an *equilibrium*, or *steady state* system. This situation is commonly encountered in the mammalian body where in a tissue, or body compartment, the total concentration of a substance may remain constant, but the individual molecules of the substance are in a continual state of flux with new molecules entering the system to replace those which are lost or destroyed. The rates of movement of molecules into or out of a system can be measured by radioactive tracer methods, for example the radionuclide ^{59}Fe can be used to measure the rates at which iron enters and leaves the plasma and is incorporated into the haemoglobin of the red blood cells.

If we inject intravenously 150 to 300 kBq of ^{59}Fe bound to the plasma protein transferrin, the radioactive iron rapidly becomes mixed with the inactive iron in the plasma. The rate of removal of the ^{59}Fe from the plasma can be determined by taking serial blood samples over a period of about 2 hours after injection and measuring the plasma radioactivity. If we plot the plasma radioactivity against time on semi-logarithmic graph paper we find that the points lie on a single straight line from which we can obtain the half-time of iron clearance and hence, from equation 13.5, the value of k. Figure 13.5. Providing we know the total ^{59}Fe activity injected we can calculate the plasma volume, and if the plasma iron concentration is determined by chemical analysis we may derive the *plasma iron turnover-rate* (PIT) from the relation:

$$PIT = \frac{\text{Plasma Volume} \times \text{Plasma iron concentration} \times 0 \cdot 693 \times 24}{T_{\frac{1}{2}} \, ^{59}Fe \text{ in Plasma}} \mu g/day$$

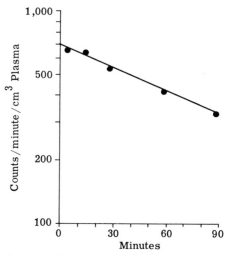

Fig. 13.5 Plasma clearance of iron-59.

After 2 to 5 days the ^{59}Fe begins to appear in the circulating red cells and the uptake reaches a maximum at 7 to 10 days. If we measure the percentage of the injected ^{59}Fe which is incorporated into the red cells we may determine the *red cell iron turnover-rate* from the expression:

Red cell iron turnover

= Plasma iron turnover × %^{59}Fe in the total Red Cell Mass

This type of study is valuable in the investigation of haematological disorders. The following example illustrates how the experimental data are handled.

A patient weighing 63 kg was given 300 kBq ^{59}Fe citrate intravenously and 5 blood samples were collected between 5 and 90 minutes after injection. An equal amount of the injected ^{59}Fe solution was diluted to 1 litre to act as a standard. The ^{59}Fe concentration in the plasma samples and standard was determined by scintillation counting and the results were as follows:

^{59}Fe Standard = 2200 counts/min/cm^3

Plasma samples	5 min	660 counts/min/cm^3
	15 min	615 counts/min/cm^3
	30 min	540 counts/min/cm^3
	60 min	420 counts/min/cm^3
	90 min	320 counts/min/cm^3

Plasma iron concentration = 1·2 mg/litre (20 μmol/dm^3).

When the plasma ^{59}Fe concentration data are plotted against time on semi logarithmic paper, Figure 13.5, the activity is found to decrease with a half time of 85 minutes and extrapolation of the straight line to zero time yields an intercept of 700 counts/min/cm^3.

$$\text{Plasma volume} = \frac{\text{Total injected } ^{59}\text{Fe activity}}{\text{Plasma } ^{59}\text{Fe/cm}^3 \text{ at } t = 0}$$

$$= \frac{2200 \times 1000}{700} = 3143 \text{ cm}^3 \text{ or } 3 \cdot 143 \text{ litres}$$

$$\text{Plasma Iron Turnover} = \frac{0 \cdot 693 \times 3 \cdot 143 \times 1 \cdot 12 \times 24}{85/60} \text{ mg Fe/day}$$

$$= 41 \cdot 3 \text{ mg/day}$$

or

0·66 mg/kg body weight/day.

Ten days after injection of the ^{59}Fe the red blood cells were found to contain 840 counts/min/cm^3 of red cells. The haematocrit was 44% and the ratio of the measured venous haematocrit to the total body haematocrit was assumed to be 0·90.

Total ^{59}Fe in the red cell mass

= Red cell ^{59}Fe (counts/min/cm^3) × Red Cell Volume (cm^3)

Red Cell Volume = Total Blood Volume − Plasma Volume

$$= \frac{\text{Plasma Volume} \times 100}{100 - (0\cdot9 \times \text{Haematocrit})} - \text{Plasma Volume}$$

$$= \left(\frac{3143 \times 100}{100 - (0\cdot9 \times 44)} \right) - 3143$$

$$= 5204 - 3143 = 2061 \text{ cm}^3$$

Percentage of the injected ^{59}Fe in the Red Cell Mass

$$= \frac{840 \times 2061 \times 100}{2200 \times 1000} = 78\cdot7\%$$

Red Cell Iron Turnover Rate

$$= \frac{41\cdot3 \times 78\cdot7}{100} \text{ mg Fe/day}$$

$$= 32\cdot5 \text{ mg/day}$$

or

0·52 mg/kg body weight/day.

13.1. Flow studies

Radionuclide techniques can be utilised to provide quantitative information on blood and lymph flow, capillary permeability and circulation times in various organs and tissues. A large number of techniques are now available for the measurement of such physiological parameters as blood flow in liver, brain, myocardium, muscle, and tumours, cardiac output, lymph flow in subcutaneous tissues, glomerular filtration rates and renal plasma flow. Such techniques now frequently involve the use of computer-coupled gamma cameras, or other imaging devices, and may measure two or more parameters simultaneously (Chapter 28). We shall consider only three of the simpler procedures which illustrate the principles of the measurement of flow *in vivo*.

Local clearance methods. In this technique a biologically inert radioactive indicator is injected locally into a tissue and the rate of clearance of the tracer is measured using a suitable scintillation detector.

One example of this method is the determination of regional blood flow in superficial tumours. The indicator used was ^{133}Xe dissolved in saline and 0·1 ml of the solution, containing 4 to 8 MBq[133]Xe, was injected into the middle of the tumour. The rate of disappearance of the radionuclide from the area was monitored with a collimated scintillation counter viewing a 10 cm diameter field. Ten second counts were made at frequent intervals over a period of 15–20 minutes following injection and the counting data were analysed using a computer. A typical disappearance curve is illustrated in Figure 13.6.

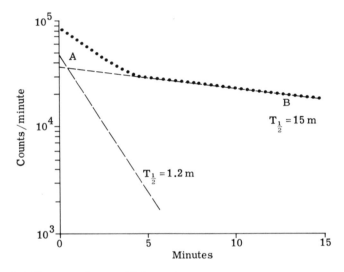

Fig. 13.6 Clearance of xenon-133 from a human tumour.

This is a two component exponential curve which can be described by the equation:

$$X = ae^{-k_1 t} + be^{-k_2 t} \tag{13.9}$$

where X is the counting rate over the tumour, k_1 and k_2 are the rate constants and a and b are the coefficients of the two exponential terms.

In order to calculate the blood flow in cm³/g tissue we need to know the partition coefficient, λ, for the indicator used. The partition coefficient is the equilibrium volume of distribution of the indicator in cm^3 of blood/g of tissue. Blood flow may then be calculated from the equation

$$F = \lambda \frac{ak_1 + bk_2}{a + b} \text{ cm}^3/\text{g} \tag{13.10}$$

The validity of the calculated value of F will depend on the accuracy of the value of λ which is used; for ^{133}Xe the value of λ can be markedly influenced by the fat content of the tissue, since the gas is soluble in fat, and to a lesser extent on the haematocrit.

For the measurement of blood flow freely diffusible indicators such as ^{133}Xe, ^{85}Kr or ^{81}Kr^m, ^{24}Na or ^{42}K are used. For studies of lymph flow a colloidal indicator such as ^{131}I-labelled human serum albumin or ^{198}Au-gold colloid is used.

Measurement of cardiac output. If a discrete source of radiation is moved at a uniform rate across the field of view of a collimated detector the recorded response will have the shape illustrated in Figure 13.7 and the rate of movement of the sources is inversely proportional to the area under the curve. This principle may be used for measurement of blood flow at a point, provided that the radioactive tracer does not diffuse out of the vessel as it passes through and that the detector is sensitive to all radiation arising within the vessel.

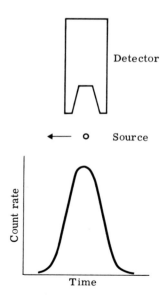

Fig. 13.7

If we consider the heart as a chamber in which mixing occurs a somewhat different picture emerges because after mixing has been completed an equilibrium level of radioactivity is established. This is illustrated in Figure 13.8 which is a diagrammatic representation of the radioactivity tracing which would be obtained by a scintillation detector, coupled to a chart recorder, placed over a patient's heart during the first few minutes following intravenous injection of about 2 MBq of ^{131}I-labelled human serum albumin.

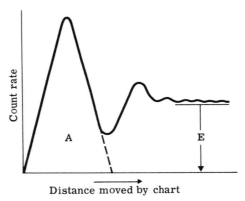

Fig. 13.8

The rate of flow of blood through the heart, the cardiac output, is inversely proportional to the area under the initial peak A, but because of the mixing fluctuations and the equilibrium level of radioactivity which is established in the blood it is necessary to deduce the area of curve A by extrapolation of the downward portion. The radioactivity tracing gives the counting rate in terms of the pen deflection, measured in mm, and in order to calculate the cardiac output in cm^3 it is necessary to count a sample of whole blood taken 5 to 10 minutes after injection of the radioactive indicator, as well as a dilution of the injected indicator solution. These latter counts may be made conveniently in a well-type scintillation counter. The cardiac output, Q, is calculated from the expression:

$$Q = \frac{E \times S \times D \times I \times R}{A \times B \times 10^3} \text{ litres/min}$$

Where E = Equilibrium Counting rate (in mm measured from the chart). S = Counting rate of the Standard in counts/min, D = Dilution of the Standard, I = Volume of solution injected, R = Recorder Chart speed in mm/min, A = Area under curve A in mm.min and B = Blood Count Rate in counts/minute.

This is a simplified description designed only to illustrate the principles of the technique. The increasingly important sub-speciality of nuclear cardiology now utilises very advanced methods of data acquisition, recording and processing which enable much more information about the function of the heart to be obtained than a simple measurement of the cardiac output (Chapter 28).

Determination of glomerular filtration rate. This is one example of a renal clearance measurement, that is the determination of the volume of a plasma which is cleared of a substance by the kidneys per minute.

For the measurement of glomerular filtration rate we need to use an indicator which is cleared from the blood by glomerular filtration without any tubular reabsorption or secretion. At the present time one of the most useful types of agent is a labelled complex of ethylenediaminetetraacetic acid (EDTA), for example ^{51}Cr-EDTA, ^{113}In^m-EDTA or ^{68}Ga-EDTA. A typical procedure using ^{51}Cr-EDTA is as follows: A priming infusion of about 2 MBq ^{51}Cr-EDTA is administered intravenously followed by the continuous infusion, at a rate of $0\cdot35$–$0\cdot5\,cm^3$/min, of a solution containing about $40\,kBq/cm^3$. After about 40 minutes the blood levels of ^{51}Cr-EDTA should be constant and urine collections are started, samples being withdrawn through a catheter every 10 to 15 minutes. Blood samples are collected at the midpoint of each urine collection period. The radioactivity in urine and plasma is assayed in a scintillation counter.

The glomerular filtration rate (GFR) is calculated from the expression

$$\text{GFR }(cm^3/\text{min}) = \frac{\text{Urinary }^{51}\text{Cr (counts/min)} \times \text{Urine Flow }(cm^3/\text{min})}{\text{Plasma }^{51}\text{Cr (counts/min)}}$$

These three examples illustrate the principles underlying the use of radionuclides for the measurement of flow rates, more detailed information on the procedures, together with consideration of their advantages and limitations will be found in the works listed in Appendix 8.

14

Basic principles of radioimmunoassay

14.1. Introduction

Many substances which control or influence biochemical or physiological processes, such as hormones or potent drugs, lack specific chemical groupings in their molecules which would permit their unequivocal determination by conventional chemical techniques at the very low concentrations which may occur in blood or body fluids. One such substance is the protein hormone insulin which is present in blood at a concentration of about 10^{-10} molar. Insulin consists of two chains of 20 to 30 amino acids (see Chapter 35) and cannot be distinguished by simple chemical methods from any other polypeptide of similar size. However, the arrangement of the amino acids in the insulin molecule does enable it to be recognised by, and to combine with, a highly specific protein antibody to form a non-covalently bound *antigen–antibody complex*. This reaction may be illustrated by the following equation:

$$Ag + Ab \underset{k_b}{\overset{k_a}{\rightleftharpoons}} Ag\text{–}Ab$$

where Ag and Ab represent unbound, or 'free', antigen and antibody respectively and Ag–Ab the antigen–antibody complex.

In 1960 S. A. Berson and Rosalyn Yallow, working in New York, described an assay for insulin in blood based on an antigen-antibody reaction using a highly-specific anti-insulin antibody and ^{131}I-labelled insulin — this technique they called *radioimmunoassay*. In the same year R. P. Ekins and his colleagues, working at the Middlesex Hospital in London, reported a technique for the determination of thyroxine in plasma which utilised ^{131}I-labelled thyroxine and a naturally occurring, non-antibody, thyroxine-binding protein — this technique was called *saturation analysis*. Subsequently similar principles have been applied to the measurement of several hundred different substances, some of which are illustrated in Table 14.1. The sensitivity of these techniques is so high that quantities in the nanogram (10^{-9} g) to the femtogram (10^{-15} g) range may be measured routinely.

Table 14.1 Some substances which may be determined by radioimmunoassay

Protein or Peptide Hormones	Insulin Human Growth Hormone Human Chorionic Gonadotrophin Oxytocin Prolactin Thyroid Stimulating Hormone Luteinising Hormone Vasopressin
Non-protein Hormones	Cortisol Testosterone Oestradiol Prostaglandins Tri-iodothyronine (T_3)
Non-hormonal substances	Folic Acid Vitamin A Vitamin D Adenosine-3',5'-monophosphate (Cyclic-AMP) Hepatitis B Antigen Ferritin Lactalbumin Carcinoembryonic Antigen-Fetoprotein
Drugs	Morphine Cannabis Lysergic Acid Diethylamide (LSD) Tubocurarine Digoxin Chlorpromazine Phenobarbitone Phenytoin Bleomycin

Various names have been used to describe these techniques including competitive binding assay, protein-binding assay and radioreceptor assay, saturation analysis and radioimmunoassay. Nowadays all such techniques are generally referred to as radioimmunoassay, or RIA, even though many of the methods for specific substances do not utilise immunological reactions.

Radioimmunoassay methods have now become of very great importance in many areas of clinical medicine, as well as in medical research, and some tens of millions of RIA assays are now carried out annually. Because the technique uses radioactively labelled indicators it has been customary to regard RIA as a branch of nuclear medicine. However, it may be argued very strongly that RIA now lies more properly in the sphere of the chemical pathologist or clinical chemist, rather than in that of the nuclear medicine physician. This argument has become stronger in recent years as for some assays the radioactive marker has been replaced by a fluorescent substance or an enzyme.

14.2.   The basic principle of radioimmunoassay

The basic principle of RIA has been aptly portrayed by Ekins in terms of a simple model involving a large jug full of water and a small glass. If we attempt to pour all the contents of the jug into the glass some will overflow. The proportions of the water in the glass and in the overflow will depend on, and reflect, the total amount of water initially present in the jug. Thus the ultimate distribution of the water between the glass, which is of a fixed and therefore limiting size, and the overflow can be used to determine the total amount of water originally present in the jug.

In general terms if the substance to be measured, S, is allowed to react with another substance, B, having a specific but limited ability to bind S, then as long as the total amount of S in the system is sufficient to saturate the binding capacity of B the substances will be partitioned into two moieties, the complex SB and free S. The ratio of these two moieties will vary as a function of the total amount of S originally present in the system. Thus an unknown amount of S may be determined by calculating the ratio SB/S and comparing this with similar ratios obtained by introducing 'standards' containing accurately known amounts of S into the system.

In order to use this principle in practice it is necessary to be able to distinguish unambiguously between S and SB and to measure the distribution of S between them. There are many ways in which these criteria may be satisfied. The most widely used technique relies on the addition of a radioactive 'marker', usually but not necessarily identical to S, to the system which is then allowed to reach equilibrium before SB and S are separated physically from each other and the relative amounts of the radioactivity contained in the free S and the SB fractions are determined. The basic steps of the procedure are illustrated in Figure 14.1. In some cases after the addition of the labelled S, but before the addition of B, it may be necessary to extract and purify the mixture of radioactivity and non-radioactive S in order to avoid interference from other substances present in the unknown sample, in this case the percentage recovery of the radioactive S in the purified extract will provide a measure of the total recovery of S.

An essential requirement for the assay when a radioactive marker is used is to be able to separate quantitatively the bound and free material and many different methods are used for this purpose including electrophoresis, chromatography, gel-filtration, ion exchange, adsorption on charcoal and a second antigen–antibody reaction. Since in practice it is often necessary to run many tens or even hundreds of samples in a single batch the chosen method of separation should be as simple as is consistent with the requirement

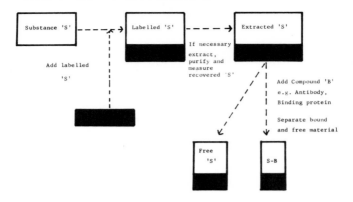

Fig. 14.1 The basic steps of radioimmunoassay

for quantitative separation. The radionuclides used in RIA indicators are commonly ^{125}I for labelling proteins and ^3H for other molecules, but other suitable nuclides may be used, for example ^{75}Se-labelled cortisol for the assay of cortisol. An essential requirement for the radioactive marker is that the specific activity should be very high in order that very small quantities of material may be measured. It is also desirable, but not essential, that the radioactive marker should have a long 'shelf-life' in order that material of known and acceptable purity should be available for reasonable periods of time before new batches must be prepared.

14.3.   Some practical aspects of radioimmunoassay

In this short account of radioimmunoassay it is not appropriate to discuss individual assay methods in detail. However, some of the practical aspects of such assays may be illustrated by a brief outline of the procedure for the assay of insulin in blood plasma.

A suitable dilution of the patients plasma, 1 in 10 or greater, is prepared and an accurately measured aliquot of this diluted plasma is mixed with an accurately known amount of ^{125}I-labelled insulin (specific activity 4 to 8 MBq/μg) and an accurately measured aliquot of a suitable dilution of a guinea-pig anti-insulin antiserum. After thorough mixing the tubes are placed in a refrigerator at 4°C for 72 hours to allow the reactions to reach equilibrium. At the end of this period the free ^{125}I-insulin is separated from the ^{125}I-insulin-antibody complex by precipitation of the complex by means of a second antibody which has been raised against the anti-insulin antiserum. This method of separation is called the 'double-antibody method'. The amounts of bound and free ^{125}I are then measured in a scintillation counter and the ratio of 'bound to free ^{125}I' is calculated. A series of standards containing accurately known amounts of insulin are run with each batch of unknown samples and from the results of these measurements a standard curve is constructed from which the amounts of insulin in the unknown plasma samples may be read.

The standard curve is constructed by plotting the ratio of free to bound radioactivity, or any other convenient expression of the radioactive content of the free or bound fractions, against the insulin content for each of the standard samples. Other forms in which the radioactivity may be expressed are bound/free, percentage of total counts bound or percentage of total counts free. The actual shape and slope of the standard curve will vary with the method of plotting and with the particular type of assay being performed. In practice the method of plotting the standard curve should be chosen to provide an 'optimum slope' for the range of quantities to be measured. Three examples of standard curves are given in Figure 14.2.

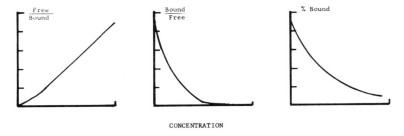

CONCENTRATION

Fig. 14.2 Three of the possible ways in which standard curves for radioimmunoassay may be plotted.

In RIA techniques, which involve the measurement of minute amounts of substances in biological materials, many problems may arise which affect the reliability of the assay. These problems may arise from the presence of unexpected interfering substances in pathological plasma or other samples, from antisera of low titre and/or poor reactivity with the antigen, inadequate specific activity of the radioactive marker, poor quantitation of the separation procedure or from poor technique on the part of the operator. A detailed discussion of these problems and their avoidance is beyond the scope of this chapter.

The increasing importance of RIA methods in modern clinical medicine and the consequent need to perform hundreds, if not thousands, of assays per week or per month has resulted in the development of many 'kits' for individual RIA methods and of automated, or semi-automated, RIA-dedicated equipment. The RIA kit offers the advantage of providing all the reagents required for a particular assay with a well controlled standard of quality and reproducibility. The use of automatic scintillation counters with dedicated computers, or operated 'on-line' to a large computer now enable the construction of the standard curve and the calculation of the individual results to be made automatically and, often, printed out in a form suitable for direct attachment to the patients report form.

PART THREE

Measurement and instrumentation

15

Measurement uncertainties

15.1. Types of uncertainty

Methods and instruments by which measurements are made in nuclear medicine form the subject of subsequent chapters. Whenever a measurement is made the result is associated with some degree of uncertainty. For example, when we weigh ourselves we might give the result as 'about 70 kg' or 'between 70 and 71 kg', accepting the fact that the figure given will not be exact. Such uncertainties need to be distinguished from mistakes, such as the recording of a wrong reading. Unfortunately the word 'error' tends to be used in both senses.

If V is the real value and X the measured value, then the error is given by $|V - X|$ where the mathematical symbol $|\text{-----}|$ means 'the absolute value of' and is called the 'modulus'. In practice the real value V is rarely known, and the best we can attain is the average $\bar{V}$ of a large number of measurements. We therefore use

$$a = |\bar{V} - X|$$

where a is called the deviation to distinguish it from the error.

Errors fall into two categories, systematic and random.

Systematic errors

These only affect the result in one direction, such as a balance which always reads high due to the zero not being correctly set. Systematic errors can be assessed by calibrating with standard weights, etc. and correction factors applied. In nuclear medicine systematic errors are likely to be associated with estimates of sample weights or volumes, or wrongly calibrated meters. This is considered in more detail with regard to the measurement of organ uptake in Sections 22.3 and 22.4.

Random errors

These can occur in either direction and may be accidental or statistical in nature. If we make a number of determinations of the same quantity we shall not always obtain the same result, but they will exhibit a spread on either side of the most likely value. This is known as a 'distribution' of values.

Random errors are very important in radiation work since radioactive decay is a random process and any measurement of counting-rate has an associated statistical uncertainty. Other sources of random error may also be significant, such as inaccuracies in pipetting.

Accuracy and precision
These words are used to distinguish between systematic and random errors. If the random errors are small then the measurement is said to be of high 'precision', in other words repeated measurements are very close to one another. The result may, however, not be the true value due to systematic errors, and if in addition the systematic errors are small then the measurement is of high 'accuracy'.

15.2. Averages
Faced with a set of measurements we frequently need to select a representative value, which in everyday life is often called an 'average'. There are a number of different types of average, and in statistical work specific terminology is used. We will consider a set of m measurements having values $x_1, x_2, x_3, \ldots, x_m$.

Arithmetic mean. This is the simplest, and is given by the sum of all the values divided by the total number of measurements:

$$\bar{x} = \frac{\sum x}{m}$$

Often $\bar{x}$ is just called the 'mean' of the set of observations.

Geometric mean. This is less frequently used, and is given by

$$G = \sqrt[m]{x_1 \times x_2 \times x_3 \times \cdots \times x_m}$$

Median. This is the value such that half of the observed values lie above and half below.

Mode is the name given to the most frequently observed value, and indicates the value of a substantial part of a set of data.

The mean, median and mode will only coincide in a symmetrical distribution, otherwise it is called 'skew' (see Fig. 15.1). Skew distributions are often encountered in medical work concerned with the results of diagnostic tests, where a particular disease causes a higher (or lower) value than normal.

Random errors usually possess a symmetrical distribution.

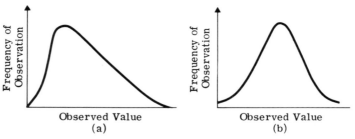

Fig. 15.1 Distributions which are (a) skew and (b) symmetrical.

15.3. Spread of results

As well as the mean we often need to know over what range the various observations occurred. This is known as the 'dispersion' and is usually measured by calculating the variance σ^2, which is the mean of the sum of the squares of the individual deviations about the arithmetic mean $\bar{x}$. The square root of the variance is called the standard deviation (S.D.) σ:

$$\text{variance} = \sigma^2 = \frac{\sum(x - \bar{x})^2}{m - 1}$$

Note that the summation $\sum(x - \bar{x})^2$ represents the total of all the squared deviations. The expression $(m - 1)$ rather than m follows from the full mathematical derivation.

15.4. The normal (or Gaussian) distribution

In the case of most sources of random errors the chance of occurrence of a positive deviation is equal to that of a negative deviation of the same magnitude, and small deviations are more likely than large ones. This gives rise to a symmetrical distribution of the type shown in Figure 15.1b and is known as the normal or Gaussian curve. It is characterised by its mean $\bar{x}$ and S.D. σ.

The normal distribution is shown in Figure 15.2, plotted this time with units of σ along the x-axis. It is a mathematical property of this curve that:

68·3 % of individual values lie between $(\bar{x} - \sigma)$ and $(\bar{x} + \sigma)$

90 % of individual values lie between $(\bar{x} - 1\cdot6\sigma)$ and $(\bar{x} + 1\cdot6\sigma)$

95·5 % of individual values lie between $(\bar{x} - 2\sigma)$ and $(\bar{x} + 2\sigma)$

99·7 % of individual values lie between $(\bar{x} - 3\sigma)$ and $(\bar{x} + 3\sigma)$

Note that it is very unlikely (a probability of 3 in 1000) that a further measurement will lie outside $\bar{x} \pm 3\sigma$.

If we have two quantities, observations on which yield the two normal distributions shown in Figure 15.2, then it is clear that they intersect at the 3σ mark. In other words, the chance of them representing the same quantity is less than 3 in 1000. This statement is known as the 'confidence limit' and if two quantities differ by more than three standard deviations it is often assumed that they are in fact different. Note that results are often quoted in the form $x \pm \sigma$, representing a confidence limit of only $68\cdot3\%$ (about 2 in 3).

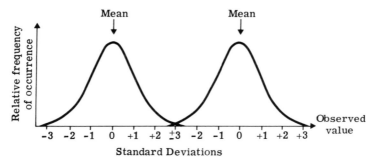

Fig. 15.2 The spread of observations for two quantities that are significantly different at the $99\cdot7\%$ (3σ) confidence level.

15.5   Standard error

The term standard deviation is reserved for the spread of a large number of measurements. We are frequently in the position of making only one observation of a quantity whose standard deviation is $\pm\sigma$. When used in this sense the S.D. is usually called the 'standard error' (S.E.) of the individual value. The 'relative S.E.' v is expressed as a percentage: $v = 100\sigma/\bar{x}$.

Many measurements in nuclear medicine require the calculation of a mean value, and if this was measured on numerous occasions the values obtained would fall on a normal curve. The 'standard deviation' of this normal distribution is the standard error in the mean.

If we take measurements $N_1, N_2, N_3, \ldots, N_m$ of the same quantity we can calculate a mean ($\bar{x}$) and a S.D. (σ_i) using the formulae in (15.2) and (15.3). The S.E. (σ_x) in this mean value is a measure of its uncertainty, and is given by

$$\sigma_x = \frac{\sigma_i}{\sqrt{m}}$$

where σ_i is the S.D. of the series of m measurements. The result is expressed in the form $\bar{x} \pm \sigma_{\bar{x}}$.

We also require the standard error of the difference (σ_{x-y}) and the sum (σ_{x+y}) of two measurements:

$$\sigma_{x-y} = \sigma_{x+y} = \sqrt{\sigma_x^2 + \sigma_y^2} \qquad (15.1)$$

When the ratio or product of two measurements is compared the standard error is given by

$$v_{x/y} = v_{xy} = \sqrt{v_x^2 + v_y^2} \qquad (15.2)$$

where v represents the relative standard error. Note that absolute standard errors are used in calculating the S.E. of a difference or sum, but relative standard errors in calculating the S.E. of a ratio or product.

15.6.   Combination of errors
The random errors connected with the statistical accuracy of counting measurements are easily quantified (see section 16.4) whilst other sources of error are less easy to assess. For this reason, in nuclear medicine the error quoted in measurements is often that due to counting statistics alone. This can be very misleading and may represent a considerable underestimate of the errors involved, although of course systematic errors, once identified, should be corrected.

If the standard errors of each of the quantities used in the final calculation can be estimated then they may be combined using equations 15.1 and 15.2.

15.7.   Example
The number of requests for tests in a nuclear medicine department over a period of 10 consecutive months was 400, 375, 420, 450, 410, 390, 470, 425, 385 and 440.

Over this period a normal distribution may be assumed. The next month a new γ-camera was installed and the number of requests rose to 510. Does this represent a significant increase?

For the first 10 values, from the equations in sections 15.2 and 15.3:

mean $\bar{x} = 416 \cdot 5$

S.D. $\sigma = \sqrt{\dfrac{\sum(-\bar{x})^2}{m-1}} = \sqrt{\dfrac{8352 \cdot 5}{9}} = 30 \cdot 5$

The deviation between 510 and $\bar{x}$ is $(510 - 416 \cdot 5) = 93 \cdot 5 = 3 \cdot 07\sigma$. Since this represents more than 3 standard deviations the chance of this happening by accident is less than 3 in 1000. The increase in requests is therefore almost certainly significant.

16

Measurement of radioactivity

In order to detect the incident radiation ionised or excited atoms must be produced within the sensitive volume of the detector. Gamma-rays are detected by the charged particles resulting from their interaction with either the detector material itself or its immediate surroundings. Here we have a twofold problem: the γ-rays should interact as little as possible before reaching the detector, but at that stage there should be a high probability of interaction. When it is required to detect charged particles, such as β-rays, the main problem is to avoid absorption before reaching the sensitive volume. This is particularly true of ^{3}H, ^{14}C, ^{35}S and ^{32}P, all of which are pure β^- emitters and are isotopes of elements which do not possess any convenient γ-emitting nuclide. Special techniques have therefore been devised for these cases (see Section 21.5).

Almost every property of radiation, such as the photographic, biological, ionising and fluorescent effects, may be utilised in detecting radiation, but the excitation and ionising effects are the basis of the most important detectors used in nuclear medicine. In this chapter the general problems of the measurement of radioactivity are considered, which are relevant to all radiation detectors. In the next chapter the most important technique — scintillation counting — is described, and chapter 18 deals with gas and semiconductor devices which are important for special purposes. Subsequently, the use of these detectors in sample (Ch. 21) and *in vivo* (Ch. 22–28) measurements is discussed.

16.1. Efficiency and sensitivity

It is necessary to distinguish between the 'intrinsic efficiency' of a radiation detector and its sensitivity. The former is the efficiency which it possesses by its very nature and measures its ability to detect the radiation reaching the device. It depends upon the type and energy spectrum of the incident radiation, and the direction(s) from which it strikes the detector. For γ-radiation the intrinsic efficiency is often quoted for a narrow parallel beam of rays incident at right angles to the detector face.

If μ is the total linear absorption coefficient of the detector material for the appropriate γ-ray energy and t the sensitive thickness, then $e^{-\mu t}$ is the proportion of the γ-rays transmitted. Thus $(1 - e^{-\mu t})$ represents the proportion of γ-rays interacting with the detector and represents the intrinsic efficiency. This is often stated as a percentage, and in the case of β^- particles is usually close to 100% due to their limited range within the detector.

More commonly encountered in practice is the sensitivity, which is the counting-rate obtained from unit activity of sample. It is dependent on factors such as the decay scheme of the radionuclide, the type of sample and the geometrical arrangement as well as the intrinsic efficiency of the detector. Usually it is measured by calibration against a standard source.

16.2. Types of measurement

Depending upon the purpose of the measurement of the activity of the sample under investigation may be determined either as an absolute quantity or relative to some other sample. Methods fall into the following categories:

Absolute. In this case the decay rate in disintegrations per unit time will be measured, from which it is a simple step to calculate absolute activity. Any radiation detector will measure counts (not disintegrations) per unit time, and it is necessary to ensure that either one pulse is recorded per disintegration or that the proportion of disintegrations recorded is known accurately. This is a specialist task and is normally restricted to centres such as the National Standardising Laboratories.

Relative to an absolute standard. Absolute activities can also be determined by comparing the count-rate with that of an absolutely calibrated sample of the same radionuclide, both being measured under identical conditions. Any factors which may affect the result, such as volume and density of sample, geometrical arrangement, absorption and back-scattering must be under strict control. This type of measurement is a determination of the counting sensitivity of the system and accuracies of $\pm 5\%$ may be easily obtained.

By means of a calibrated instrument. The above method does, in fact, calibrate the instrument which can then be used for subsequent measurements. It is common practice to calibrate equipment using absolute standards of appropriate radionuclides which are obtained from National Standardising Laboratories at convenient intervals, such as every six months. In this way routine deliveries of radioactive materials may be measured before administration to a patient. It is necessary to check the constancy of the calibration at frequent intervals; this may be done using a convenient long lived nuclide such as ^{60}Co or ^{137}Cs as a reference source.

Relative to an aliquot. In clinical investigations it is often customary to set aside a small part (aliquot) of the radionuclide before administration to the patient. The activity in any subsequent samples, such as blood or urine, is then compared to the aliquot. Dilution analysis techniques (see Ch. 12) are frequently undertaken in this way. Since only comparative measurements are required the absolute activities of individual samples need not be determined.

Relative to other samples measured at the same time. When radioisotope scanning is undertaken to determine the distribution of activity within a patient the results are often expressed relative to the maximum, as in a colour scan. A similar situation exists in studies such as radiochromatography.

16.3.   Counts due to background

Whenever counting apparatus is used it will be observed that a count-rate is recorded even in the absence of a sample. This is known as the background count-rate and must be measured whenever sample counting is undertaken. If possible it should be small compared with the sample counting-rate and, if significant, constant during the period of sample counting. Background counts are due to the following causes:

External radiation. Nearby radioactive sources will affect the count-rate in a sample counter and so care should be taken to provide adequate shielding (typically 2 to 5 cm lead) around the counter, and to store sources well away from counting equipment. External radiation may also arise from nearby X-ray generators, or from naturally occurring radioactive elements within building materials or in the air. When *in vivo* counting is undertaken parts of the patient outside the region of interest constitute a source of background radiation, as indeed do waiting patients who have already received injections of radioactive material.

Internal contamination. The material used in constructing the counter may contain small amounts of radioactive materials, such as thorium or fission products, which affect the background due to their close proximity to the detecting volume. A more usual cause is accidental contamination of the counter from samples that are counted; this will be discovered by frequent checks of the background count-rate and can be avoided by careful housekeeping. It is a wise precaution to cover detectors, when possible, with a thin covering of plastic which is easily removed if contaminated.

Cosmic radiation. This is natural radiation which is extraterrestrial in origin, and consists of highly penetrating charged particles as well as photons and neutrons. It is extremely difficult to shield against but fortunately the count-rate is usually low and varies only very slowly with time.

Electrical interference. A proportion of the background count-rate may originate in the electronic part of the apparatus due to bad connections or pick-up of noise pulses from other equipment in the vicinity. It can be largely avoided by routine attention to cables and sockets, and by care in the earthing arrangements.

Noise is also generated in electronic components and photo-multipliers. This can be troublesome when low energy radiation such as that from ^{3}H or ^{125}I is to be measured. In these cases special procedures may be required, as with liquid scintillation counting (Section 21.5).

16.4.   Statistics of counting

In nuclear medicine we are normally concerned with the detection of individual events, representing the decay of individual nuclei. This is a random process and so repeated observations of the count-rate for a sample of constant activity will not, in fact, give exactly the same result. The laws of radioactive decay are governed by the Poisson distribution. Unlike the normal distribution this deals only with whole numbers and describes all random processes whose probability of occurrence is both small and constant. It therefore applies to the disintegration of atomic nuclei provided the mean life is long compared with the total period of the observation.

For small numbers of counts the distribution is very skew since negative counts cannot be observed. When the number of counts is large (in practice > 100) the Poisson distribution approximates to a particular normal distribution of mean $\bar{N}$ and whose variance is also $\bar{N}$, where $\bar{N}$ is the mean value of many determinations of the number of counts $N_1, N_2, N_3, \ldots$. Thus

$$\text{standard deviation in } \bar{N} = \sigma_N = \sqrt{\bar{N}}.$$

The standard deviation σ_N provides an indication of the spread to be found in a given series of measurements (Fig. 16.1). What we often need to know is the confidence that we can place in a single measurement. If we know $\bar{N}$ through taking a very large number of measurements then $\sigma_N = \sqrt{\bar{N}}$ and we can predict the confidence in taking one additional measurement. We call σ_N for a single estimate

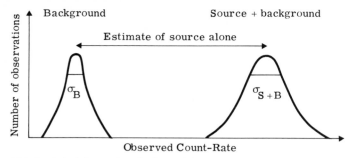

Fig. 16.1 Statistical fluctuations in determining a count-rate.

the standard error, and when expressed as a percentage the relative standard error v_N. In practice we often make just one single measurement whose significance we require. In this case we do not know $\bar{N}$, but the use of N instead is approximately correct. Thus:

$$\text{relative standard error } v_N \approx \frac{100\sqrt{N}}{N}\%$$

and for 100 counts $\quad v_N = 10\%$
for 1000 counts $\quad v_N = 3\%$
for 10 000 counts $v_N = 1\%$
for 10^6 counts $\quad v_N = 0.1\%$.

16.5. The effect of the background count-rate

Measurements of radioactivity require the subtraction of the background count-rate (R_b) from that of the sample plus background (R_{s+b}). Thus the sample count-rate R_s is given by

$$R_s = R_{s+b} - R_b \tag{16.1}$$

Both R_{s+b} and R_b are subject to statistical variations (Fig. 16.1). Let a time T_{s+b} be spent in measuring the sample plus background: then the total number of counts accumulated will be $R_{s+b}T_{s+b}$. Similarly the total number of background counts in time T_b will be R_bT_b. Then

S.E. in observed count rate $\quad \sigma_{s+b} = (R_{s+b}T_{s+b})^{1/2}/T_{s+b}$
$$= (R_{s+b}/T_{s+b})^{1/2}$$

S.E. in background count-rate $\quad \sigma_b = (R_bT_b)^{1/2}T_b = (R_b/T_b)^{1/2}$

and S.E. in sample count-rate $\quad \sigma_s = (\sigma_{s+b}^2 + \sigma_b^2)^{1/2}$

$$\therefore \quad \sigma_s = (R_{s+b}/T_{s+b} + R_b/T_b)^{1/2} \tag{16.2}$$

If the total time available for counting is T then it can be shown that the minimum standard error in an estimate of the sample count-rate will be obtained when T is divided between the two measurements in proportion to the square roots of the individual count-rates, namely

$$\frac{T_b}{T_{s+b}} = \left(\frac{R_b}{R_{s+b}}\right)^{1/2} \tag{16.3}$$

Example: Suppose quick approximate observations indicate that $R_{s+b} = 400 \, \text{ct/sec}$ and $R_b = 25 \, \text{ct/sec}$. If the total time available is 50 seconds, (a) how should the time be apportioned, (b) what will be the sample count-rate and (c) what will be its relative standard error?

(a)   From eqn. 16.3 $\quad \dfrac{T_b}{T_{s+b}} = \left(\dfrac{25}{400}\right)^{1/2} = \dfrac{5}{20} = \dfrac{1}{4}$

Thus as the total time available is 50 sec, 10 sec should be spent counting the background and 40 sec the source plus background. Note that in this case the background is counted for less time than the sample.

(b)   From eqn. 16.1, $R_s = 400 - 25 = 375 \, \text{ct/sec}$

(c)   From eqn. 16.2, $\sigma_s = (400/40 + 25/10)^{1/2}$

$$= (10 + 2\cdot5)^{1/2} = \sqrt{12\cdot5}$$

$$= 3\cdot5$$

and the relative standard error $v_s = \dfrac{100\sigma_s}{R_s} = \dfrac{100 \times 3\cdot5}{375}$

$$= 0\cdot9\%$$

16.6. Detection limits

A sample of extremely low activity will not exhibit a count-rate significantly above background. This is due to the random fluctuation in the background and so all estimates of the detection limit are based on the standard deviation of the background count-rate. In general the criterion chosen for the 'minimum detectable activity' is that it yields a count-rate equal to three standard deviations of the background count-rate. The 'background equivalent activity' is the activity of a sample which will give a count-rate equal to background. If the detector sensitivity is ε and the background count-rate R_b when measured over a time T_b, then the standard error in R_b will be $\sqrt{R_b T_b}/T_b$, or $(R_b/T_b)^{1/2}$.

Thus

minimum detectable activity (MDA) $= 3(R_b/T_b)^{1/2}$ counts per unit time

$= 3(R_b/T_b)^{1/2}/\varepsilon$ dis per unit time

and the background equivalent activity (BEA) $= R_b/\varepsilon$ dis per unit time.

Example: If $R_b = 100$ ct/s and it is measured over 100 seconds with a counting sensitivity of 10^6 ct/s per MBq, then

$$\text{BEA} = 100/10^6 = 10^{-4}\,\text{MBq} = 0\cdot1\,\text{kBq}$$

and $\quad \text{MDA} = 3(100/100)^{1/2}/10^6 = 3 \times 10^{-6}\,\text{MBq}$

$$= 3\,\text{Bq}$$

16.7.   Choice of optimum detector and measuring technique

We are often faced with the necessity of deciding between a number of different counting techniques, all of which have different values for ε and R_b. These can be combined into a 'figure of merit' based on the best statistical accuracy that can be achieved in a given time. Then

for high activities $(R_s \gg R_b)$ optimise R_s/R_b

for low activities $(R_s \leq R_b)$ optimise R_s^2/R_b

In both cases it is important to pay attention to R_s and so a high sensitivity is important. Note that if the amount of sample is unrestricted R_s can be increased by enlarging the volume of the sample, keeping the specific activity constant.

As an example, consider two counting systems suitable for measuring γ-ray emitters. The first has a sensitivity of 200 ct/s per MBq and a background count rate of 20 ct/s, whilst the other has the higher sensitivity of 4000 ct/s per MBq and a higher background of 2000 ct/s.

For a sample of 100 MBq $(R_s \gg R_b)$ then the figures of merit are $2 \times 10^4/20$ and $4 \times 10^5/2000$, that is 10^3 and 200 respectively. Thus the lower sensitivity system is best since it has a very low background. On the other hand, if the sample is only 10^{-2} MBq $(R_s \ll R_b)$ then we use the criterion R_s^2/R_b and obtain figures of merit of $(2^2/20)$ and $(40^2/2000)$, that is 0·2 and 0·8 respectively. In this case the higher sensitivity system is preferable even though it has the higher background.

17

Scintillation counting and
γ-spectrometry

When they absorb energy from ionising radiation a number of substances emit a weak flash of visible light. This is due to excitation, and the intensity of the light is proportional to the total energy absorbed within the material, or 'scintillator' as it is called.

In his classical experiments on the scattering of α-particles Rutherford used zinc sulphide as the scintillator, observing the light flashes with the dark-adapted naked eye. However, the scintillation detector was not really developed until after 1944, when Curran and Baker invented the photomultiplier. This converts the light flashes into electrical pulses capable of operating various items of electronic equipment. Many other scintillators have been developed and the scintillation counter is the most important type of radiation detector used in nuclear medicine. It is capable of detecting both β- and γ-radiation with high efficiency and information can be obtained regarding both the type and energy of the incident radiation. Figure 17.1 shows a scintillation counter in diagrammatic form.

17.1.   The scintillator
In order to behave satisfactorily as a scintillator the material must possess certain properties:

1. It must be a good absorber of the incident radiation. For β-particles it must therefore be greater in size than the β-range, which is not often a serious restriction. In the case of γ-rays it should be as large as possible and of high atomic number so as to increase the probability of total absorption of the γ-ray photon.

2. The energy absorbed is obtained from the intensity of the light emitted. To facilitate detection the conversion to light should be efficient, and the light intensity should be proportional to the energy absorbed over a wide range in order to permit the measurement of energy.

3. The scintillator needs to be transparent to the visible light emitted so that only a small amount is absorbed before reaching the

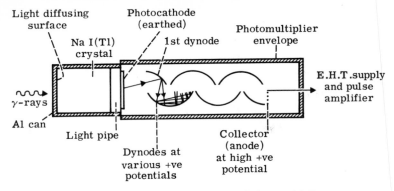

Fig. 17.1 Construction of a scintillation counter and photomultiplier.

photomultiplier. This restricts the optical properties of the material and single crystals are normally used.

4. The wavelengths of the light emitted from the scintillator should correspond to those at which the photomultiplier is most sensitive. Most scintillators emit light in the blue-green part of the spectrum.

5. The intensity of the light flash builds up quickly but dies away more slowly. This decay time should be as short as possible (preferably $< 1\ \mu s$) since it restricts the maximum count-rates that can be handled.

No material is perfect in all these respects, but a number have been found satisfactory and are listed in Table 17.1. The elements in brackets (e.g. T1) represent small amounts of impurities, about 0·1 to 0·5%, the addition of which is found to increase greatly the light output. This table also gives information on the main applications and features of the materials.

The scintillator is contained in a light-tight can usually constructed from aluminium (see Fig. 17.1). A window is on the side facing the photomultiplier so as to permit the exit of the light. The inside of the can is fitted with a diffuse reflector, such as powdered titanium dioxide, in order to direct the light towards the photomultiplier. In the case of NaI(T1), which is hygroscopic, the whole assembly has to be airtight. Good optical coupling between the scintillator and the face of the photomultiplier is obtained using silicone grease and in some cases a specially shaped light pipe constructed from a non-scintillating material such as transparent plastic is placed between the scintillator and the photomultiplier.

17.2. The photomultiplier

This may be regarded as a two-stage device (see Fig. 17.1). At the

Table 17.1 Scintillators in common use

Material	Type	Density g cm^{-3}	Decay constant ns	Light output relative to sodium iodide	Main uses	Comments
NaI(Tl)	Inorganic	3·67	250	100	γ-ray detection and spectrometry	Available in large single crystals Hygroscopic—must be sealed in airtight can Very widely used
CsI(Na)	Inorganic	4·51	650	70–90	γ-ray detection and spectrometry	Available in large single crystals which are not hydroscopic. Higher detection efficiency than NaI(Tl) but poorer light output
Liquid Scintillators	Organic	0·86	2–8	20	Measurement of β-particles from ^{3}H, ^{14}C etc.	Wide range available for specific types of sample
Plastic Scintillators	Organic	1·04	2–5	30	Large detectors when energy information is not required	Easily machinable. Very fast. Inexpensive

photocathode the photons of visible light knock out low energy photoelectrons, which are then amplified in number within the multiplier section.

The photocathode is a very thin semitransparent coating of caesium antimonide or similar material, which absorbs the energy of the light photons with the emission of a few low energy electrons. These are then accelerated towards the first dynode by the electric field existing between the photocathode (at earth potential) and dynode 1 (at around $+200$ V). The dynode is a metal electrode coated with a similar type of material to the photocathode, only this time it is the arrival of an accelerated electron that stimulates the emission of a number of low energy electrons. These in turn are accelerated to dynode 2 and the process is repeated for perhaps thirteen stages before the resulting bunch of electrons is collected at the anode, resulting in a pulse of electric charge.

The photocathode has a low quantum efficiency, that is only about 10–20% of the incident light photons cause the emission of a photoelectron. At the dynodes it is normal for 2 to 3 electrons to be emitted for every electron arriving — for illustration suppose it is only 2. Then when an electron arrives at dynode 1, two will be produced. In turn these will each produce two further electrons at dynode 2, resulting in 2^2 ($=4$) electrons in all. The gain of 13 stages will therefore be $2^{13} = 8192$. In fact gains of 10^6 can be obtained and it must be noted that the gain is very dependent on the voltage between the dynodes. The total potential across the photomultiplier may be 1000–2000 V, and is distributed to the appropriate dynodes by means of a resistor chain.

A vacuum envelope contains the photocathode and dynodes. Even in the absence of light there will be a certain number of photoelectrons emitted (called the dark current) due to thermionic effects, which can be reduced by cooling. This is only necessary in liquid scintillation counting (see Section 21.5). The overall gain of the photomultiplier also depends on the ambient temperature, which can cause practical problems within a nuclear medicine department.

17.3. Energy resolution

In a typical scintillator about 30 eV are required to produce a photon of visible light. Thus in the case of a ^{99}Tc^m γ-ray (140 keV) about $(140 \times 10^3)/30 = 4700$ photons are produced. Due to optical losses perhaps only 4000 will reach the photocathode. If this has a quantum efficiency of 10% then only 400 photoelectrons will be emitted. All these processes are statistical and the standard deviation in this number will be $\sqrt{400} = 20$, or 5%.

Thus if monoenergetic γ-rays are totally absorbed in the scintillator the resulting pulses from the photomultiplier will not all be of the same size, but will be distributed as shown in Fig. 17.2. The range of pulse sizes is a measure of the accuracy with which pulse size (and therefore energy absorbed) may be measured. A convenient quantity for his purpose is the full-width at half-maximum (FWHM) of the curve, marked 'a' in the figure. For a Gaussian shaped curve $a = 2 \cdot 3 \times$ (S.D.). The FWHM is often expressed as a percentage of the peak position, namely $100\,a/b$. It depends upon many factors, including both the efficiency of the scintillator in converting absorbed energy to emitted light, and the total energy absorbed. The energy resolution will improve as the energy increases, being approximately proportional to (energy)$^{-1/2}$. For the example of 140 keV γ-rays considered above $\sigma = 5\%$, so FWHM $= 2 \cdot 3 \times 5 = 11 \cdot 5\%$. In practice the light losses will probably be greater and additional fluctuations will be introduced due to the statistical nature of electron multiplication within the photomultiplier. Typical values for NaI(T1) are 7% for ^{137}Cs (662 keV) and 15% for ^{99}Tc^{m} (140 keV).

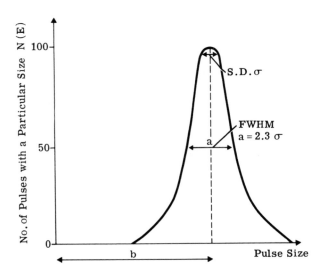

Fig. 17.2 Meaning of full width at half maximum (FWHM).

17.4. Gamma-spectrometry

It must be emphasised that the *intensity* of the light flash is directly proportional to the amount of energy *absorbed* in the scintillator and that the overall process is statistical, contributing a spread in pulse height. This pulse of light is converted to an electrical pulse and it is the height of this that is invariably measured. The distribution of pulse-heights is known as the γ-spectrum and is frequently drawn with γ-ray energy along the x-axis. In fact, pulse height and γ-ray energy may not be strictly proportional due to non-linearities produced within the apparatus.

Gamma rays interact with the scintillator by one of the processes described in Chapter 7, namely the photoelectric, Compton or pair production processes. Electrons are set free by the first two, and electron-positron pairs created by the third. It is part of the energy lost by these charged particles which excites the scintillator, producing light photons. Thus the pulse height distribution (that is the number of pulses of a particular size plotted against pulse size) depends on the relative importance of these three interaction processes.

In order to understand the various features of a γ-spectrum we shall consider a detector in which there is no statistical spread in pulse height. Various interactions will be described and in this way a complex γ-spectrum built up. In each case the energy of the incident γ-ray is E_{in}.

Interaction of γ-rays with energy $< 1 \cdot 02 \, MeV$

In this case the incident γ-ray may interact with the scintillator by the photoelectric or Compton effect: the energy is too low for pair production.

Figure 17.3a represents the situation for a single, photoelectric interaction. If we assume that both the photoelectron and the resulting characteristic X-rays are totally absorbed then energy E_{in} is absorbed, and the spectrum consists of a single line corresponding to energy E_{in}. This peak is referred to as the 'total absorption peak'. Should the characteristic X-rays escape without interacting within the scintillator then a second, lower energy, peak will appear corresponding to the kinetic energy given to the photoelectron. The energy of the K X-rays of iodine is 29 keV and escape is significant only for small detectors and is particularly noticeable when low energy γ-rays (< 100 keV) are being counted.

In Figure 17.3b there is a single Compton interaction with the Compton electron totally absorbed and the scattered Compton γ-ray escaping without further interaction. The pulse-height spectrum obtained for a number of such interactions is as shown; the energy given to the Compton electron can extend from zero up to a maximum energy which is less than E_{in} (see Ch. 7). Multiple Compton interactions are shown in Figure 17.3c. Since they occur virtually simultaneously, in far less time than the decay time of the scintillator,

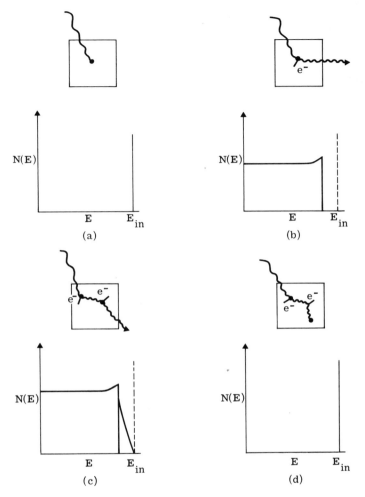

Fig. 17.3 Pulse height distributions for monoenergetic γ-ray source, energy E_{in}.

the intensity of light emitted by the various Compton electrons will be additive and the resulting pulse height represents the total energy loss in the scintillator. This can now extend from zero up to almost E_{in}.

Single or multiple Compton interactions which culminate in a photoelectric interaction within the scintillator result in total absorption of energy E_{in} (see Fig. 17.3d). The γ-spectrum is therefore identical with that in Figure 17.3a, but the total absorption peak includes both multiple events and single photoelectric events. It is for this reason that the popular name 'photopeak' is a misnomer. In large crystals, particularly with high energy γ-rays, multiple effects are a very important contributor to the total absorption peak.

Figure 17.4 illustrates a typical γ-spectrum obtained with 140 keV monoenergetic γ-rays. All of the effects described above are represented and the features are broadened out due to statistical spread. Note the total absorption peak (A), the Compton continuum (B), the Compton edge (C) and the valley due to multiple Compton interactions (D).

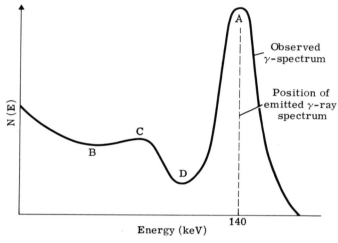

Fig. 17.4 Experimentally obtained γ-spectrum for $^{99}Tc^m$ γ-rays.

Interactions of γ-rays with energy $\geqq 1 \cdot 02$ MeV

When $E_{in} \geqq 1 \cdot 02$ MeV pair production may take place, and in Figure 17.5 the additional features are illustrated. An energy of $1 \cdot 02$ MeV is utilised in forming the electron-positron pair, whose total kinetic energy is thus $(E_{in} - 1 \cdot 02)$MeV. When the positron has lost its kinetic energy it is annihilated with the emission of two $0 \cdot 51$ MeV γ-rays at 180° to each other.

Both annihilation quanta, each of energy $0 \cdot 51$ MeV, may escape without interacting with the scintillator (Fig. 17.5a). Thus the spectrum consists of a single line $1 \cdot 02$ MeV below E_{in}: it is called the 'double escape peak' since both annihilation quanta escape. Alternatively only one $0 \cdot 51$ MeV γ-ray may escape, giving rise to the single escape peak, $0 \cdot 51$ MeV below E_{in}, shown in Figure 17.5b. If both annihilation quanta are totally absorbed as in Figure 17.4c there will be a single peak corresponding to the total absorption peak at E_{in}.

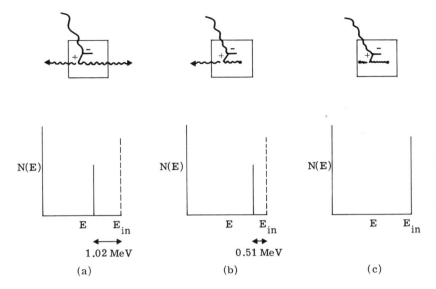

Fig. 17.5 Pulse height distributions due to pair-production interactions

In practice, of course, the annihilation quanta can interact by the Compton effect providing additional features in the spectrum.

Interaction of γ-rays with the source material
Gamma-rays will also interact with the source material itself, particularly if it is large as in *in vivo* studies. Back-scatter within the source itself results in scattered photons all of which are of approximately the same energy. There is therefore a wide, but well-defined peak in the γ-spectrum which may be pronounced if the source is deep within a scattering medium (Fig. 17.6a).

Many γ-rays will undergo small angle scatter. This may result in only a small energy loss, particularly in the case of lower energy γ-rays. For example, with 140 keV radiation scatter through 50° results in a loss of only 15 keV. This produces a low energy distortion to the total absorption peak illustrated in Figure 17.6b.

Interactions of γ-rays with shielding material and collimators
Photons undergoing photoelectric absorption within the surroundings will cause the emission of fluorescent X-rays which may be detected (Fig. 17.6c). This is particularly noticeable with lead collimators which produce a strong peak at 88 keV, the energy of the K fluorescent X-radiation.

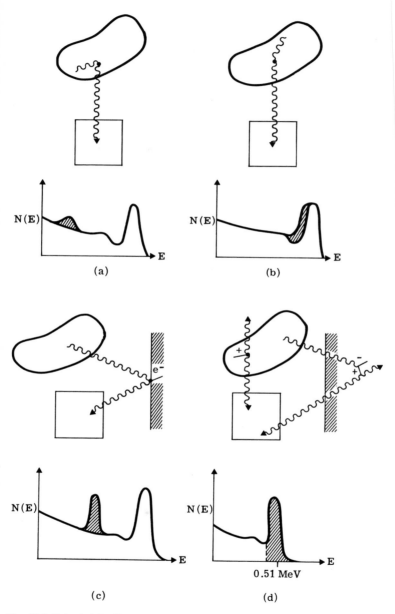

Fig. 17.6 Pulse height distributions resulting from interactions by γ-rays with the source and its surroundings.

If positrons are annihilated either within the source or the surroundings they will produce a 0·51 MeV peak in the γ-spectrum (Fig. 17.6d). This can happen if the γ-rays are originally $\geq 1\cdot02$ MeV in energy.

Electrons and positron-emitting sources

Electrons emitted within the source will produce bremmstrahlung, which in turn will be detected. This provides a useful, although very inefficient method of determining β-emitters such as ^{32}P.

Positrons will be annihilated within the source, emitting 0·51 MeV γ-rays which can be detected by an external scintillation counter. In this way counting and scanning of positron emitters such as ^{18}F is achieved (see Fig. 17.6d).

Complex γ-spectra

Radionuclides emitting more than one γ-ray, or mixtures of different radionuclides, will exhibit γ-spectra corresponding to each γ-ray superimposed on one another. Nevertheless, the basic shape of Figure 17.4 will be retained and is usually easily picked out. In practice, one is often concerned only with the total absorption peak, which is usually the most obvious part of the γ-spectrum.

If a γ-emitting radionuclide emits two γ-rays in cascade (as with the 1·17 MeV and 1·33 MeV γ-rays of ^{60}Co) then it is possible for both γ-rays to be detected simultaneously. This will produce a 'sum peak' in this case of $1\cdot17 + 1\cdot33 = 2\cdot50$ MeV. The likelihood of detecting both γ-rays from the same disintegration is greatest if 4π geometry is used, as in a well counter.

18

Gas and semiconductor detectors

The ability to cause ionisation in a gas is a well-known property of γ-rays and β-particles which has been widely used in their detection since the early part of the century. The energy required to produce an ion pair, that is an electron and a positive ion, depends primarily upon the gas, but is fairly constant at around 34 eV. Thus the total absorption of a 100 keV β-particle will result in $(100 \times 10^3/34) = 3000$ ion pairs.

If an electric field is applied across the gas volume these ions may be collected and in this way the radiation detected. The characteristics of the collection process are very dependent on the strength of the applied electric field.

18.1. General properties of gas counters

Consider a volume of gas contained within an outer cylindrical electrode with a potential difference applied between this electrode and a central wire (Fig. 18.1). When an ionizing event occurs within the gas volume the electrons are attracted to the positive central anode, whilst the heavy positive ions migrate towards the outer

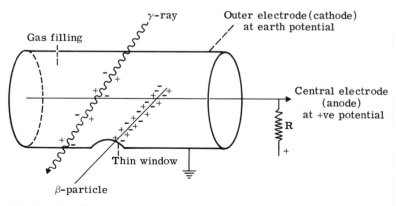

Fig. 18.1 Gas-filled radiation detector.

cathode. The electrons collected on the anode will flow through the resistor R and produce a voltage pulse which can be used to operate subsequent electronic equipment such as scalers.

In Figure 18.2 the relationship between the size of the pulse and the applied voltage is shown for two types of radiation, namely 100 keV and 200 keV β-rays: in the latter case twice as many ions will be created initially if complete absorption is assumed.

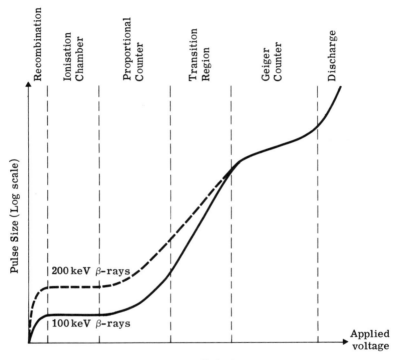

Fig. 18.2 Variation of pulse size with applied voltage.

At very low electric fields some of the ion pairs created will recombine before collection. As the field is increased so the likelihood of recombination diminishes and in the *ionization chamber* region separation and collection of all the ions is achieved. The pulse size is then independent of the applied voltage until the *proportional counter* region is reached. At this stage the electric field is high enough to give an ion sufficient energy to ionise gas atoms thus bringing about an increase in the number of ions produced. This gas amplification is at first restricted to the close vicinity of the original ion track and the secondary ions do not therefore produce additional ions by collision.

Thus the pulse size is proportional to the original number of ions created, as in the ionization chamber region.

This is no longer true when the applied voltage is raised still further. The secondary ions themselves produce additional ionization and the proportionality is gradually lost (*transition* region). When the gas amplification becomes very high no proportionality exists and we have 'avalanche multiplication' where ionization is not restricted to the neighbourhood of the original ion track. This is the *Geiger* region. Finally if the voltage is still further increased then electrical discharge will occur and there will be sparking.

We shall now consider the ionization chamber and Geiger regions in more detail. Proportional counters are rarely encountered in nuclear medicine although they are being developed for specialised applications such as positron imaging.

18.2.   Ionization chambers

These are commonly employed in radiation work for the measurement of Exposure, which is a measure of the ionising ability of the radiation. The special unit of Exposure is the roentgen (R), which has undergone a number of definitions the final one being

$$1 \text{ roentgen} = 2 \cdot 58 \times 10^{-4} \text{ C kg}^{-1} \text{ of air}$$

Since 1980 the unit of Exposure is the SI unit $C \, kg^{-1}$, but the roentgen can be used temporarily and is defined as above.

Note that Exposure refers to the amount of ionization produced in air, and is not directly related to the energy absorbed in other materials such as tissue. Nevertheless it is widely used, primarily due to convenience of measurement. Ionization chambers are the basis of many radiation protection instruments (see Ch. 40) which are therefore calibrated in roentgens.

In general the number of ions liberated is too small to permit the measurement of individual particles; the only exception is for heavy charged particles such as α-particles. However, the interaction of a large number of particles per unit time will result in a measurable ionization current flowing across the chamber. Thus it is a useful instrument for measuring relatively high activity sources, for example on delivery, or when checking the source strength in a syringe before administration to patients. Figure 18.3 shows a re-entrant ionization chamber constructed for this purpose. By placing the sample in the well variations in sensitivity due to differences in sample volume and shape are reduced. Both β- and γ- emitters down to about 1 MBq in activity may be measured and the sensitivity of the instrument can be

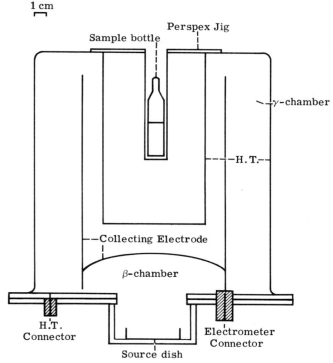

Fig. 18.3 Cut-away view of re-entrant ionization chamber N.P.L. Type 1383A (Crown Copyright).

increased by using air or another suitable gas under pressure (typically 20 atmospheres, 2×10^6 Pa).

18.3.   Geiger–Muller counters

Ionization chambers are unsuitable for detecting individual photons or β-particles due to the small number of ions produced. In the Geiger region this number is increased by as much as $\times 10^8$ due to avalanche multiplication. The resultant pulse of electric charge is of nearly uniform amplitude irrespective of the number of ions initiating the discharge. Unlike the scintillation counter it does not provide information on the amount of energy absorbed, but the size of the pulse is sufficient to operate registering circuitry such as scalers.

Construction and operation

Figure 18.4 illustrates the construction of a Geiger counter provided with an end-window to permit the entry of β-particles. The glass bead

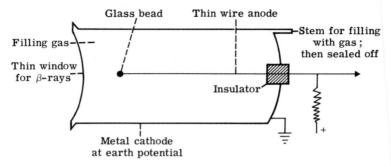

Fig. 18.4 Construction of an end-window Geiger counter.

on the end of the central wire is to stop electrical discharges, and the counter is normally filled with argon at below atmospheric pressure, about 10 cm Hg (1·3 kPa).

The electric field varies across the diameter of the counter, being much greater close to the central wire. It is in this region that the negative ions (electrons) acquire sufficient energy to bring about avalanche multiplication and take only a few microseconds to reach the anode. The heavy positive ions migrate slowly to the cathode where, on arrival, they may stimulate photon or electron emission from the metal. These can initiate a further discharge.

The migration time of the positive ions can be several hundred microseconds, during which period the counter may be unable to produce further pulses — this is known as the 'dead time' and will vary between individual pulses depending on where they were initiated. It is advisable to stabilise the dead time electronically by reducing the electric field below the threshold for avalanche multiplication over a period of 100–300 μs, triggered by the arrival of the mobile electrons at the anode. In addition such an electronic circuit will quench any spurious discharges initiated at the cathode by the arrival of positive ions. Quenching is also achieved by the addition of polyatomic molecules such as ethyl alcohol vapour or halogens to the counter gas; the molecules are dissociated rather than ionized.

The performance of a Geiger counter is characterised by the variation of count-rate with anode voltage when exposed to a source of constant activity (Fig. 18.5). Over the 'plateau' region shown all the pulses are counted but there are few spurious discharges. The slope and length of the plateau is an index of the counter performance; slopes of between 1 and 5 % per 100 V can be achieved over a plateau length of 100–300 V, but will deteriorate with time. Periodic checks should therefore be made of the counting rate characteristic.

Operation at a point on the plateau achieves reproducible performance without undue reliance on the stability of the high voltage supply. Organic quenched counters normally operate at 1000–1500 V, whilst halogen quenching results in lower operating voltages, around 300–800 V.

Measurement of γ-radiation
The probability of γ-rays interacting directly with the counting gas is very small. More likely are photoelectric or Compton interactions in the counter wall sufficiently close to the sensitive volume for the secondary particles to enter and ionize the gas. The efficiency of Geiger counters to γ-radiation can be increased by using high atomic number cathodes, such as copper or lead, but is at the best less than 2 per cent for γ-rays below 3 MeV. This efficiency is dependent on both the photon energy and the atomic number of the wall material, being greatest at around 100 keV where photoelectric interactions are important and the secondary electron energies still appreciable.

Uses in nuclear medicine
The Geiger counter is a simple, inexpensive and rugged detector whose β-efficiency can be high but whose γ-efficiency is low. Due to its size and the large output pulse the whole device can be easily carried, but no information on the nature or energy of the incident radiation can be obtained directly, nor can it cope with high count-rates (in excess of around 100 ct/s, depending on the counter and associated

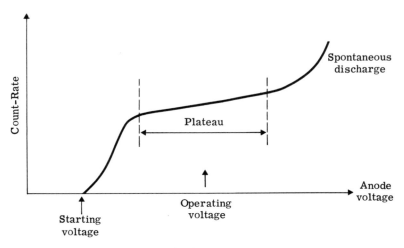

Fig. 18.5 Counting characteristic of a Geiger counter.

circuitry). Portable battery-operated counters are often used for contamination monitoring. A shielded, circular array of tubular counters provides a cheap and convenient method of measuring large γ-emitting samples such as urine and faeces. For most other applications Geiger-counters have been superseded by scintillation detectors.

18.4.   Semiconductor detectors

Whilst scintillation counters are in widespread use as γ-ray detectors they suffer from restricted energy resolution. As we have seen, this is due to the indirect and inefficient manner by which energy is transformed first to visible light then photoelectrons. Recently semiconductor detectors constructed from silicon or germanium have

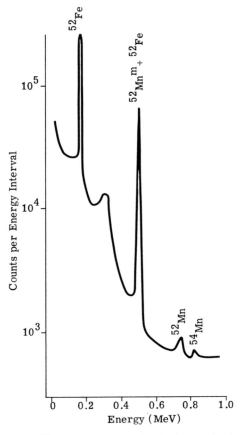

Fig. 18.6. γ-spectrum of ^{52}Fe sample measured 24 h after production using a Ge semiconductor detector, showing small amounts of radiochemical contaminants.

become available. In many respects they are similar to an ionization chamber constructed from a solid material. The photon energy absorbed is transformed directly into electrical charge carriers, only about 3 eV being required, which is about one hundredth of that needed in a scintillation counter. The energy resolution is therefore significantly better, being in the range 1–4 keV for photons of energies up to several MeV.

The benefits of the improved energy resolution are shown in Fig. 18.6 and are of considerable value in separating out mixtures of γ-emitters without the need for chemical separations. As shown in the Figure this is of help in identifying unknown sources, such as radionuclidic contaminants, by an accurate determination of photon energy. Their application to *in vivo* studies is under development and the clinical results obtained show some promise, particularly for fluorescent scanning (Section 27.4). Nevertheless at the present stage of evolution, they are expensive, less efficient than NaI(T1) due to their lower atomic number and smaller size, and require more complex associated equipment.

19

Electronic equipment associated with radiation detectors

The instrumentation of nuclear medicine is primarily involved with detecting and registering individual photons or particles. In the previous two chapters the basic operation of the detectors has been considered; this chapter deals with the handling of the resultant electrical pulses as a prelude to a consideration of complete systems for sample counting and *in vivo* studies.

No attempt is made here to explain the working of electronic circuits. On the contrary an essentially 'black box' approach is adopted with the aim of providing the student with a knowledge of the purpose of the various items of electronic equipment, an understanding of the function of the various controls and an ability to decide what equipment might be needed for a specific job and how it should be connected together.

19.1. Equipment ancillary to the detector

The detector assembly is often some distance from the rest of the electronic equipment and long cable lengths are likely to distort or attenuate the pulses. The preamplifier is a small unit, frequently built into the base of the detector assembly, which matches the electrical characteristics of the detector to those of the cable and subsequent instrumentation. If the cable runs are short (<1 metre) the preamplifier is unnecessary, except in the case of semiconductor detectors which produce only very small pulses.

As explained in Section 18.3 Geiger counters are equipped with an electronic quench unit. This has three functions. Firstly it decreases the voltage on the counter for a set period in order to quench the discharge. Secondly it provides a definite preset dead time, and thirdly it matches the counter to the cable and subsequent equipment. The pulse at the output is usually of sufficient size to operate registering equipment directly.

198

19.2.   Treatment of the pulses

Amplifiers

Both scintillation and semiconductor detectors provide pulses which are too small to operate recording equipment directly without conversion to pulses of sufficient amplitude and suitable shape. This is achieved in the main amplifier which has the following requirements:

1. A variable gain of 50–1000 times, providing output pulses in the range 1–10 V. Normally both coarse (switched) and fine (continuously variable) controls are fitted. In some equipments an amplifier of fixed gain is provided, with a variable attenuator to alter the size of the pulses produced.

2. Linearity, so that the size of the input pulse is directly proportional to that of the output pulse, thus preserving information on pulse height. Very large pulses need to be limited in size without causing distortions in other parts of the γ-spectrum.

3. Stability. The gain should not vary significantly with changes in ambient temperature or small variations in supply voltage.

4. Pulse shaping. The amplitude of the electrical pulse from a radiation detector first increases rapidly with time (rise time) and then slowly decreases (fall time), the overall period being at least several microseconds. This pulse requires shaping, that is the rise time is standardised and the decay time is trimmed so that the next pulse is unlikely to be superimposed on the tail of the old one. This is achieved by circuits selected using the controls marked 'time constants'. The integrating time constant (I.T.C.) governs the rise time and the differentiation time constant (D.T.C.) the fall time. The rule is that these are set equal at a value somewhat longer than the decay time of the detector used: $0.8–1\,\mu s$ is suitable for NaI(T1). Other, more complicated, methods of pulse shaping are available and many manufacturers now adjust this internally so that no separate control is provided.

Pulse-height discriminators and analysers

The pulses from the main amplifier should retain the proportionality between pulse size and energy absorbed in the detector. We normally need to select a particular part of the γ-spectrum, such as the total absorption peak, in order to discriminate against low energy scatter.

Figure 19.1 illustrates the variable sized pulses, corresponding to different energy losses within the scintillator, which are observed at the output terminals of the amplifier. These pulses may be treated in various ways:

1. All pulses greater than a preset size V_1 are accepted (marked (D) in the figure). This is known as pulse height discrimination.

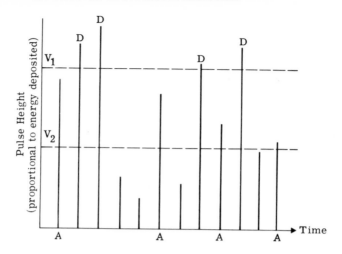

Fig. 19.1 Principle of pulse-height analysis.

2. All pulses within the preset range (V_1 to V_2) are selected (marked (A) in the figure.) This operation is called 'pulse height analysis', the acceptance range (V_1 to V_2) being the analyser window.

These tasks are carried out by a pulse height analyser (P.H.A.) which provides a constant sized output pulse for every selected input pulse, whatever its original size. In some equipments the window adjustment is marked ΔV in others it is calibrated as a percentage, usually (but not always) of the lower discriminator level V_2. Frequently the discriminator level is calibrated directly in keV, but this requires correct adjustment of the amplifier or high voltage supply which controls the sizes of the incoming pulses—the operation referred to as 'peaking'. Since manufacturers differ in their methods it is essential that the equipment manual is consulted.

If measurements corresponding to a number of different energy windows are required, as in a determination of the complete γ-spectrum, the use of a single channel analyser of the above type is very laborious. Multichannel analysers are invariably used which are effectively a hundred or more single channel analysers connected in parallel. The results are displayed on a cathode ray tube.

19.3. Data recording

The pulses which pass the discriminator or pulse height analyser are of a constant size and may be recorded in a variety of ways.

Scalers and timers

The simplest method of recording is to count the pulses and display the result, usually on a number display. If count-rate is required then the scaler can be automatically operated by a preset timer, which is really another scaler counting pulses from a built-in electronic clock. Counting equipment is generally designed to stop automatically after either a preset time or at a preset count. In automatic sample changers the results are printed out or transmitted to a computer, after which the next sample is placed in position.

Scalers do, of course, have a dead time during which they cannot respond to an incoming pulse, but count rates of 10^5–10^6 cts/sec can usually be handled.

Ratemeters

A continuous indication of counting rate is provided by the analogue ratemeter, in which each incoming pulse charges a capacitor of value C which is allowed to leak through a shunt resistance R. At equilibrium the voltage across the resistor will be proportional to the count-rate.

The performance is governed by the time constant which is equal to the product RC and which can be controlled by the operator. It effectively governs the time over which counts are integrated; a short time constant will respond quickly to fluctuations in count-rate and will thus show random statistical fluctuations. Alternatively long time constants provide a steady output signal but respond only slowly to changes in count-rate (see Fig. 19.2).

Since ratemeters are usually employed to follow variations in count-rate the time constant must be carefully chosen. A steady reading will be reached in a period of 5 to 7 times the RC value set. If the count-rate is then obtained from a single reading (I) of the meter the standard error is given by

$$\sigma = \sqrt{\frac{I}{2RC}}.$$

For example, if the count-rate is suddenly increased from zero to 200 cts/s and the time constant setting is 1 s, then after about 7 seconds the count-rate can be estimated with a standard error of $(200/2)^{1/2} = 10$, that is to $\pm 5\%$.

The memory effect of analogue ratemeters can be a distinct disadvantage, and digital ratemeters are now often used in dynamic studies such as renography. They consist of a scaler which after a preset time (the 'memory time') resets to zero and starts counting again. At the

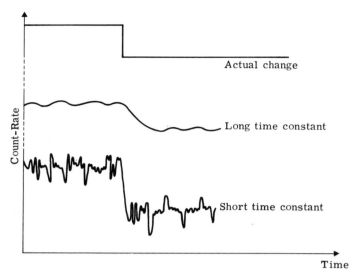

Fig. 19.2 Effect of time constants on the rate-meter response.

end of each counting period the accumulated counts are divided by the appropriate time and the count-rate displayed. There is thus no time lag, and the results are in a suitable form for subsequent computer processing.

Recorders
Count-rates may be conveniently recorded by a pen recorder and ratemeters are often provided with a special output socket for this purpose. The response of the pen recorder must be at least as fast as that of the ratemeter and if necessary fast recorders using ink jets or heat sensitive paper must be used.

Alternatively, data may be recorded by a variety of ways suitable for subsequent data processing, such as on magnetic tape. Further details are given in Chapter 20.

19.4.   Power supplies
All electronic equipment requires power, conventionally at a low D.C. voltage. This can be provided by one unit which feeds all the other items in the system.

Geiger counters require an extra high tension (EHT) supply in the range 0–3000 V but provided the detector is operated on the plateau stability is not important. Scintillation counters also require an EHT supply but in this case it must be stable to about $\pm 0.01 \%$ due to the dependence of the photomultiplier gain on the applied voltage. A change of EHT of 1 % would produce a 10 % change in pulse size!

19.5.   Systems

The individual items considered above may be supplied as separate items on a modular basis. Alternatively a complete instrument will be provided, such as a γ-spectrometer. In the latter case it will still be made up of individual items, but these will be located as separate circuit boards inside the apparatus rather than as physically distinct components.

Whilst great advances are being made in electronic design with the use of integrated circuits and microprocessors, the same basic principles apply from the point of view of the user. The units required and their manner of connection depends on the purpose for which they are needed. In subsequent chapters schematic diagrams will be given illustrating this. Figure 19.3 shows the requirements for a Geiger contamination monitor and a straight forward γ-spectrometer.

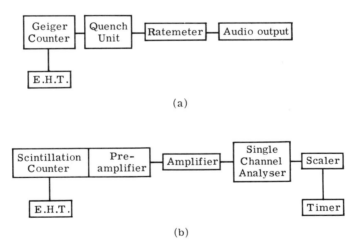

(a)

(b)

Fig. 19.3 Schematic diagram of (a) a Geiger contamination monitor and (b) a γ-spectrometer.

20

An introduction to computers

Computers are used increasingly in nuclear medicine departments, particularly to cope with the vast amounts of data produced in dynamic studies and emission tomography. In this chapter the basic concepts of computers will be presented in order to explain the specialised terminology of the subject and to indicate the variety of tasks for which computers are suited. The main applications in nuclear medicine will then be summarised. No attempt is made to teach computer programming and the reader requiring more advanced knowledge should consult one of the texts listed in Appendix 8.

Computer technology is advancing at such a rapid rate that parts of this chapter will be outdated rapidly. Nevertheless the basic concepts are unlikely to alter.

20.1. Digital and analogue computers

As their name implies, digital computers carry out calculations using numbers in the form of digits, in the same way as one uses a pencil and paper or a simple pocket calculator. Analogue computers rely on the construction of a model which is mathematically equivalent to the problem requiring solution. This model is usually electrical or mechanical, an example of the latter being the slide rule where the relative positions of two scales represent addition and subtraction. Digital computers are limited in their accuracy by the number of digits used in the calculation whilst analogue computers are limited by the accuracy with which the model represents the real problem and with which the corresponding variables can be measured.

Analogue computers can be cheap and are very suitable for certain specialised tasks. Examples in nuclear medicine are the subtraction scanning unit (see Section 23.6) and the position computer in most Anger γ-cameras (Section 24.1). The great advantages of digital computers are their potential accuracy and versatility. For these reasons they are more important and form the subject of the remainder of this chapter.

When using a simple pocket calculator the operator has to intercede at each stage of the calculation. With a computer a sequence of instructions called the program is constructed beforehand and the calculation thus proceeds automatically. The magnitude of the task can vary enormously, ranging from the calculation of the mean of a few numbers using a pocket programmable calculator to a large computation requiring millions of arithmetical operations within a large computer.

20.2.   The binary system and computers

In everyday life we use a system of numbers based on powers of 10 — the decimal system. Digital computers operate by electrical signals which basically exist in two states denoting the presence or absence of an electrical signal. As a result they can count only two numbers: 1 for 'on' and 0 for 'off'. This is the 2-based, or 'binary' system of arithmetic and the two binary digits are called 'bits'. Decimal numbers can be easily converted to binary. Fortunately modern computers carry out this conversion automatically and to operate a computer the user can usually ignore its use of binary arithmetic.

Nevertheless the binary nature is important when assessing the size of a computer installation required for a particular task. Each item of data, such as a number of counts, is converted into a group of bits called a 'word', often consisting of 8 bits (a 'byte') arranged so as to represent a binary number of alphabetic character. Long words may contain several bytes and obviously require more storage space but provide a high degree of accuracy.

In order to carry out a calculation the computer requires the necessary data in digital form. This may be straightforward: the presence of an electrical pulse at the output terminals of a single channel analyser represents one count in an uptake measurement. In other cases the data are initially available in analogue form, as with the position pulses from an Anger γ-camera where the sizes of the X and Y pulses may have any value between predetermined limits. In the latter case an analogue-to-digital converter (A.D.C.) is required to convert the pulse size into the appropriate arrangement of bits. Similarly digital-to-analogue converters (D.A.C.) are used when a byte is required in analogue form, as with the voltage applied to a graph plotter.

Frequently the size, polarity and shape of the electrical pulse produced by an item of equipment are unsuitable for direct connection to a computer. The special circuitry (possibly including an A.D.C. or D.A.C.) which matches equipment to the computer is called an 'interface'.

20.3.   Principal components of a computer system

A diagrammatic lay-out of a digital computer installation is shown in Figure 20.1. The input and output devices are peripheral equipment which are considered in Section 7. Backing store consists of storage devices which hold information required during the processing, or arising out of it, but which are not immediately needed (see Section 6). The heart of the computer is the central processor unit (C.P.U.)

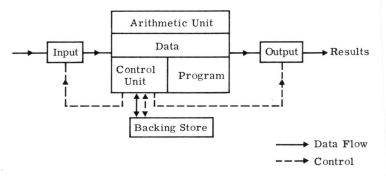

Fig. 20.1 The components of a typical computer installation.

consisting of the control and arithmetic units together with storage space which is immediately available. The latter contains both the data undergoing processing and the program. The program itself is stored as a series of binary numbers (words) which are translated in turn by the control unit and initiate the necessary logical operations by opening or closing the appropriate electronic switches. The actual calculations are performed as a series of binary operations within the arithmetic unit, which may be capable of several million operations per second.

The electronic circuits, storage and peripheral devices are known as computer hardware, whilst the term software is concerned with the specification and instructions which govern the operation of the computer and how, when, and in what sequence, the data shall be processed. A special program called the 'operating system' controls the running of the various programs together with the input and output functions.

20.4.   Flow-charts and programs

A computer program is a set of instructions which tell the machine what to do in detail. The first programmers had to address their computers directly in 'machine language' which as we have seen consists of long strings of binary digits. Later 'assembly codes' were introduced in which every machine operation still has to be itemised but mnemonics are used for convenience. Nowadays all but the smallest computers can be programmed using a 'high-level language' such as FORTRAN or BASIC. Whole blocks of machine instructions are gathered into recognisable phrases such as READ, GO TO. A special program — the compiler — converts this into machine code for a particular computer.

A particular problem is first analysed into a series of steps called a flow-chart. Figure 20.2 illustrates this for the everyday experience of preparing to drive to work. Some of the operations (switch on ignition) are straightforward; others require a decision based on the result of a previous operation (engine fires?). Yet others involve repetitive operations, either a preset number of times or for a number dependent on previous results. It is due to the computer's capacity to carry out rapidly these types of task that it is so efficient at involved and repetitive mathematical operations. An example of a simple flow chart in nuclear medicine is shown in Figure 24.3.

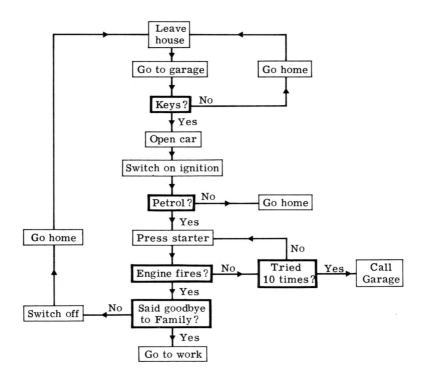

Fig. 20.2 The flow chart for a person driving to work.

A complete program can be stored in the computer before use and the whole process may proceed automatically without human intervention. Alternatively the program can cause the computer to stop at certain times for the entry of information such as a patient's name, or for instructions based on the progress of the investigations. This interactive mode of use is very suitable in clinical applications.

20.5. Microprocessors

Since the 1950s there have been enormous advances in the miniaturisation of electronic components. The old radio valve, which resembled an electric light bulb, has been superseded by the transistor based on a very small wafer of semiconducting material such as silicon. The miniaturisation process then progressed to the design of integrated circuits (I.C's) consisting of complete electronic units (such as amplifiers) on one piece of silicon. Technology advanced still further until there were as many as 10 000 transistors on one small silicon chip, and eventually the stage has been reached where a complete digital computer can be microminiaturised. The so-called microprocessor incorporates the whole of the central processor unit of the computer, including internal storage, the control unit and arithmetic unit, together with interfaces to peripheral units, on one silicon chip. This, together with a certain amount of additional storage facility for programs and data, forms a microcomputer. (The name microprocessor is increasingly used as a synonym for microcomputer).

The high degree of miniaturisation also results in a very considerable decrease in cost. It is now possible to use digital computers of this type for a wide variety of tasks; they are commonplace in industry, business and the home, and are the 'brains' of home computers and video games.

Nuclear medicine instrumentation is rapidly incorporating such devices. The use of integrated circuits has considerably reduced the size of electronic units and complex equipment can be accommodated on a few printed circuit boards; nevertheless the basic functions remain those outlined in Chapter 19. Microprocessors are used for control tasks and for the correction of data as in the digital Anger γ-camera (see Section 24.3).

20.6. Storage

Computer storage is basically of two types, memory and backing store, capable of accepting data and retaining it so that it can be retrieved and used when required. In the central processor or microcomputer data must be stored and retrieved very rapidly (less than $1\,\mu s$ per byte) and similarly stored programs and operating systems must be capable of fast access. On the other hand processed images from a γ-camera need to be stored for long periods of time, but speed of access is relatively unimportant. Types of store are also called 'volatile' or 'non-volatile' respectively, depending on whether they lose or retain the stored information when the electric supply is cut off.

Table 20.1 lists the main types of storage media in current use.

Table 20.1 Types of computer store

(a)	Memory — solid state	
	RAM	Random access memory
	ROM	Read-only memory
	PROM	Programmable read-only memory
	EPROM	Erasable read-only memory
(b)	Backing store — magnetic media	
	Floppy disk	
	Hard, or cartridge, disk	
	Magnetic tape	

A unique characteristic of most microcomputer-based systems is that the operating system and any compilers and associated programs are stored in 'READ-ONLY' memories. The information is stored in a fixed pattern of bits in the silicon chip and will not be lost when the power is disconnected. In system operation it is impossible for the processor to cause data to be stored in the device — it can only read that stored during the manufacturing process. The programmable read-only memory (PROM) can be programmed by the user after manufacture, using a special programmer unit, and thus he can create his own ROM. The EPROM can be both erased and programmed by the user, normally by erasure of existing data through exposure to ultra-violet light followed by electrical programming; some types are also electrically erasable.

For temporary storage of data, the results of arithmetic operations and similar operations, a 'READ/WRITE' memory is used — the RAM. The retrieval speed is independent of where on the chip the data are stored, but turning off the power to the chip will cause the loss of all data stored there.

Semiconductor memory is expensive compared to backing memory and is restricted in size. Magnetic media in the form of tapes or disks are very suitable for long-term storage, but are slower in access time. The floppy disk is somewhat similar to a small gramophone record and can store several scan images with a fairly fast access time. Much greater capacity is provided by the larger and more expensive hard disks, on which several hundred scans can be held. Magnetic tape is very convenient for long-term, high capacity storage due to its relative cheapness, but can have a long access time if the data required are at the wrong end of the tape.

Over the next few years it is likely that video disks will come into widespread use for storing large numbers of images.

20.7. Input and output

There are a wide variety of methods used to read data into a computer and to communicate the results in the most suitable form, either for immediate display or for subsequent reprocessing. They are summarised in Tables 20.2 and 20.3.

Table 20.2 Details of input devices

Name	Remarks
Keyboard	Operator can interact
Direct transfer	Very fast
Magnetic disks	Suitable for stored data
Magnetic tape	
Tape cassette	
Paper tape	Less used
Punched cards	

Table 20.3 Details of output devices

Name	Remarks
Visual display unit (VDU)	Display of images
Line printer	Alphanumeric information
Electrostatic printer	Grey-scale display and printing
Storage media	
Direct transfer	Connection to another computer

When data are stored and later processed by a machine, we call it 'off-line' usage. For many applications in nuclear medicine the results are required as rapidly as possible. It is therefore more usual to use a dedicated computer system in which data are transferred directly down an electric cable to the computer, a process known as 'on-line'. This does, of course, limit the use of the computer by other people, but is the quickest way of getting results, particularly when the amount of data is large, as in dynamic studies.

The keyboard, attached to a visual display unit (VDU), permits control of the system by the operator together with display of the results. These may then be photographed or stored digitally. The various types of printer are very suitable for alphabetic and numeric characters, but are rather limited when a grey-scale or colour image is to be reproduced. It must never be forgotten that the end-point of many nuclear medicine procedures is a high-quality image on which the clinician can report.

In addition to those methods listed in Tables 20.2 and 20.3 certain specialised equipment such as optical character readers are available for particular purposes, for example reading preprinted request forms.

20.8.   Computer installations and usage

In many cases we are concerned with the processing of scans, usually from a γ-camera. The position pulses require digitisation using two A.D.C.'s and the field of view is divided into a matrix of square elements, usually 64×64 or 128×128. For example, a field of view 32 cm in diameter would be divided into 64^2 (4096) square elements each 5×5 mm. A larger matrix is really necessary with good resolution cameras and large fields of view, but requires four times as much storage and an accompanying increase in computing time and cost.

There are many suitable computer systems on the market, mostly based on minicomputers which are dedicated to the task. Systems vary according to requirements but are likely to include at least 16 000 words (16 K) of memory as well as magnetic discs and tape as backing store. It is most important that the system is straightforward for a non-specialist to use and that the display facilities are adequate for clinical reporting.

Certain tasks require large computers. These are usually shared between many users, a number of whom can be connected at the same time, a mode of operation known as multiaccess. Users can either interact with the computer as their program is being run, or hand it in as a 'batch' job and collect the results at a later time.

20.9.   Applications of computers in nuclear medicine

In nuclear medicine computers perform four main functions. Firstly they act as *recorders*, both for the storage of scans for subsequent reporting and analysis, and of the statistics of patients examined. Secondly, they are able to carry out repetitive calculations and thus *analyse* large amounts of data, such as those produced in a dynamic study. They also permit the use of *displays* such as colour T.V. with facilities for interaction by the clinician reporting the scans. Lastly, they can *control* instruments as illustrated by their increasing use in departments dealing with large numbers of radioimmunoassay specimens.

Subsequent chapters will deal with these uses in more detail, but the main areas of application are as follows:

Static imaging

Uniformity corrections may be applied routinely to γ-camera scans, using the results from the measurement of a uniform flood source to provide the correction factors. Smoothing of the data can also be carried out to reduce the effects of noise, and much effort has gone into complex techniques for improving the quality of the pictures by mathematical operations; their clinical value is, however, open to some dispute.

Various types of display are available and using, for example, a colour T.V. the number of levels displayed can be much greater than in a Polaroid print. Contrast enhancement and background suppression can be applied as desired by the clinician at the time of reporting the scan, without destroying the original data. Special scanning techniques such as dual isotope studies, quantitative scanning, whole body counting and tomography rely heavily on computers to carry out the calculations required.

Dynamic studies

A dynamic study may produce 50 separate images, all of which require storing, usually by a computer connected on-line. These may be played back rapidly, as in a cine film, or analysed in order to condense the useful data. Corrections can be applied for effects such as blood background. It is also possible to control the computer from an ECG machine so that data are only collected at certain parts of the cardiac cycle, thus achieving an effectively static image of a moving organ. Dynamic studies have proved to be one of the most useful applications of digital computers in nuclear medicine.

Sample counting

In automatic sample counting systems computers are used to analyse the spectra of individual sampoles, apply any necessary corrections for decay, background and quenching, and calculate the results using standards as in radioimmunoassay techniques. An almost automatic service can be provided in which samples are loaded into the counter and the computer prints the results onto suitable forms for sending to the clinician concerned.

General calculations

Many minor calculations are necessary in nuclear medicine, particularly in relation to radionuclide dispensing. These are increasingly carried out using pocket calculators, some of which can be programmed for specific tasks. Larger computers are required for research applications as well as the routine and tedious task of updating the statistical records of a department.

21

Sample and whole body counting

For the majority of sample counting carried out in Departments of Nuclear Medicine, such as that connected with radioimmunoassay investigations, the background count rate is steady and small compared with that due to the sample. It is therefore important to employ a detector which has as large a sensitivity as is practicable (Section 16.7).

The sensitivity is primarily determined by the intrinsic efficiency of the detector and its geometrical configuration with respect to the sample. In most cases high intrinsic efficiency can be obtained only by the use of scintillation counters. The geometric arrangement affects the number of photons or particles which traverse the detector and are thus liable to detection. Ideally the detector should totally surround the sample, a situation referred to as '4π counting' since the solid angle subtended by the detector at the source is 4π steradians. This is attained in the liquid scintillation counting of β-emitters where the sample is intimately mixed with the scintillator (see Section 21.5). Gamma-emitting samples, such as specimens of blood, are best counted in a re-entrant well type scintillation counter, where the solid angle is close to 4π.

21.1. Ways by which the sensitivity is affected

Efficiency of detector
The total detection efficiency measures the probability of an interaction (of any type) between the incident γ-rays or particles and the detector. For a given energy and material it will depend on detector thickness and encapsulation, the latter being important only for β-particles and low energy photon emitters such as [125]I. With γ-emitting samples calculated data are usually satisfactory to within $\pm 5\%$ for scintillation counters of standard dimensions. They are frequently given for point sources at different distances from the detector, and some typical values are given in Table 21.1.

In γ-spectrometry the ratio of the counts observed in the total absorption peak to those under the whole of the γ-spectrum is known

Table 21.1 Detection efficiency for point sources at centre of face of 5 cm dia. × 5 cm high cylindrical NaI(T1) crystal, and within the 2·5 cm dia. × 5·0 cm deep well of a 7·6 cm dia. × 7·6 cm high NaI(T1) well crystal

Detector	Total detection efficiency (%)		Pk/Total ratio		Total absorption efficiency (%)	
	5 × 5 cm	well	5 × 5 cm	well	5 × 5 cm	well
Energy (MeV)						
0·279	43	80	0·84	0·87	36	70
0·661	30	51	0·49	0·49	15	25
1·33	22	39	0·30	0·34	7	13
2·62	18	32	0·18	0·23	3	7

as the 'peak-to-total-ratio' and may also be obtained by calculation. It is very dependent on γ-energy and detector size, but does not vary rapidly with position of source. By multiplying the total detection efficiency for a point source by the peak-to-total ratio we obtain the total absorption efficiency (Table 21.1).

Geometrical arrangement

In practice volume, not point, sources are encountered and these will subtend a variety of angles at the detector. It is clearly wise to subtend as large an angle as possible: thus with a cylindrical detector the source should be as close as possible. The angle subtended (and therefore the sensitivity) will, however, be very dependent on the position and volume of the source, providing the possibility of considerable error. Where possible re-entrant well type detectors should be used: the angle subtended will be greater than 2π and so the sensitivity is much improved. Table 21.1 illustrates this. It is also an advantage that the sensitivity is fairly independent of sample volume, at least for small volumes.

Care must be taken that the geometric arrangement does not vary during the counting period, which will happen if the sample slowly precipitates out or is adsorbed onto the sides of the container.

Scatter

Gamma-rays will be scattered from the material surrounding the detector and may thus be deflected and enter the detector. Therefore measurements should always be carried out with the surrounding shielding (particularly the lid) in the same position.

Self-absorption

At low γ-energies absorption within the sample may be serious. For example, the half-value thickness of 140 keV γ-rays in water is less than 5 cm, and for the 27–35 keV emission from ^{125}I below 2 cm (see Table 7.1). Since absorption will depend on the physical and chemical nature of the sample these should be standardised in any one investigation.

21.2. Measurement of γ-emitters

The importance of geometrical arrangement has been emphasised previously, since this affects both the overall sensitivity and the reproducibility of measurements. Whenever possible an approximation to 4π geometry is used in routine γ-counting procedures.

Small samples are most commonly blood or other body fluids amounting to a few ml in volume. They are most conveniently assayed in a well-type scintillation counter of 5 cm or 7·5 cm diameter. A number of manufacturers supply automatic sample changing equipment in conjunction with these detectors, results being either printed out or fed into a digital computer. It is usual for such systems to incorporate at least one single channel analyser. If low energy measurements are to be made such as ^{125}I determinations for radioimmunoassay procedures, then an NaI(T1) crystal with a thin encapsulation should be used to reduce absorption losses.

Large samples normally consist of urine or faecal collections, which are most conveniently assayed in the original container. Since it is not easy to standardise volumes — or even the distribution of material within the container — then a counting system is required whose

Table 21.2 Some comparative data for sample measurement systems (γ- or X-ray emitters)

Sensitivity	ct/MBq s		pA/GBq	
	NaI(T1)* 7·5 × 7·5 cm	16GM† counter	Well type ionisation chamber NPL 1383A	TPA
Radionuclide	(well type)	ring	(1 atmos.)	(20 atmos.)
^{51}Cr	5×10^4	700	25	800
^{59}Fe	2×10^5	6000	700	2×10^4
^{67}Ga	7×10^5	—	150	5000
^{99}Tc^{m}	7×10^5	3000	150	5000
^{125}I	8×10^5	—	—	—
^{131}I	5×10^5	7000	300	1×10^4
Background	1 to 3ct/s	25ct/s	0·01pA	0·1pA

* 4 ml sample
† 2 litre sample

sensitivity is relatively independent of sample position. Large NaI(T1) crystals may be used, but a cheaper and usually satisfactory method for moderately active specimens is to use a ring of perhaps sixteen shielded lead-cathode GM counters which surround the sample. Volumes up to 2 litres may be accommodated. Table 21.2 gives data pertaining to γ-counting systems in common use. High activities, in excess of 5 to 50 MBq, are most conveniently measured using the well-type ionisation chamber described in Section 18.2.

21.3.   Corrections and errors

Whenever the counting rate from a sample is measured certain corrections must be applied. These are considered below: liquid scintillation counting represents a special case and is discussed in Section 21.5.

Background

This should always be measured when a series of samples is assayed and has been discussed in Sections 16.3 and 16.5.

Radioactive decay

Since many short-lived radionuclides are used clinically this can be an important correction. A note should always be made of the time and date when a measurement is made; it is normally sufficient to correct for decay to the mid-point of the counting period for any one sample. Note that when samples are compared with an aliquot or with others measured at the same time decay corrections may cancel out.

Dilution and chemical losses

Dilutions need to be corrected for in the usual manner and considerable care taken since they can be a significant source of error. Certain radionuclides (e.g. ^{32}P) are particularly prone to preferential absorption on the walls of vessels and small amounts of inactive carriers need to be added.

Geometry, self-absorption and detector efficiency

These were discussed in Section 21.1. It is important that all samples and reference standards are measured under identical conditions, particularly as regards sample volume.

Lost counts

Since radiation detecting equipment normally takes a significant time t to detect and process an event (the 'dead time') they will not respond to any new events for this period. A significant number of counts may therefore be lost.

If N_0 = observed count-rate per second

N_c = correct count-rate per second

t = dead time in seconds

then the total insensitive time in each second will be $N_0 t$ seconds. In this period $N_0 t \times N_c$ counts will be missed.

$$\therefore \quad N_c = N_0 + N_0 N_c t$$

$$\text{i.e. } N_c = \frac{N_0}{1 - N_0 t}$$

It is important for long dead times (as in the Geiger counter) and high count-rates (as with scintillation counting). This is illustrated in Table 21.3. Some apparatus automatically corrects for lost counts by measuring for a longer time. In this case the controls are set to 'live time' so that the timer controlling the count is rendered inoperative during the dead time. Conventional timing can be carried out by selecting 'clock time'.

Table 21.3 Lost counts corrections

Observed count-rate	Dead time 1 μs	10 μs	300 μs
100 ct/s	<0·1 %	0·1 %	3 %
1000 ct/s	0·1 %	1 %	43 %
10 000 ct/s	1 %	11 %	—

21.4.   Multiple radionuclide studies

On occasions two radionuclides require measuring simultaneously in the same sample. In most cases each nuclide has one prominent total absorption peak, as shown in Figure 21.1.

Two single channel analysers are set to encompass the energy bands (1) and (2) corresponding to the two total absorption peaks.

First a sample of B alone is measured, and the proportion (b) of counts in channel (1) due to B alone determined. Then the nuclide B can be measured directly in channel (2) — let this be N_2 counts. Channel A will register counts (N_1) due to A alone together with a contribution ($b N_2$) from nuclide B. The true counting rate in (1) due to A alone will therefore be ($N_1 - b N_2$).

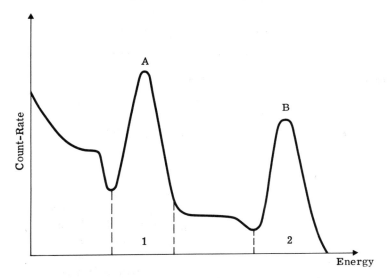

Fig. 21.1 γ-Spectrum of two radionuclides present in the same sample.

As an example consider the case where a measurement of ^{51}Cr gave 1000 counts in the ^{51}Cr channel and 200 counts in the (lower) ^{99}Tc^m channel. When a mixed sample was assayed the ^{51}Cr channel contained 5000 counts and the ^{99}Tc^m channel 8000 counts.

In this case the contribution from the ^{51}Cr to the ^{99}Tc^m channel is $200/1000 = 20\%$. Thus the ^{51}Cr contributes 20% of 5000, i.e. 1000 counts, to the ^{99}Tc^m channel. It follows that the corrected ^{99}Tc^m counts are $8000 - 1000 = 7000$ counts, whilst the ^{51}Cr channel will be unaffected since it would be wholly above the ^{99}Tc^m channel.

More complex situations can be solved using simultaneous equations. A similar technique may be used when there are not clearly defined photopeaks, as in the measurement of two or more β-emitters by liquid scintillation counting (see next section).

21.5.   Liquid scintillation counting

The only convenient radioactive isotopes of hydrogen, carbon and sulphur (^{3}H, ^{14}C and ^{35}S) are all low energy β^- emitters (Table 21.4). Since the β-particles are easily absorbed they are conveniently detected by intimately mixing the sample with a scintillator which is in solution. This is the basis of liquid scintillation counting, which may also be used with low energy X- and γ-ray emitters such as ^{55}Fe and ^{125}I as well as high energy β^- emitters like ^{32}P. Due to the

Table 21.4 Low energy β^- emitting radionuclides

Nuclide	Half-life	Max. β^- energy (MeV)
^{3}H	12·3 y	0·018
^{14}C	5730 y	0·155
^{35}S	87 d	0·167

effectively 4π geometry and lack of self or window absorption counting efficiencies of 50–60 % for ^{3}H and 95 % for ^{14}C can be achieved.

Method

The sample to be counted is made up of three components: the radioactive material, an organic solvent and a liquid scintillator. The passage of an electron causes excitation of molecules along its path; some of this energy is transferred to a molecule of the scintillator which is in turn excited and emits photons of ultraviolet or visible light. The sample is contained in a transparent counting vial of glass or plastic, usually 20 ml in capacity, which is placed between two photomultipliers.

Owing to the low energy of the β-particles the light flashes from the scintillator are of very low intensity — on the average one β^- particle from ^{3}H will cause the emission of only a few electrons from the photocathode. This is comparable with the number of photoelectrons emitted by the photocathode due to thermal effects. However, the light photons from the scintillator are likely to emit electrons from the photocathodes of both photomultipliers simultaneously, whilst thermal effects will cause the emission of electrons randomly with time. The photomultipliers are therefore connected in coincidence, that is only photoelectrons emitted simultaneously at both photocathodes are recorded. In this way the background count rate for ^{3}H is reduced by orders of magnitude, and may be still further reduced by cooling the sample and photomultipliers to around 4°C. The resulting background for ^{3}H counting is about 40–60 ct/min. Figure 21.2 shows a schematic diagram of a modern liquid scintillation counter. In addition to the normal amplifier and pulse height analysers a coincidence circuit is provided which 'gates' the scalers so that only coincident pulses are recorded. The pulses from the two photomultipliers are summed so as to improve energy resolution. In the case shown two counting channels are provided to enable dual isotope studies to be carried out. A liquid scintillation counter will normally include facilities for automatic sample changing and the printing out of results.

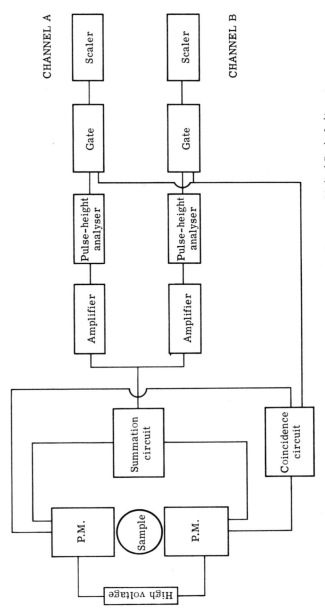

Fig. 21.2 Schematic diagram of a liquid scintillation counter (*Courtesy William Heinemann Medical Books Ltd.*).

Liquid scintillators and solvents

The purpose of the solvent is to ensure intimate contact between the sample and the scintillator and also to aid in transfer of energy between the two. Toluene is the most widely used, together with xylene and dioxane. The solvent forms the largest part of the scintillator mix and is chosen for its ability to incorporate the particular type of sample required.

The scintillators most commonly used are complex organic molecules known by their abbreviated chemical names; amongst those widely employed are PPO, POPOP and butyl-PBD.

A number of substances may absorb the excitation energy before it is transferred to the scintillator. This is known as 'chemical quenching' and is particularly important with aqueous samples. In addition 'colour quenching' can occur, in which the visible light photons are absorbed by the solution before they reach the photocathodes. In both cases there is a reduction in the observed pulse height spectrum (see Fig. 21.3). In the case of ^{3}H fewer β^- particles may be detected since none of the few photons produced may reach the photocathodes.

Samples and sample preparation

Samples may be prepared both rapidly and simply, and they can consist of solids, gases and plant or animal tissues as well as liquids. Some materials such as fatty acids are readily soluble in scintillator solvents such as toluene. In other cases chemical treatment is required: for example, the sample can be oxidised and the products directly dissolved in the scintillator solvent.

For biological materials such as tissues, aminoacids and RNA, solubilizers like hyamine are used to facilitate incorporation in toluene. For water and aqueous solutions it is now normal to use emulsion counting, in which the water is introduced after a detergent such as Triton-X100 has been mixed with the scintillator. Up to 40 % of water by volume can be incorporated and the method is so versatile that many biological substances can be measured in this way with little or no sample preparation.

High energy β-emitters (above 0·26 MeV and preferably above 1 MeV) can be detected using the liquid scintillation counter to detect the visible light (Cerenkov radiation) which is emitted when an electron of sufficient energy passes through a medium such as water. In this case no scintillator is required and sample preparation is particularly easy. Phosphorus-32 can be counted in this way with an efficiency of 25 %.

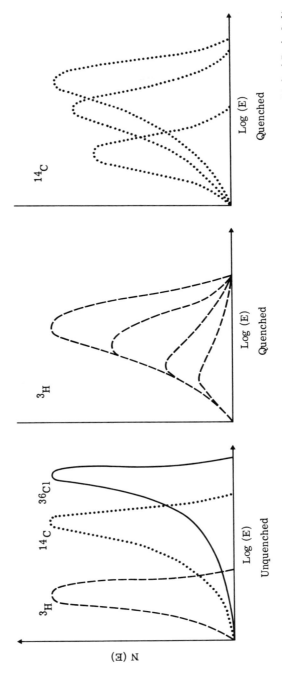

Fig. 21.3 Quenched and unquenched β^- spectra as obtained using a liquid scintillation counter (*Courtesy William Heinemann Medical Books Ltd.*).

Quench corrections

Since chemical and colour quenching affect the counting efficiency it is important to estimate and correct the amount of quenching, which may even vary between samples in the same batch. Three main methods are in use.

Internal standard. The specimen is first counted and is then recounted after the addition of a known amount of the radionuclide. From the increase in count-rate the counting efficiency can be calculated, and this in turn used to correct the initial reading from the sample alone.

Channels ratio. The measured spectrum is divided into two counting channels, covering different ranges of pulse height. Quenching which causes a shift to lower energies (see Fig. 21.3) will alter the ratio of the counts in the two channels. Since this depends only on the shape of the pulse height spectrum and is independent of the activity it can be used to measure the amount of quenching. Calibration curves need to be prepared using a range of samples exhibiting different degrees of quenching and whose activity has been measured by the internal standard method.

External standard. This uses a γ-emitting source such as ^{137}Cs which can be placed close to the sample vial. Gamma-rays will interact with the scintillator and the count-rate obtained will depend on the degree of quenching. Thus the correction factor can be estimated after this additional measurement is carried out. Again calibration curves must be constructed using samples of known activity.

Facilities for the last two methods are usually provided in commercial apparatus and data processing equipment can be used to apply the corrections automatically to each sample. The channels-ratio is usually more accurate than the external standard method, but a combination of the two methods can be used.

21.6. Whole body counting

In certain clinical studies such as metabolic tests involving ^{58}Co-Vitamin B-12 the retention of labelled material must be determined over a period of several days or even weeks. Such data can be obtained by the collection and measurement of all excreta, but the practical problems are formidable and the errors usually large when substantial activity is lost from the body. In these cases it is far better to use a whole body counter for measuring directly the activity retained by the patient. If, however, only a few per cent of activity is lost, as in red blood cell loss studies, excreta measurements must be used.

Since the radioactivity present is likely to redistribute in the body during the course of the investigation the response of the whole body counter should be independent of the distribution of activity within the body. This may be achieved either by placing detectors in carefully chosen positions around the body or by using a scanning technique in which the patient is moved past a detector array. Shielding requirements depend on the amount of activity to be measured.

Many configurations have been developed and only the ones likely to be encountered in clinical work are described here. Each represents a balance between sensitivity and uniformity of response to various distributions of activity within the body. The simplest can be used for the measurement of only high activities, such as ^{131}I retention in patients being treated with radioiodine for carcinoma of the thyroid. With the most sensitive counter radioactivity body burdens following accidental exposure can be identified and measured.

Single detector systems

For measurements of around 5 MBq upwards a very simple and cheap counter can be used which consists of a single 2·5 cm dia. × 2·5 cm thick plastic scintillator sited at a height of about 2 m above the centre of the patient (Fig. 21.4a). Since the detector is approximately equidistant from all parts of the body errors due to redistribution are at an acceptable level although the sensitivity is poor. Shielding is unnecessary provided the background is stable. For example, using a detector fixed to the ceiling the retention following a therapeutic dose of ^{131}I can be measured to within $\pm 25\%$ without disturbing the patient.

Shadow shield systems

Two shielded NaI(T1) counters of about 10 cm diameter are mounted opposite each other and partially collimated so that a strip about 30 cm wide across the patient is in the field of view (Fig. 21.4b). The patient is moved slowly between the two detectors and both the count-rate and total counts recorded. In this way the total activity can be measured to about $\pm 20\%$ and additional useful data on localization obtained from the profile scan. The total length of traverse is about 2·5 m and with a measurement time of 15 min a total body activity in the range 0·05 MBq–500 MBq can be conveniently measured. This is sufficient for most diagnostic tests.

Multiple fixed detectors in shielded rooms

An alternative but usually more expensive arrangement is a fixed detector system placed around a couch within a shielded room.

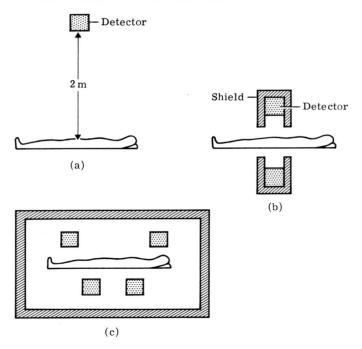

Fig. 21.4 Types of whole body counter. (a) Single detector, (b) Shadow shield, (c) Shielded room with fixed detectors.

Typically four 10 cm dia. × 7·5 cm thick NaI(T1) detectors are arranged in the positions shown in Figure 21.4c, which provides a response independent of distribution to within ±20 %. The overall sensitivity is improved by using massive shielding such as 10–20 cm of steel, in which case whole body potassium can be readily measured through the natural ^{40}K content and in addition cases of accidental contamination studied. The minimum detectable activity is very dependent on the nuclide and the system used, but can be below 10 Bq.

Calibrations
Whole body counters can, of course, be calibrated by carrying out measurements of excreta as well as whole body determinations. More convenient is the use of suitable phantoms containing known amounts of activity or the measurement of the subjects themselves after administration of a known amount of activity but before significant excretion has occurred.

22

Measurement of organ uptake

So far we have restricted the discussion to measurements of total radioactive content, mainly in samples but also in the whole body. An important part of the work of a nuclear medicine department is, however, the measurement of the activity in a selected organ of the body, such as the thyroid, kidneys or heart. This may be determined just once, as in 24 h thyroid uptake studies, or more frequently as a function of time as in renography.

These studies are invariably carried out using radionuclides emitting γ- or X-rays, usually in the range of $0 \cdot 1 - 0 \cdot 4$ MeV although ^{125}I (27 keV) and ^{24}Na (2·75 MeV) may be encountered. Scintillation detectors are therefore used and it is necessary to restrict the field of view of the detector so that ideally only the region of interest is seen. This is achieved using a collimator, usually of lead, which permits the entry of radiation from only one region of the body whilst preventing radiation from other areas being detected.

Many departments use γ-cameras coupled to digital computers in order to determine uptake as a function of time. This is dealt with in Chapters 24 and 28.

22.1. Single-hole collimators

The simplest collimator consists of a single cylindrical hole in a lead block (Fig. 22.1). We shall study this in some detail as it illustrates the basic principles of collimator design.

Spatial resolution
Ideally the field of view is restricted to that immediately below the hole marked diameter D in Figure 22.1a and referred to as the 'visual field'. However, an additional area of the source outside the visual field is viewed by a restricted area of the detector. This is known as the penumbra. Thus if a point source is moved beneath the collimator and the count-rate recorded as a function of position then a curve of the general shape shown at the bottom of Figure 22.1a will be obtained. It is called the 'point source response'.

For measurements on individual organs we require constant sensitivity over the visual field and a narrow penumbra so as to minimise the contribution of activity within neighbouring tissues. Note that the penumbra increases with distance from the collimator whilst the visual field is of constant size. Thus the collimator should be as close to the organ as possible; in practice there are restrictions due to anatomical problems and the depth within tissue of the organ.

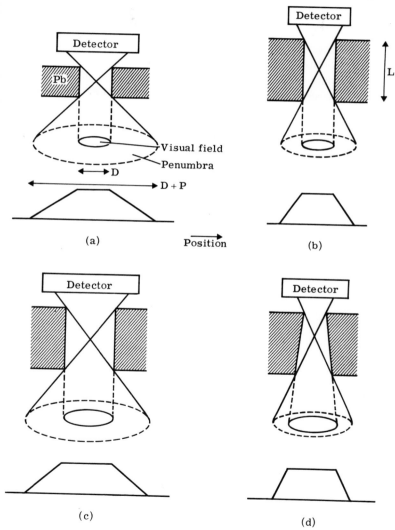

Fig. 22.1 Characteristics of single hole collimators.

If the hole length L is increased (Fig. 22.1b) whilst keeping D constant then the visual field is unaltered but the penumbra at a given distance is decreased. This is desirable in terms of physical characteristics but requires a more exact placement of the collimator.

The diameter D of the hole may also be increased (Fig. 22.1c). For example, the Figure shows an increase of 60% resulting in a penumbra diameter similar to that of Figure 22.1a but with improved visual field.

'Spatial resolution' refers to the ability of a collimated detector to distinguish between two radioisotope sources placed close together, and is clearly related to the point source response. The further apart the sources need to be the worse (larger) the spatial resolution. The term 'resolution' is often used loosely, but may be defined as the distance on a point source response curve between the two positions where the response is half the maximum. It is analogous to the full width at half maximum (FWHM) concept encountered previously in connection with energy resolution (Section 17.3). Note that the best resolution is obtained with a long, narrow hole (Fig. 22.1b).

Sensitivity

This term refers to the ability of the collimator to accept radiation from the source and is closely related to the field of view. Two distinct situations must be considered.

Source smaller than the field of view. In this case the sensitivity will decrease with distance from the detector according to the inverse square law. Reproducible measurements will be obtained only if the distance is fixed. This is the situation applying to most organ uptake measurements.

Source larger than the field of view. Again the inverse square law will apply, but as the distance is increased so the area of source which is viewed will increase, and in air the two effects will exactly compensate provided there is no penetration of γ-rays through the lead.

Summary

The characteristics of a single cylindrical hole collimator are governed by the diameter and length of the hole, and by the source area and its distance from the collimator. The spatial resolution depends on the diameter D and falls off with distance from collimator. Increasing the length improves the resolution at a depth, but with some loss in sensitivity due to the smaller penumbra. For organs smaller than the resolution distance the sensitivity is approximately governed by the inverse square law.

The design of collimators is seen to be a compromise between sensitivity and spatial resolution.

22.2.   Diverging-hole collimators

For a given visual field size the penumbra may be reduced by using a wide angle collimator with a diverging hole. In Figure 22.1d the visual field is the same size as in Figure 22.1c, but the penumbra is reduced. However, with diverging holes the visual field will get larger with increase in distance from the detector. Again the source should be as close as possible to the end of the collimator.

High energy γ-rays such as those from ^{131}I may penetrate the edges of the collimator to a significant degree increasing both the size and importance of the penumbral region. Diverging holes are better than cylindrical ones in this respect and are normally used for measurements of the radioactive content of particular organs.

22.3.   Measurement of thyroid uptake

Even though it is now largely supplanted by *in vitro* tests the measurement of thyroid uptake is an important illustration of the use of a single scintillation detector fitted with a diverging hole collimator.

A certain amount of radioiodine, usually 0·2 to 1 MBq ^{131}I is administered and after a suitable interval of time the fraction present in the thyroid is determined. A schematic diagram of a suitable system is shown in Fig. 22.2. The detector is preferably a 5 cm dia. × 2·5 cm thick NaI(T1) detector which provides reasonable sensitivity, and is set up on the 364 keV total absorption peak so as to exclude the effects of scattered radiation. The collimator has a visual field of about 12 cm

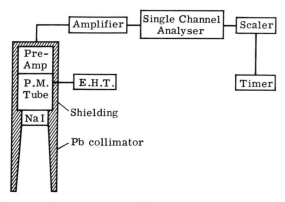

Fig. 22.2 Apparatus for measurement of thyroid uptake.

at the working distance of 20–30 cm, which must be carefully and reproducibly set up whenever measurements are taken. Additional shielding is provided at the sides and rear of the detector to guard against radiation emitted from other regions in the patient or from other sources that may be present.

The radioiodine is administered orally and an equal quantity retained as a reference standard. After the required time (normally 24 h) the radioiodine in the thyroid is determined, and immediately afterwards the reference standard is also measured. In order to simulate the attenuating and scattering properties of tissue the bottle containing the standard is placed in a suitable neck phantom which is set up in the same way as the patient. After correction for background counts the thyroidal uptake is calculated as a percentage of the standard (which was made equal to the administered dose). Note that a decay correction is not required since both the standard and the administered dose have decayed by the same amount.

Statistical errors due to counting are usually small ($<3\%$) but there are systematic errors inherent in this technique. Thus the neck phantom may not be truly representative of the patient, and the collimator may not be correctly positioned over the gland at the correct distance. In addition extrathyroidal iodine within the field of view of the collimator will contribute counts. This is not usually serious at 24 h, but for early uptake measurements allowance must be made. For example, the thigh may be used to simulate an athyreotic neck provided correction factors have been carefully determined.

It is clear that considerable errors can occur due to poor positioning, extrathyroidal activity and non-representative neck phantom. In addition, the uptake may be affected by clinical factors such as medication and dietary intake.

22.4. Renography

The passage through each kidney of a suitable radioactive material such as ^{131}I hippuran is monitored by two scintillation detectors, one placed over each kidney. In this case the count rate is required as a function of time, digital ratemeters connected to a pen-recorder being convenient for this purpose. No attempt is made to measure absolute uptake so the type of calibrations described in the previous section are not required. Suitable equipment is shown diagrammatically in Figure 22.3. Each scintillation detector is fitted with a diverging hole collimator adjusted so that the whole kidney is within the field of view.

The digital ratemeter is set for a suitable cycle time, such as 1 min, and the pen recorder started just prior to injection of approximately 10 MBq ^{131}I-hippuran. Over the first few minutes the count rate

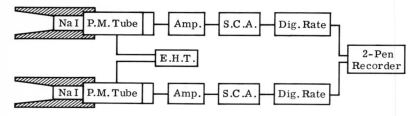

Fig. 22.3 Apparatus for renography using twin probes and a chart recorder.

increases rapidly due to the activity in the blood and its subsequent appearance within the kidney. In the normal patient the readings then fall to a low value within 30 min. Information on renal function is obtained from an analysis of the curve.

Three important sources of error should be noted:

1. Counting errors: The activity of ^{131}I administered is restricted due to dose considerations so that the number of counts recorded per minute is likely to be small, particularly with poorly functioning kidneys. The time cannot be increased without losing information on the dynamic behaviour of the radiopharmaceutical.

2. The collimators should be designed and adjusted so that the kidney is completely within the field of view, but a minimum of other tissue. This can be very difficult without some means of localisation such as X-rays or small tracer doses of ^{131}I hippuran.

3. Even with correctly adjusted collimators activity within under- and over-lying tissues will contribute significantly to the count-rate, particularly in the early stages of the study. Corrections can be applied if the blood levels are also monitored using, for example, a third probe situated over the heart. Alternatively a second radiopharmaceutical, such as ^{131}I-HSA, can be used to determine the blood background.

If a γ-camera equipped with a digital computer system is available then errors (2) and (3) may be reduced or avoided altogether, as described later (section 28.2). Other radioactive labels are also now being used which are better from the point of view of dosimetry. Thus ^{99}Tc^{m}-DPTA delivers a much lower patient dose per study than ^{131}I-hippuran.

23

Radioisotope scanners

The distribution of a radiopharmaceutical within the body can provide important diagnostic information. Localization studies of this type are carried out using γ-ray emitters with the object of determining the relative count-rate distribution over the region under examination and provide what is an essentially two-dimensional picture of a three-dimensional situation. Early work was carried out by moving a hand-held Geiger tube over the body. The sensitivity was greatly improved by the use of scintillation counters and the process became automated around 1950; commercial machines became available in the late 1950's. These early machines were all of a scanning type although γ-cameras, as described in the next chapter, are now much more common. Scanners are less used, but are required for certain special purposes such as imaging with high energy γ-emitters, quantitative studies, and certain types of tomographic methods. In this book they also form a convenient introduction to many of the features of both 'in vivo' imaging techniques and collimator design.

23.1. The rectilinear scanner

Normally the detector is moved in a rectilinear manner over the patient (Fig. 23.1) the recording of the count-rate being synchronised to the position of the detector by a mechanical linkage. A block

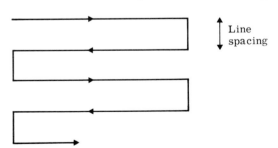

Fig. 23.1 The path of the detector in a rectilinear scanner.

diagram showing the main components is shown in Figure 23.2. The purpose of the collimator is to restrict the field of view at any one time to a small part of the organ under examination, and is dealt with in detail in the next section. A 7·5 cm or 10·0 cm diameter × 5 cm thick NaI(T1) detector is usual and often two are provided, one on each side of the patient, to reduce the overall time of examination. The detectors are connected via the usual amplifier and pulse height analyser to both a ratemeter and a scaler. These in turn operate the display which provides a pictorial representation of the radioisotope distribution and frequently gives quantitative data as well (see Section 23.5).

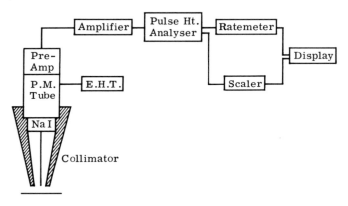

Fig. 23.2 The elements of a rectilinear scanner.

In the past only analogue ratemeters were used. These provide a continuous record of the count-rate but there is a 'memory' effect (see Section 19.3) which distorts the picture. This is particularly noticeable at the end of a line which may appear to continue past the end of the scan, an effect known as 'scalloping'. It may be overcome using digital ratemeters which recycle after a fixed distance (e.g. 2 mm) has been traversed. The total number of counts accumulated over that path interval is then displayed. In both types of scanner the head is moved by a motor whose speed can be adjusted over a wide range. Variations in speed will appear as variations in counts recorded per unit distance and thus lead to non-uniformity. Fortunately, this is rarely a problem except at the ends of lines.

23.2. Focussing collimators for use with scanners

The purpose of the collimator in radionuclide scanning is to restrict the field of view to a small area at any one time, with a minimum of penumbra. The parallel and diverging hole collimators considered previously (Sections 22.1 and 22.2) are very limited in sensitivity if good spatial resolution is required. If the hole is tapered (Fig. 23.3) then at a particular distance from the collimator face, known as the focal distance, the visual field is a point. However, in the focal plane as it is called, there is considerable penumbra.

The sensitivity can be improved without appreciably affecting the penumbra if a number of tapered holes are used, whose fields of view superimpose only in the focal plane (Fig. 23.4). Collimators are normally made of lead, with the holes packed closely together in a circular pattern, resulting in a total of 7, 13, 19, 25, 31 ... holes. Their closeness is related to the amount of lead remaining between, called the septal thickness; this is required to stop penetration of γ-rays

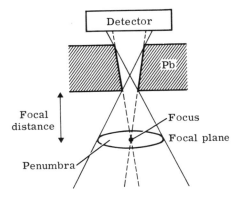

Fig. 23.3 Single tapering hole collimator.

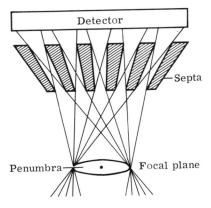

Fig. 23.4 Focussing collimator made up of many tapering holes.

between the holes. The higher the γ-ray energy the greater the septal thickness required.

In the focal plane there is a rapid fall-off of sensitivity as we go away from the focus. Other planes have lower sensitivity on the axis, and the fall-off is not so rapid. This is shown in Figure 23.5a where isocount contours (lines of equal sensitivity) are plotted for a 199 hole low energy collimator. If the source is in tissue the attenuation of the γ-rays will bring the point of maximum sensitivity nearer the surface (Figure 23.5b). It is usual to display the characteristics of a collimator as a series of cross-sections through the isocount contours. It will be remembered that the cross-section corresponds to the point source response function (Section 22.1). In Figure 23.6 a set of collimator characteristics in air are given for the same collimator as in Figure 23.5.

The detector must be of sufficient diameter to cover all the holes. It might be expected that very large diameters could be used to gain in number of holes, and therefore in sensitivity. In practice there is little

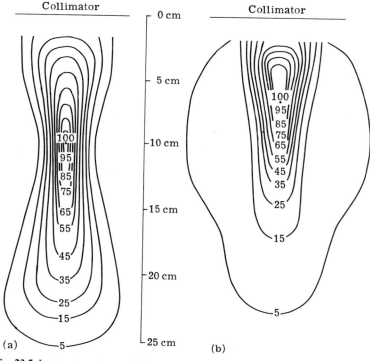

Fig. 23.5 Isocount contours of a low energy collimator and $^{99}Tc^m$: (a) in air, and (b) in water.

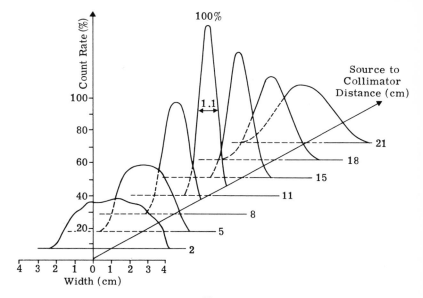

Fig. 23.6 Response curves for a typical $^{99}Tc^m$ focussing collimator in air.

gain in going above 12·5 cm diameter since the rays are then very oblique and, except at high energies, are likely to be absorbed in tissue before they reach the detector.

23.3. Effect of scatter and penetration

It is clear from Figure 23.6 that the point source response of a focussing collimator to a low energy γ-ray emitter in air is approximately Gaussian in shape, decreasing to zero outside the penumbra (Fig. 23.7A). If the same collimator is used with a high energy γ-ray emitter then some of the rays will penetrate the lead septa. Thus a point source outside the field of view will still contribute counts and the point source response will have 'wings' as shown in Figure 23.7B.

Scatter of low energy γ-rays within the patient has a similar result although for a different reason. Low energy γ-rays can be scattered through large angles with only a small loss in energy (see Fig. 7.5 and 7.6), and so it is likely that such photons will be included within the pulse height analyser window selected. Therefore we will again have counts recorded when the source is outside the penumbral region.

Notice that the FWHM is hardly affected, although there is appreciable broadening at the 1% level. This may appear insignificant but in practice is important since a large volume of tissue

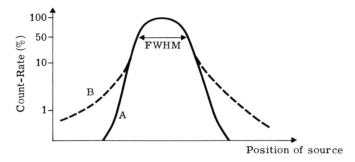

Fig. 23.7 Point source response functions (A) for a low energy γ-ray emitter in air, and (B) in the presence of scatter or penetration.

may be contributing at this level. The point source response curve of a nearby source will be superimposed on the 'wings' and the source will therefore be seen with reduced contrast. This reduction in contrast is similar in its effects to the omission of a grid in diagnostic radiology and is particularly important when a low contrast situation is being investigated; a good example is the detection of regions of low uptake in liver scanning using $^{99}Tc^m$-sulphur colloid.

23.4.   Modulation transfer function
Clearly the FWHM is not a totally satisfactory description of the spatial resolution capability of an imaging system. It is insensitive to the effects of scatter and penetration and furthermore even the complete point source response curve does not immediately convey the resolution of the system. In an attempt to overcome these problems the concept of modulation transfer function (MTF) has been introduced into nuclear medicine. It can be used to describe the behaviour of any imaging device, including both scanners and γ-cameras.

Consider the imaging of a radioactive source whose activity varies with position as a mathematical sine wave function (Fig. 23.8). The modulation is a measure of contrast and is given by the ratio of the sinusoidal amplitude to the average background level:

$$\text{Amplitude} = \frac{\text{max. value} - \text{min. value}}{2}$$

$$\text{Thus source modulation } M_S = \frac{S_{max} - S_{min}}{S_{max} + S_{min}}$$

$$\text{image modulation } M_I = \frac{I_{max} - I_{min}}{I_{max} + I_{min}}$$

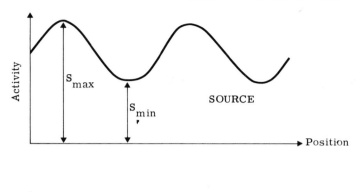

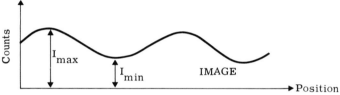

Fig. 23.8 Concept of modulation transfer function.

whence $\text{MTF} = M_I/M_S$. The MTF is normally presented as a function of spatial frequency.

In clinical practice the source will not be sinusoidal, but will consist of different structures with a range of sizes. Some of these will be resolved in the image, others will not. Any object can be considered as a superposition of a set of different objects, each of a separate size. The situation is analogous to white light which can be split up into light of different wavelengths or frequencies. Similarly, the object may be represented by a set of different 'spatial frequencies', a concept known as Fourier analysis (see Section 28.4). Due to limitations in the resolving power of the system not all spatial frequencies present in the object will be transferred to the image. Poor resolution causes flattening of the image, or loss of modulation. This results in a proportionate decrease in the MTF.

Thus the MTF measured the ability of an imaging system to transfer modulation from a source to its image. Any imaging system is made up of various components, such as the collimator and display, each of which will affect the MTF. External factors like scatter and penetration are also involved. Each of these components possesses its own MTF, and the overall system MTF is the product of the individual components. Note that the component with the worst MTF may have the most influence on the total system resolution. It is no use seeking to improve the resolution significantly by using a high resolution γ-camera if the collimator has very poor resolution.

An estimate of the MTF can be obtained by imaging a source containing a number of sinusoidal components. However, sources of different frequencies would have to be used and this is tedious and difficult in practice. Accurate determinations are normally based on an analysis of the shape of the response function to a line source, and is outside the scope of this book.

23.5. Displays

Whilst a rectilinear scanner is capable of providing a purely numerical presentation of the variations in radioactive distribution this is very difficult to interpret. It is normal to provide a pictorial representation, which may take a variety of forms.

Black and white dots

The outgoing pulses from the pulse-height analyser may be used to operate a metal stylus which prints dots onto paper every time a pulse arrives. The dots will be close together at high count-rates and far apart at low count-rates. Printers of this type frequently cannot operate fast enough for the count-rates normally encountered in nuclear medicine so a recycling scaler is used. If this is set to N counts, where $1/N$ is called the 'dot factor' then a dot will be printed only every N counts. The main disadvantage of this system is the restricted dynamic range — that is only a few easily recognisable levels can be discerned.

Photoscan

A much wider dynamic range is available if an image of the organ being scanned is also produced on a photographic film. In this case the blackening of a film is used as a measure of the count-rate at the corresponding point over the patient.

Various versions of the technique exist but the basic principle is as follows. The film (often a standard X-ray film) is contained in a light-tight holder and is 'scanned' by a light source attached to the scanner arm. In this case no division by a dot factor is required. The intensity of the light is controlled by the ratemeter (either analogue or digital), and so a picture is built up whose density, after development, depends on the count-rate distribution. The higher the count-rate the brighter the light thus producing a higher number of dots and a blacker film at that point. Both the intensity and the duration of the individual flashes can be adjusted so as to achieve a suitable range of densities on the developed film.

Colour scan

This provides a useful method of introducing count-rate information into the dot picture. A multi-coloured ribbon is moved between the dotting stylus and the paper in such a way that the colour printed is proportional to the count-rate reading. It is normal to have 7 or 8 colours, which are usually set up so that the highest (normally red) corresponds to the region of greatest activity.

Contrast enhancement

The response of the display used is not necessarily directly proportional to the count-rate. In Figure 23.9 curve A refers to the linear case, whilst in curve B the response is accentuated at the higher count-rates. Quite often the response to low count-rates is completely cut off, as in C. This is called background suppression and is particularly useful in displaying areas of high count-rate super-imposed on a general level of low count-rate, as in brain scans.

23.6. Double isotope scanning

In certain cases uptake in the organ to be imaged is not specific to the radiopharmaceutical used. For example, ^{75}Se-methionine is the most commonly used radiopharmaceutical for pancreas imaging, but is also localised in the liver which frequently overlies part of the pancreas. A way round this problem is to administer ^{99}Tc^m colloid as well: this is localised by the liver but not by the pancreas and by subtraction the view of the pancreas alone may be obtained. A similar problem exists when seeking to image labelled antibodies in the presence of a considerable blood-pool activity.

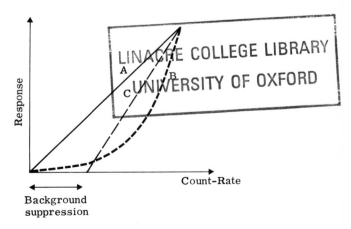

Fig. 23.9 Contrast enhancement.

It is neither necessary nor desirable to carry out two separate scans. The pulses from the amplifier may be fed into two pulse height analysers, in the case of pancreas scanning one is set for ^{75}Se and the other for ^{99}Tc^m. Suppose the count-rate in these two channels is S and T respectively. Then the count-rate due to the pancreas alone is given by $(\alpha S - \beta T)$ where α and β are constants whose values depend on the relative uptake of the two nuclides in the particular patient. The calculation of $(\alpha S - \beta T)$ can be achieved either by a special electronic circuit (as in many commercial scanners) or with a digital computer. Suitable values for α and β are determined when setting up the scan by measurements over non-overlapping areas of the liver and pancreas. Similar methods apply when subtracting the blood background.

23.7.   Quantitative scanning

The response of the ordinary focussing collimator is very depth-dependent as shown in Figure 23.6. If the responses of two opposed detectors, each fitted with a suitable focussing collimator, are added together then the total response can be independent of depth. It is therefore possible to determine the total activity contained in the volume directly between the two collimators. This is of assistance in comparing scans taken at one time with those at another, for example to examine the effect of treatment.

Allowance must be made for the activity in under- and over-lying tissue. This can be done by double isotope techniques, or by comparison with the contralateral view of the patient. Neither method is very satisfactory and it is best to use tomographic methods (see Chapter 26).

24

Gamma cameras

Rectilinear scanners are restricted in their application due to the time required to carry out a study, which is frequently 20–30 minutes. Instead of scanning the patient point by point γ-cameras utilise a stationary detector which views all parts of the field simultaneously. Images can be taken in a short interval of time, thus permitting investigations of fast dynamic processes.

Whilst there are many types of γ-camera the most commonly used is the scintillation camera, first developed by Anger in 1956. This chapter is therefore primarily concerned with this device.

24.1. The Anger γ-camera

A single, large area, scintillation crystal is viewed by an array of photomultipliers as shown in Figure 24.1(a). When a scintillation occurs within the crystal the light is divided between the photomultipliers, the relative pulse sizes giving the position of the scintillation. The pulses from the individual photomultipliers are also summed and passed to a pulse-height analyser in order to measure the total energy loss in the interaction.

The original Anger camera used a crystal 10 cm in diameter: recently developed large field of view (LFOV) cameras are over 50 cm in diameter. The collimator ensures that each part of the crystal looks at only a small area of the patient, so that a γ-ray image of the subject exists at the exit side of the collimator (see Section 24.2). The crystal is viewed by a hexagonal array of photomultipliers (Fig. 24.1b) connected to the crystal by light-pipes; the total number of photomultipliers is often 19 or 37, but the trend is to larger numbers. Lead shielding is provided both at the sides and rear of the camera.

From the preamplifiers and amplifiers situated near the base of each photomultiplier the pulses pass to the position computer consisting of circuits which compare the relative pulse heights from the individual tubes. Four signals are provided by the position computer: X^-, X^+, Y^- and Y^+, which together give the x, y coordinates of the scintillation. The total light intensity is examined

243

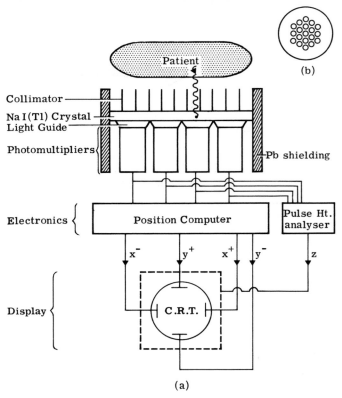

Fig. 24.1 The Anger γ-camera.

by a pulse height analyser and if it falls within the window set a Z pulse is also created.

The X and Y pulses are fed to the deflection plates of a cathode ray tube (CRT). If the Z pulse is also present then the beam of the CRT is switched on for a short time and a flash of light appears on the face of the CRT. The position of this flash depends on the x, y coordinates of the scintillation within the crystal, and in turn upon the point within the patient from which the detected γ-ray originated. As individual γ-rays are detected short flashes occur at different places on the CRT screen. These flashes are photographed over a period of time, the pattern of dots providing an image of the activity distribution within the patient. Polaroid film is convenient but conventional film and multiformat imagers are widely used; monochrome and colour TV displays are also common. Frequently the X, Y, and Z pulses are fed directly into a digital computer for storage and subsequent analysis, as described in the next chapter. A storage oscilloscope is of assistance when positioning a patient under the γ-camera.

The thickness of the crystal is restricted, usually to 12·7 mm (0·5 inch) of NaI(T1). If it were too thick two effects would cause degradation of the image. Firstly multiple Compton events are more likely, particularly with higher energy γ-rays: simultaneous light flashes at different parts of the crystal will produce X and Y pulses corresponding to the position of the average luminous intensity rather than the true position. Secondly, in a thick crystal the depth of the light flash within the crystal will affect the relative light intensity received by the photomultipliers. On the other hand very thin crystals will have poor detection efficiency for the γ-rays. A thickness of 12·7 mm is a convenient compromise and is particularly suited to imaging γ-rays between 100 and 200 keV in energy. Table 24.1 gives values of the total absorption detection efficiency of such a crystal.

In an effort to improve the intrinsic spatial resolution, some manufacturers are now employing thinner crystals of sodium iodide. Such cameras are only slightly less efficient for the 140 keV γ-radiation from ^{99}Tc^{m}, but are somewhat unsatisfactory when used with higher energy γ-emitters.

Due to the statistical nature of the scintillation process and its method of detection there will be an uncertainty associated with the recorded position of a γ-ray. This may be represented by the FWHM of the point source response curve obtained when a narrow parallel γ-ray beam is incident on a small area of the crystal. The intrinsic resolution measured in this way depends on the γ-ray energy being approximately inversely proportional to the square root of the energy. The actual values obtained vary with the type of photomultiplier and light guide system employed 4 to 6 mm at 140 keV being typical.

24.2. Collimators for γ-cameras

The purpose of a γ-camera collimator is to project an image of the radioactive distribution on to the scintillator. With one exception (the

Table 24.1 Total absorption efficiencies of 12·7 mm thick NaI(T1) crystal

γ-ray energy (keV)	Total absorption detection efficiency (%)
100	98
150	90
200	69
360	26
500	15

pinhole collimator) this is achieved by using multihole collimators in which each hole projects γ-rays from different areas of the object onto the corresponding area of the scintillator. As we saw with scanner collimators, the requirements of resolution and sensitivity are conflicting and compromises are required. The different types are shown diagrammatically in Figure 24.2.

Parallel-hole collimator
This is the most commonly used and there is a 1:1 correspondence between the object and its projection onto the scintillator. Thus the size of the image is independent of distance from collimator face. Thus the size of the image is independent of distance from collimator face. The collimator consists of a large number — possible several thousand — of parallel-sided holes, each of which acts as a single hole collimator similar to that described in Section 22.1. The thickness of the septa, and hence the number of holes, is governed by the γ-ray

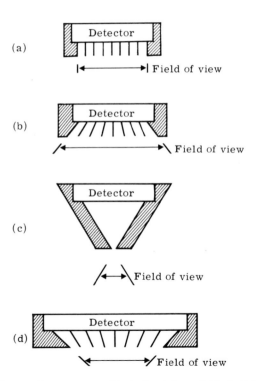

Fig. 24.2 Collimators for a γ-camera, illustrating (a) parallel-hole, (b) diverging-hole (c) pin-hole and (d) converging.

energy to be used: low energy collimators have thin septa and hence many holes.

As discussed in Section 22.1 the spatial resolution falls off with distance from the end of the collimator and for this reason the collimator should be close to the patient. Provided the source is in air, and is imaged completely within the field of view, then the sensitivity is independent of distance. Both high sensitivity and high resolution collimators are often available for a particular energy: the two may well possess the same hole structure, but the high resolution have twice the hole-length of the high sensitivity collimator. In this case the resolution at a depth will be twice as good, but the sensitivity decreased by a factor of four.

Diverging-hole collimator

If objects larger than the crystal size are to be imaged (such as both lungs) then a collimator with slightly diverging holes is used. The object is therefore demagnified and since not all parts will be affected equally a certain amount of distortion is introduced. Again the resolution will fall off slowly with distance, but this time there will be an accompanying reduction in sensitivity.

Pin-hole collimator

This consists of a small hole at the end of a lead shield (Fig. 24.2c) and is similar in concept to an old-fashioned pin-hole camera. Objects close to the aperture are magnified, whilst those far away are demagnified. Thus considerable distortion can be introduced and it is only suitable for relatively thin objects.

Due to the small solid angle subtended by the detector this collimator is very insensitive and furthermore the sensitivity falls off with distance. Whilst the resolution also falls off with distance due to the magnification effect, objects close to the pin-hole are effectively imaged with a resolution close to the inherent resolution of the γ-camera. Pin-hole collimators are best suited for imaging small objects close to the collimator and are very suitable for eyes and thyroids. In the latter case, their overall shape permits them to be placed under the chin and close to the thyroid.

Converging collimator

This is almost opposite in its properties to the diverging collimator, and has much in common with the pin-hole but with much improved sensitivity. The resolution improves with distance until the 'focus' is reached, and the sensitivity may be three to four times that of the equivalent parallel-hole collimator. However, distortion is introduced which limits the degree of convergence used in practice. Normally they are restricted to use with large field of view cameras where the reduction in field of view may be acceptable and the improved resolution and sensitivity is advantageous, particularly in dynamic studies where the overall counting time is limited.

Collimator characteristics
As with scanner collimators, the modulation transfer function may be used to describe the overall performance of the system, although the FWHM of the point source response curve is helpful when choosing a collimator for a particular patient.

Table 24.2 lists the characteristics of some commercially available collimators; these are constantly being improved but an idea of average performance can be obtained. Note that whatever the intrinsic resolution of the γ-camera the performance at a depth is usually governed by the collimator, and in practice the resolution (FWHM) obtained at a depth within a scattering medium is 10–20 mm. The collimator also introduces a considerable loss in sensitivity: the fraction of γ-rays emitted by the subject which pass through a parallel-hole collimator is in the range 0·01–0·1 %.

24.3.   Inherent distortion and uniformity of response
In theory a uniform γ-ray intensity incident upon the crystal will produce a uniform intensity in the resultant image. In practice the measured sensitivity per unit area is not constant over the field of view for a number of reasons which are discussed in turn.   Systematic errors exist in the calculation of the point of interaction within the crystal since the distance of these points from the photomultipliers are not constant. This geometric distortion is most severe close to the photomultipliers since the recorded positions of events close to the photocathode tend to crowd into its centre. The energy response of the various photomultipliers will also vary across the field of view and so the pulse height analyser window must be wide enough to encompass the full range encountered; this is unlikely to be optimum for any one phototube. All these sources of error depend on the photomultiplier size and arrangement and will affect the response over the full field of view. Such spatial distortion frequently results in 'hot spots' corresponding to the positions of the photomultipliers. This effect is particularly pronounced at the periphery of the detector since the photomultiplier arrangement is no longer symmetrical and the situation is further complicated by reflections from the crystal sides. For this reason the outermost part of the crystal is usually blanked out.

Table 24.2 Characteristics of some collimators suitable for a large field of view γ-camera

Collimator	Type	Energy limit keV	No. of holes	Hole length mm	Septal thickness mm	Hole diam. mm	Relative sensitivity (%)	System resolution at: (FWHM (mm)) 0 cm	10 cm
High resolution	P	140	41 000	32	0·25	1·5	100	7·5	10·8
High sensitivity	P	140	41 000	17	0·25	1·5	330	7·7	15·6
Converging	C	140	20 000	26·5	0·25	2·4	0 cm–270 10 cm–460	7·5	11·6
Medium energy	P	280	8 600	38	0·84	3·1	180	7·9	15·1
High energy	P	400	3 400	64	1·6	6·4	120	9·2	16·3
Pin-hole	PH	400	1	—	—	3·0	10 cm–40	—	4·1

Notes: P = parallel hole, C = converging hole, PH = pin hole.
Relative sensitivity of $100\% = 150\,\mathrm{ct/s}$ per MBq for $^{99}\mathrm{Tc^m}$.

The energy response of the phototubes will also vary with time since it depends on their gain (which is EHT and temperature dependent) and the pulse height and other settings. Again this will give rise to non-uniformity of response, as will mechanical imperfections in the collimator and distortion due to both scattered and fluorescent radiation from the collimator septa.

When a γ-camera is exposed to a large area uniform source (a 'flood phantom'), these spatial shifts and variations in sensitivity give rise to a non-uniformity of response that may well amount to ± 10 per cent over the central area. A first-order correction can be applied using a digital computer: the results from a measurement of a uniform flood source provide a series of correction factors for each matrix element. This method does not, however, correct for the spatial distortion which is the prime cause of the non-uniformity, nor does it cope with non-uniform energy response. Such corrections are possible in recently designed digital Anger cameras. For example, the energy may be measured over the whole field-of-view and each matrix element of the crystal is assigned to a suitable energy window, which will be selected by its X and Y signals. Similarly, a source in the form of a square grid can be imaged and each matrix element is given a displacement correction factor which is a measure of the amount of distortion at that particular point on the crystal. All these correction factors are stored in a microcomputer and applied on-line.

Using such methods it is possible to reduce non-uniformity and spatial distortion to a very low level. Nevertheless, the uniformity should be checked each day using a suitable flood phantom; it is wise for the clinician to have this 'uniformity picture' in front of him when reporting.

24.4.   The use of a γ-camera for dynamic studies

Since images of the whole field-of-view can be taken in a short interval of time it is possible to record a series of such images to provide a kind of cine-film showing how the radioactive distribution changes with time. Such dynamic studies have already been described in principle in Chapter 13, and form one of the major applications of modern nuclear medicine. More details are given in Chapter 28.

Such a study may produce 50 separate images, all of which require storing, invariably by a computer connected on-line. These may be analysed in order to condense the useful data. Figure 24.3 illustrates the simplified flow-chart of a typical dynamic imaging study program in which the variation in activity with time is computed for a specific area which was chosen after the study was terminated, and is referred to as a 'region of interest' (ROI). Corrections can be applied for effects

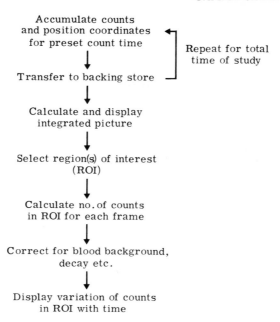

Fig. 24.3 Simplified flow-chart illustrating the sequence of calculation in a dynamic study computer program.

such as blood background. It is also possible to control the computer from an ECG machine so that data are only collected at certain parts of the cardiac cycle, thus achieving an effectively static image of the heart, corresponding to one particular section of the ECG.

Dynamic studies are proving to be one of the most useful applications of digital computing in nuclear medicine, particularly for studies concerned with cerebral blood flow, regional respiratory function, cardiac investigations and renography. Such studies are limited by the small number of photons that can be recorded in a short space of time and it is often necessary to use a much smaller image matrix such as 16×16 instead of the more common 64×64 or 128×128 used in static imaging. In this way spatial resolution is sacrificed for improvements in statistical accuracy.

Notwithstanding these problems of statistical accuracy, the actual counting-rate over a small area of the crystal may be very high at a particular time during a dynamic study. For example, in cardiac investigations the actual count rate for a scintillation camera over the precordium may be as high as 500 000 per second. If the system cannot respond accurately to such high count-rates loss of statistics, distortion of uptake-washout curves and degradation of spatial resolution will result. It is therefore necessary to examine the high count rate performance of a γ-camera, which is characterised by its dead-time (see Section 21.3). It has been shown that the dead-time is not constant, but varies with count-rate and possibly with position. It is wise to choose a system capable of high count-rate performance if such studies are to be undertaken. The count-rate behaviour of the whole system must be considered since it is quite possible for the computer and its peripherals to be the limiting factor.

Further consideration is given to dynamic studies in Chapter 28.

24.5. The digital autofluoroscope

One way of overcoming this count-rate problem is to utilise a large number of scintillator crystals, each viewed separately, instead of one large crystal as in the Anger γ-camera.

This is done in the autofluoroscope invented by Bender and Blau in the early 1960s. About 300 separate sodium iodide crystals are used, arranged in a rectangular matrix and with each optically isolated from its neighbours. Each crystal is opposite its own hole in the parallel-hole collimator. In principle, every crystal has its own photomultiplier, but in practice one photomultiplier is used for each row and one for each column. The light from each crystal is divided between two plastic light guides, one leading to a 'row' and the other to the appropriate 'column'. Thus the crystal in which a gamma-ray is detected is identified by the simultaneous detection of a light flash in a row and a column phototube.

The main advantage of the system is its ability to cope with high counting rates since each crystal acts as its own independent detector. In addition it is possible to use thicker crystals than in an Anger camera, which is of value for use with higher energy γ-emitters. However, the energy resolution is not as good which makes it difficult to exclude scattered photons.

The advantages of the autofluoroscope are, for most applications, small compared with the less complex Anger camera, and it is not therefore widely used.

25

Selection of operating parameters and choice of equipment

Previous chapters have described the basic types of imaging equipment encountered in nuclear medicine departments. It is obvious that even the best equipment can give poor results if misapplied. In this chapter general guidance is given as to the selection of operating parameters, and some comments made on the choice between different types of equipment.

There are many factors which influence whether a 'good' or a 'bad' final picture is obtained. Some are outside the control of the radiographer or technician, such as the quality of the radiopharmaceutical, whilst others are due to inherent limitations in the equipment or in the procedure itself. Patient positioning and management are of great importance but discussion of them is inappropriate to this book. The main technical considerations are listed in Table 25.1. To achieve the best results each imaging procedure should be examined separately and all aspects, clinical as well as technical, taken into account. It should be noted that a 'good' scan is not necessarily the most aesthetically pleasing or even the one which shows the normal anatomy best, but that which most clearly provides the required diagnostic information.

Some of the technical considerations listed in Table 25.1 are dealt with in detail in other chapters and will be mentioned only briefly. For

Table 25.1 Operating parameters of scanners and γ-cameras

1. Collimators:
   energy
   depth-of-focus
   resolution
   sensitivity

2. Setting of pulse height analyser

3. Information density:
   scanning speed   (scanner)
   total counts   (γ-camera)

4. Display

convenience scanners and γ-cameras are treated together. The various parameters are not generally independent and the correct setting or choice of one will depend on the value selected for another.

25.1. Choice of collimator

Most manufacturers market collimators optimised for different energies and a frequent classification is low ($<150\,$keV), medium ($<375\,$keV) and high energy ($<525\,$keV). The higher the energy the thicker the septa required, and the effect is marked due to the change, by more than a factor of ten between $150\,$keV and $500\,$keV, in the attenuation of γ-rays by lead (see Table 7.1). Thicker septa lead to considerable reductions in sensitivity (see Table 25.2) and for this

Table 25.2 Relative sensitivities of collimators. The collimators selected have similar resolution but those for the scanner and camera are compared separately.

Energy (keV)	Scanner	Camera
150	1	1
360	0·57	0·57
500	0·29	0·36

reason the collimator should, if possible, be matched to the energy of the γ-ray being imaged. One restriction must be borne in mind, that there are no appreciable higher energy γ-rays emitted by the nuclide being used or from any radionuclide impurity that may be present. These will cause degradation of the image due to septal penetration, an effect which can be particularly noticeable in the case of γ-cameras. For work with unusually high energy γ-rays, such as those from ^{59}Fe ($1\cdot1$–$1\cdot3\,$MeV), very thick septa are required which are not readily obtainable commercially.

The sensitivity and resolution of collimators are intimately linked, usually by an approximately square law. Thus if the resolution is improved by a factor of 2 only a quarter of the area will be viewed by the collimator, resulting in a decrease in sensitivity by a factor of four. A compromise is required to optimise the information obtained. If too good a resolution is used then the count-rate will be very low and the object to be imaged will not be optimally visualized due to statistical fluctuations. At the other extreme the use of a collimator with inadequate resolution results in high sensitivity but detail will be lost. For dynamic studies, where the number of counts acquired is limited, it can be advisable to use a coarse resolution, high-sensitivity collimator.

In the case of a rectilinear scanner the focal length of the collimator should be chosen bearing in mind the depth of the organ, the clearance needed between the collimator and the skin whilst scanning, and the shortening effect due to attenuation by tissue (Figure 23.5). The variation in resolution with depth is particularly important and rescanning a patient with a different collimator to skin distance can sometimes be of assistance in clarifying an equivocal area. With a γ-camera equipped with the usual parallel-hole collimator it should be positioned as close as possible to the patient since the resolution decreases continuously with depth. The differences in behaviour between focussing parallel-hole collimators are illustrated in Figure 25.1.

Due to the limited range of collimators normally purchased for a particular imaging device by a department the optimum collimator is not always available. For common procedures additional collimators which maximise the information gained can often provide considerable saving in imaging time and lead to improvements in picture quality.

25.2. Selection of analyser window
Radiation which is scattered in tissue degrades the image, as discussed in Sections 17.4 and 23.3. To reduce its effect the lower edge of the pulse height analyser window should be set as high as possible consistent with not excluding too much unscattered radiation. In

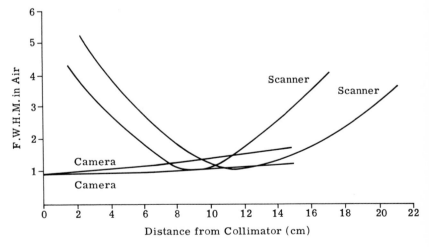

Fig. 25.1 Variation of resolution (FWHM) with distance in air for several typical scanner and camera collimators. The two focussing collimators are for 12·5 cm diameter crystals. All collimators are designed for use with $^{99}\mathrm{Tc^m}$.

most situations the optimum level for $^{99}Tc^m$ lies between 125 and 133 keV. With scanners an asymmetric window can be used but for γ-cameras this may lead to non-uniformity of response.

When multiple γ-rays are emitted, as with ^{67}Ga, a very wide window will encompass several total absorption peaks. A better solution is to use two or more analysers in parallel. However, there will be the problem of scattered radiation from the higher energy emission entering the lower energy window and, with γ-cameras, differences in uniformity at the various energies.

25.3. Information density

In the previous sections it has been pointed out that the pulse height analyser setting, and particularly the choice of collimator, will affect the sensitivity and hence the number of counts registered within the available scan time. If this number is too low statistical fluctuations will bring about unacceptable degradation of the picture and possibly lead to false diagnoses.

This concept is quantified by the information density, which is the number of counts recorded per unit area imaged, often expressed in counts per square centimetre. With some scanners the information density is displayed in terms of other units, such as counts per cell, where the size of the cell is dependent on the line spacing. In such cases the counts per square centimetre should be calculated.

The information density is most useful in effecting the compromise between choice of collimator resolution and overall counting time (scan speed in the case of rectilinear scanners). Consider the case where a collimator has a resolution (FWHM) of 1 cm: here we are looking for significant changes in counts between areas greater than about 1 cm^2. Let N = No. of counts required per cm^2 so that a change ΔN in counts compared with another equal area is just significant. The standard error of the difference between the number of counts from the two areas, σ_s, is given by equation (15.1):

$$\sigma_s^2 = N + (N + \Delta N)$$

$$\therefore \quad \sigma_s = \sqrt{2N + \Delta N}.$$

If $\Delta N \ll N$ this may be approximated to

$$\sigma_s \simeq \sqrt{2N}.$$

Now for most display systems a change of about 10 % in count density is required before it can be reliably detected by eye. If we take a 10 % change then

$$\Delta N = 0 \cdot 1 N.$$

Thus for one standard error to equal $0.1\,N$ there will be a 68.3% chance that the change is significant, and

$$\sigma_s = 0.1N = \sqrt{2N} \qquad \text{i.e. } N = 200.$$

For a 95.5% probability the difference should equal two standard errors, and

$$2\sigma_s = 0.1\,N = 2\sqrt{2\,N} \qquad \text{i.e. } N = 800.$$

Therefore in setting up a scanner or camera in this situation it would be desirable to aim for an information density of $500-1000\,\mathrm{cts\,cm}^{-2}$ over the critical areas. Crude calculations of this type can be helpful, but are limited and the other factors involved in interpreting an image, such as pattern recognition, need to be taken into account.

In the case of a radioisotope scanner the information density required, together with a quick measurement of the count-rate over the region of interest, will enable a suitable scan speed to be selected. Should this not permit an acceptable total scan time then the collimator may have to be changed or a lower information density accepted. For γ-cameras the relevant parameter is the total number of counts accumulated. If a reasonably homogeneous image is obtained which fills the whole area of the crystal then the average information density can be estimated by dividing the total counts by the crystal area. For example, a 24 cm diameter crystal and 250×10^3 cts gives an average information density of about $550\,\mathrm{cts\,cm}^{-2}$. If a computer is connected on-line to the γ-camera then the scan can be set to terminate when a preset information density is reached at a selected part of the image.

25.4. Effect of display

The usual display systems encountered have been described in previous chapters. It is important that the function of each control on a particular display system is understood in terms of its effect on the response–count rate characteristic (Fig. 23.9). Often the aim is to spread the restricted dynamic range of the display device over the relevant range of count-rates. Thus that part of the count-rate scale is enhanced where it is anticipated that the significant changes are likely to occur. Two restrictions must be borne in mind. Firstly the number of counts must be sufficiently great for the extra contrast to provide significant results, and secondly by enhancing the contrast in one part the contrast is reduced in another. Deciding the optimum settings for a display system requires close cooperation between the person carrying out the procedure and the clinician responsible for interpreting the picture. If the numerical data are stored then the display settings can be selected at the time of reporting rather than before scanning. This is most readily achieved when reporting is carried out on a display attached to a dedicated computer system.

25.5.   Quality control of γ-cameras

On delivery any piece of nuclear medicine equipment should be subjected to an extensive series of tests to ensure that it is up to specification. Fortunately internationally agreed standards, such as those drawn up by the IEC and NEMA, are now available, together with details as to how such type tests should be carried out. Studies of this kind are also of value in comparing different models under similar conditions.

In operation various quality control checks should be carried out on a regular basis to ensure that the equipment is working optimally. This is particularly necessary with γ-cameras. It is recommended that as a minimum the following tests are performed:

1. *Daily checks*
   a. Uniformity response using flood source
   b. Energy settings of pulse height analysers
   c. Visual inspection of image quality
   d. Electrical and mechanical safety inspection
2. *Monthly checks*
   a. Spatial resolution using bar phantom (Fig. 25.2)
   b. Electrical and mechanical safety tests

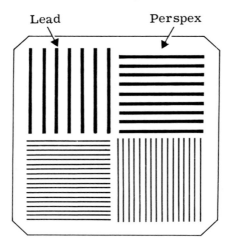

Fig. 25.2 Bar phantom for spatial resolution measurements over field of view

3. *Quarterly checks*
   a. Sensitivity to a calibrated γ source
   b. Count-rate capability
   c. Image distortion

In addition staff should be encouraged to examine the clinical images and report any deterioration in image quality.

25.6. Comparison between a γ-camera and a scanner

Nowadays a nuclear medicine department is likely to purchase a γ-camera in preference to a rectilinear scanner. It is however helpful to compare the two types of instrument, particularly since hybrid devices are now available (Chapter 27).

The final choice of equipment will be strongly influenced by clinical requirements. For example, if dynamic studies are to be undertaken, the γ-camera is obligatory; a cardiac department may even wish to consider the purchase of a multicrystal camera to facilitate first-pass studies. Conversely a whole-body scanner or hybrid device should be considered if many bone studies are performed. In Table 25.3 the main differences between γ-cameras and scanners are summarised.

Table 25.3 Comparison of γ-camera and scanner

	γ-camera	Rectilinear scanner
Clinical		
Dynamic studies	Excellent	Long term only
Views obtainable	Good	Restricted
Patient movement	Affects whole picture	Affects remainder of scan
Immobilisation devices	Poor	Fair
Setting up	Good if suitable display available	More difficult
Ease of operation	Straightforward	Requires skill
Anatomical markers	Acceptable	Good
Physical		
Area of scan	Up to ∼ 50 cm dia.	Whole body possible
Resolution	1–2 cm at a depth	> 0·5 cm at focus
Collimators	Reasonable range available, but changing takes time	Wide range, easily changed
Field uniformity	Requires correction	Very good
Display	Usually by film or VDU	Full size or minified, of various types; easily selected
Energy range	80–400 keV, best at 100–200 keV	> 25 keV
Dual isotope studies	Possible	Easily achieved
Data processing	On-line connection common	Off-line connection possible

Table 25.3—(*Contd.*)

	γ-camera	Rectilinear scanner
Quantitative studies	Poor	Satisfactory
Longitudinal tomography	Possible for small organs	One plane at a time
Transverse axial tomography	Practicable	Limited by statistics
Logistics		
Purchase cost	Usually more expensive than scanner	Can be cheaper, but not always
Running costs	Comparable	Comparable
Reliability	Good apart from uniformity	Good
No. of views/day	>100	10–15
No. of patients/day	>15	5–10
Maintenance	PM tubes require adjustment	Little required
Transportability	Small ones available	Unsuitable

26

Emission tomography

26.1. Introduction

When a γ-camera equipped with a parallel-hole collimator views a patient, a two-dimensional image is obtained which portrays a three-dimensional object, the human body. This image is clearly of great value, but there are three drawbacks to this simple imaging process. Firstly, no depth information is provided, secondly tissues are superimposed resulting in loss of image contrast, and thirdly no allowance is made for the effects of γ-ray attenuation by the tissues.

Depth information is normally obtained by taking a number of views, e.g. AP- and lateral. Focussed collimators can also be of help, particularly with rectilinear scanners; the image is only sharply in focus at the focal plane, the images of sources in other planes being blurred out to varying degrees. A tomographic effect is therefore achieved similar to that of longitudinal tomography in diagnostic radiology, but with a much greater depth of focus amounting to several centimetres. Longitudinal tomography is discussed in section 26.4, but basically suffers from problems of reduced image contrast, and artefacts due to contributions from activity in superimposed tissues which are difficult to remove. A more successful approach is transverse axial tomography, analogous to X-ray computerised tomography, which has developed so rapidly over the past 10–15 years. A large number of one-dimensional views are taken of a two-dimensional transverse axial slice and the activity distribution within that slice reconstructed mathematically (see section 26.2). Thus there is no superposition problem and depth information can be obtained directly from the image. Information in the longitudinal direction is provided by imaging contiguous slices.

Instrumentation for emission tomography has been developed using two separate approaches depending on the type of radionuclide being imaged. Single photon emission tomography (SPET) is used with single photon emitters such as $^{99}Tc^m$ whilst, with positron emitters such as ^{11}C and ^{13}N, coincidence detection of the annihilation photons is utilised (positron emission tomography, PET, section 26.5).

These techniques are currently under investigation in many centres and the areas of clinical usefulness are slowly emerging. The biggest problem is the rather poor utilisation of the γ-quanta emitted by the patient. For example, the nuclide is continuously emitting significant numbers of photons over a period of several hours, if not days, whilst they are only utilised by the tomographic device for a small proportion of this time. In addition, many of the emitted photons are not detected due to the small solid angle subtended by the detectors, and the effects of tissue absorption. By contrast, in X-ray computerised axial tomography the X-ray tube only emits quanta during the period of measurement and these are detected efficiently. Thus, for comparable radiation dose to the patient, an emission computerised axial tomographic examination (ECAT) will have much poorer resolution and image quality than an X-ray transmission CT scan (TCAT).

26.2. Principles of computerised axial tomography (CAT)

In CAT views are taken from various directions around the periphery of the transverse axial slice — these views are called 'projections'. Since image reconstruction is performed mathematically the object is effectively divided into a matrix of squares ('pixels'), perhaps 128 × 128. In its simplest form each view is taken by moving a highly collimated detector along a line at the side of a slice and recording the count-rate (see Fig. 26.1). A series of projections is built up, taken at regular angles such as every 10° around the slice; for simplicity, only two are shown, 90° apart, in Fig. 26.1.

The reconstruction process may be posed as a question: 'Given a set of projections, how can the activity distribution within the slice be

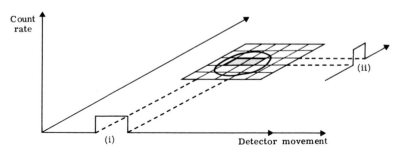

Fig. 26.1 Profiles of count rate measured by a detector scanning an area of radioactivity (shaded) within an object

calculated?' Consider profile (i) in Fig. 26.1. This tells us only the direction from which the γ-rays have come and their total intensity — no information is provided on the distribution of the activity. The most basic reconstruction method simply projects these data back along the individual rays, distributing the numbers equally between the pixels along the beam (Fig. 26.2). The process is repeated for all the other projections and the count-rate per pixel obtained by simple addition of the different values. Such a reconstruction method is called 'back projection' and was first used for radionuclide imaging.

It can be seen from Fig. 26.2 that the original distribution is reconstructed at A, but there is a surrounding background, B. The simple back projection method does not give a true representation because each point is, in fact, blurred out. It can be shown that this surrounding background falls off with distance, r, from the centre of a point object with a 1/r dependence. To obtain a true reconstruction the blurring must be removed. This is normally achieved by multiplying each projection by a mathematical function — called a 'filter' — before back projecting (Fig. 26.3). The filter has central positive components together with negative components at the sides, the overall effect being to cancel out the blurring and leave only the object itself.

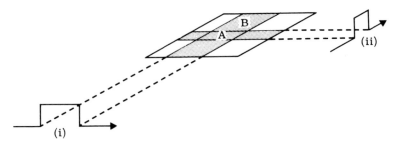

Fig. 26.2 Reconstructed image using only back projection

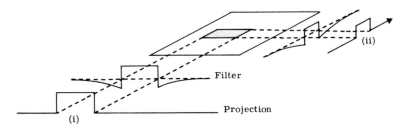

Fig. 26.3 Reconstructed image using filtered back projection technique

This process of filtered back projection (FBP) is used in most commercial tomography systems and can be carried out almost instantaneously if sufficient computing power is available. In practice, a choice of filters is provided which contribute a certain amount of image processing such as smoothing or edge enhancement.

So far in this discussion, we have ignored the effects of γ-ray absorption. In the practical situation photons emitted from the interior of the object will be attenuated before detection, and the resulting activity distribution requires correction. This is a difficult task, requiring some 'a priori' information on the shape and nature of the object. Considerable effort is currently devoted to devising methods which overcome this source of error, many based on iterative reconstruction techniques. In these the back projected image is continually refined by comparing the simulated projection values provided by the image with those actually measured, which obviously include the effects of γ-ray absorption. This process is very demanding on computer time.

26.3. Equipment for ECAT

The early work on ECAT with single photon γ-emitters such as $^{99}Tc^m$ was carried out using rectilinear scanners which could be moved around the patient to provide views at various angles. Studies were predominantly of the brain with scan times of many minutes, and only one slice could be measured at a time.

Gamma-cameras, together with dedicated digital computers, are now widespread and of recent years their tomographic potential has been exploited. It is now possible to obtain commercially a system in which a LFOV γ-camera, fitted with parallel-hole collimators, rotates around the patient at any desired radius. Images are recorded digitally at each of a series of angles and since a number of slices (typically 32) are viewed simultaneously it is possible to obtain many reconstructed slices from one set of measurements. However, great demands are made on the mechanical accuracy, electronic and count-rate performance and uniformity of the camera as otherwise artefacts are easily produced. The reconstruction programs are run on the dedicated computer and take several minutes, although the necessary software is not yet fully developed.

The overriding problem in any kind of emission tomography is sensitivity. From this viewpoint the γ-camera is not an ideal instrument: however, the rotating camera method makes economic sense and, of course, the camera system can be used at any time for conventional views (from any angle) and for dynamic studies. Other workers have examined multicrystal systems. These are more sensitive for single slices but for multiple slice studies the rotating camera becomes more competitive since many slices are measured simultaneously.

26.4.   Longitudinal tomography with single photon emitters

Here we are concerned with planes parallel to the long axis of the body. Images in such planes can be obtained by selecting the relevant data from a series of contiguous transverse axial slices, but it is also possible to determine the activity distribution directly.

A rectilinear scanner fitted with focussing collimators produces longitudinal tomograms in the focal plane and in the 1970s Anger developed an instrument which simultaneously imaged separate planes. This tomographic scanner consists of two small γ-cameras fitted with focussing collimators, one above and one below the patient. The cameras move across the patient with a scanning motion and up to 12 planes can be obtained simultaneously.

It is also possible to adapt a γ-camera for longitudinal tomography. One of the most promising techniques is the 7-pinhole method introduced by Vogel and Kirch in 1978. The camera collimator contains 7 pinholes which produce 7 non-overlapping images of the object, taken from different directions and projected on to non overlapping regions of the crystal. After correction for non-uniformity and distortion the images are reconstructed at a planar separation of 1–2 cm using an iterative process. The field of view is very limited (12–14 cm diameter) and so only small organs are imaged, mainly the heart. Again the system is available commercially but success is dependent on using state-of-the-art γ-cameras and, as with all tomographic techniques, artefacts are common. A variant on the 7 pinhole is the rotating slant-hole collimator which has parallel holes slanted at 20–30° from the vertical. This is rotated beneath the camera crystal. Iterative reconstruction methods are used, rather similar to those employed in multi-pinhole tomography. Although the rotating slit is more complicated than the multiple-pinhole collimator, the field of view and depth resolution are better.

26.5.   Positron tomography

In section 5.4 it was explained that when a radionuclide emits a positron the latter loses its kinetic energy whilst traversing a few millimetres of tissue and is then annihilated forming two 0·51 MeV photons emitted at 180° to one another. If these photons are detected simultaneously then their origin will lie on the line joining the two detectors. By taking a number of views a series of intersecting lines are obtained which identify the point of origin in three dimensions.

Such a tomographic system has advantages over SPET in that no lead collimators are required. Thus the sensitivity can be greater, although it is still desirable to surround the patient with detectors. It has also been shown that attenuation corrections are easier to apply than with SPET.

Most of the commercially available units are transverse axial systems using rings of detectors to image one or more slices simultaneously. There is also a certain amount of interest in the use of large area detectors placed around the patient which enable either transverse axial or longitudinal images to be reconstructed directly.

Positron tomographic units usually depend solely on the coincidence detection of the two annihilation γ-quanta. However there will normally be a very small time difference between the time of arrival of the two quanta, since γ-rays travel at the speed of light. Recently developed fast scintillators and photomultipliers enable this time difference to be determined to a few hundred picoseconds, corresponding to an uncertainty in position of several centimetres.

Normally the reconstructed image is obtained by using the whole field of view. Time-of-flight measurements permit considerable reduction in the size of the object area which is used in the reconstruction process of each pixel, thus improving signal to noise.

All positron tomographic systems are very expensive and in order to be exploited fully they require a cyclotron on-site to produce short-lived positron emitters such as ^{11}C, ^{13}N and ^{15}O. These are very important since they are the only radioisotopes of these biologically important elements that can be used for imaging. It is also possible to utilise the longer-lived β^+-emitter ^{18}F and the generator-produced ^{68}Ga.

26.6. Applications of emission tomography

A great deal of effort is being injected into the development of instrumentation for emission tomography since better image contrast will result and thus detectability should be improved. In addition the depth information is useful particularly for lesions close to other sources of activity such as the scalp. The possibilities of carrying out quantitative studies are also improved considerably since the contributions of overlying tissue are removed.

It is too early to give a balanced view on the clinical usefulness of emission tomography although useful clinical results are being obtained. Transverse axial tomography, using rotating γ-cameras, is receiving considerable attention for brain and liver imaging, whilst the chest is better suited to longitudinal methods. Tomographic scanners are arousing particular interest in providing depth information for whole body scans. Positron tomography is only carried out in a few research centres and the main stimulus is the development of better pharmaceuticals, such as $^{15}CO_2$, $^{13}NH_3$ and ^{18}F-deoxyglucose which hold promise in the imaging of regional physiology and organ function.

27

Special techniques and instruments

Certain nuclear medicine procedures are of great value for a particular purpose, and may thus justify the development of special dedicated equipment. In this chapter mention is made of some of these which may be encountered in specialised departments. The main emphasis is given to whole-body imaging, since the use of skeletal imaging for the detection of neoplastic disease is one of the most successful clinical tests in nuclear medicine.

27.1. Rectilinear scanners for whole-body imaging

Most rectilinear scanners are limited in imaging area to the size of a large X-ray film ($420 \times 350 \, \text{mm}^2$), as described in Ch. 23. In order to cover a larger area they are fitted with a minification feature, typically 5:1, which enables a whole-body image to be recorded on a single sheet of X-ray film. The information is therefore compressed and the resulting dot density in the image for a 5:1 minification will be 25 times as high as in a 1:1 scan. The image appears less noisy, but in fact the actual count density per unit area of patient will be unchanged. In addition mechanical inaccuracies are magnified five times, which is particularly important since the minification is frequently obtained by moving the patient relative to the scanner by mechanical means.

Such a system can be readily available if a rectilinear scanner is already sited within the department, but the sensitivity is poor, as with all scanners. The use of focussing collimators results in a limited depth of focus which may result in lesions being missed through being situated in off-focus planes.

To some extent these problems are overcome in the multicrystal whole-body scanner. This is similar to a rectilinear scanner, with detectors above and below the patient, but each detector head contains an array of scintillation detectors, each with its own collimator, phototube, amplifier and pulse-height analyser.

In one commercial instrument 10 crystals are situated in each head providing very high sensitivity. Nevertheless the problem of focal depth remains. Since the device is a dedicated instrument it is best suited for departments undertaking a large number of bone scans.

The Anger tomoscanner (see section 26.4) is a hybrid scanner-camera, but retains many of the characteristics of a scanner. It is a dedicated instrument capable of simultaneously producing images in a number of planes and overcomes the problem of focal depth. Oblique view imaging is also possible, but the equipment is expensive and is limited in count-rate capability.

27.2.   Whole-body imaging using γ-cameras

The resolution characteristics of γ-camera collimators avoid some of the problems of rectilinear scanners, and in addition the large crystal area increases sensitivity considerably. A LFOV γ-camera can be used to take multiple spot views of the body, thus obtaining a number of high-resolution images with good sensitivity.

However a LFOV camera, particularly if fitted with a slightly diverging collimator, can image the whole width of the patient in one view. Two methods have been adopted to obtain whole-body images automatically; in one the detector moves over the patient and in the other the patient's couch moves under the detector. As the table or camera head is moved, so the image is electronically moved across the cathode ray tube in the display, thus producing a minified whole-body image. In order to obtain the same sensitivity over the entire scan area, each portion of the body is viewed for the same amount of time. This is achieved by overscanning the head and feet, electronically masking the edges of the crystal so as to obtain a rectangular sensitive area, and paying great attention to mechanical reproducibility of movement. If the γ-camera used has too small a field of view to image the total width of the patient in one exposure then multiple passes will be required.

As with all electromechanical systems artefacts are possible, but a whole-body scanning attachment may well be a very useful accessory for a LFOV camera.

27.3.   Transmission imaging

The basic principle is the same as in X-radiography, but the γ-rays emitted from a radionuclide replace the X-ray source and a γ-camera takes the place of the X-ray film. Radionuclides that can be used are ^{125}I, ^{241}Am and ^{57}Co. The images obtained are poor compared with X-radiographs, but can be used to identify the patient anatomy in conjunction with the ordinary emission taken in the same position. Transmission images are also of value in applying attenuation corrections to ECAT images.

27.4. Fluorescent scanning

When X or γ-radiation interacts with an atom characteristic, or fluorescent, X-rays may be emitted (Ch. 7). The energy and intensity of these X-rays may be used to measure the quantity of the stable element present, provided the conditions are carefully controlled.

The sensitivity is such that an ^{241}Am source (60 keV γ-rays) of about 50 GBq can be used to excite the K X-rays (27 keV) from the stable iodine present in the thyroid gland. In order to reject scattered radiation a good energy resolution semiconductor detector must be used. If this is mounted on the arm of a rectilinear scanner the distribution of stable iodine may be determined, which is of use in the study of thyroid disease. The disadvantage is that only elements of high atomic number can be used due to the energy of the K X-rays; iodine is the only suitable element occurring naturally *in vivo*.

Alternatively fluorescent excitation can be used to measure the total amount of stable element present in a sample, for example, iodine in the blood following administration of a stable contrast agent such as meglumine iothalamate. In this way glomerular filtration rate can be determined without any radiation dose to the patient.

27.5. Neutron activation analysis

If an object is subjected to neutron irradiation then radioactivity will be induced; this in turn can be detected and using γ-spectrometry the elemental composition may be determined. This method — neutron activation analysis — is only suitable with elements which possess both a high neutron cross-section for the irradiating beam, and suitable γ-ray emissions. As a method of analysis the technique is very sensitive, and can be used for *in vivo* measurements of stable element concentration.

The neutrons used for this purpose are usually several MeV in energy and are produced by a cyclotron, neutron generator or fission source such as ^{252}Cf. A number of reactions are possible, such as ^{14}N (n, 2n) ^{13}N, ^{23}Na (n, γ) ^{24}Na, ^{31}P (n, α) ^{28}Al, ^{37}Cl (n, γ) ^{38}Cl and ^{48}Ca (n, γ) ^{49}Ca. The activation products decay emitting γ-rays, and with an irradiation time of a few minutes and a whole-body dose of less than 10 mSv the activity induced in a patient is easily detectable using a whole body counter (section 21.6). In this way total body nitrogen, sodium, potassium, chlorine and calcium may be determined, which is very difficult by other means and of great value in metabolic investigations.

28

Dynamic imaging

Dynamic imaging adds an extra dimension, that of time, to simple static imaging performed with a gamma camera. It allows a sequence of images of the distribution of a radiopharmaceutical in, and passage through, an organ to be obtained. However, the technique is greatly enhanced if the images are available in digital form, thereby allowing quantitative information about organ function to be obtained. The basic hardware required is a gamma camera (Ch. 24) and an on-line computer (Ch. 20).

Two branches of Nuclear Medicine are combined in dynamic imaging, kinetic tracer studies (Ch. 13) and imaging. The first essentially gives information about physiology (and patho-physiology) and the latter about anatomy. The approach of this chapter will be to illustrate some of the features and techniques of dynamic imaging by reference to studies of two organs, the kidney and the heart. It is not possible to describe all types of processing and manipulation of images currently available, nor to go into the details of the mathematics involved. However, brief mention will be made of one type of mathematical approach—Fourier analysis—which is used in a number of procedures. Finally the value of modelling in the interpretation of the results of dynamic studies will be discussed.

28.1.   Digital imaging — is it quantitative?

A clear distinction must be made between absolute quantitative studies, where the aim is to determine the actual activity, or radioactive concentration, in an organ or particular volume of tissue, for example a tumour, and the studies considered in this chapter. The former have been discussed in Chapter 22 and whilst the ultimate aim must be to combine absolute quantitation with dynamic studies this is not feasible with equipment commonly available.

A digital image is a two-dimensional array of numbers. Each number is proportional to the number of gamma rays (photons) detected by the camera in a certain time (the frame time) and from a small element of crystal. If the digital image is a 128 × 128 array and the diameter of the field of view of the camera is 40 cm then each element of the array represents approximately $3 \times 3\,mm^2$. An element of the array is often referred to as a 'pixel' (picture element).

A gamma ray arriving at a particular location on the camera crystal can originate from three sources:

1. Activity in the organ being investigated.

2. Activity in the tissue above or below the organ.

3. Activity outside the field of view due to scattering.

The absolute number of gamma rays detected will depend on many factors including injected activity, position of the patient and thickness of tissue overlying the organ of interest (Ch. 22). However, a number of these factors are constant during a particular study and therefore useful information can be extracted by comparing one frame with another.

It should always be borne in mind that conventional images are two-dimensional, whereas the activity distribution is three-dimensional. Care must therefore be exercised in attributing a specific pattern of counts to a particular activity distribution. For example, a certain number of counts can be due to a small volume of tissue with a high radioactive concentration or a large volume of tissue with a low radioactive concentration. One reason why more counts may be detected from one part of an organ than another is that the activity may just be nearer the surface and thus the gamma rays suffer less attenuation. It should be remembered that the half-value thickness in tissue of the 140 keV photons of $^{99}Tc^m$ is approximately 4 cm.

Background subtraction
In order to minimise the effect of the contribution to the counts detected from radioactivity in tissue above and below the organ of interest the technique of background subtraction is often used. An area or region of interest (ROI) adjacent to the organ is selected and the counts from that area is subtracted from the counts collected from a region of interest (ROI) over the organ. The two areas must either be the same size or a proportionate correction must be made.

$C_S = C_O - C$ $\qquad C_S$ = Counts in ROI of organ after subtraction.
$\qquad\qquad\qquad C_O$ = Counts in ROI of organ before subtraction.

where

$$C = \frac{A_O}{A_B} \times C_B$$

C_B = Counts in background ROI.

A_O = Number of pixels of organ ROI.

A_B = Number of pixels of background ROI.

The background area must be selected with care so that the time-activity curve of the activity in the background ROI closely matches that of the over and underlying tissue. ROIs may either be rectangular or any desired shape, depending on the computer facilities available.

ECAT (emission computerised axial tomography) is an effective approach to the problem of background activity; however, as was discussed in Chapter 26, sensitivity considerations limit the use of these techniques for dynamic studies.

28.2. Dynamic imaging studies of the kidneys

If a radiopharmaceutical such as ^{123}I o-iodohippurate (hippuran) (Section 34.5) were injected directly as a small bolus into the renal artery of a patient, most of it would be taken up by the kidneys, pass through the tubular system into the pelvis and from thence, via the ureter, to the bladder. The transit time is the time taken for the radiopharmaceutical to pass through the kidney and for a normal person is in the range of 2–3 minutes. An idealised time–activity curve of the activity in the kidney is shown in Figure 28.1 — this curve could

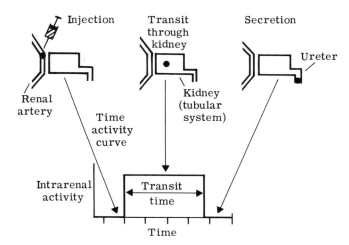

Fig. 28.1 Schematic illustration of injection of activity into renal artery and subsequent passage through the kidney.

be obtained if a sequence of digital images were taken (say every 20 seconds) and the total counts within the area of the kidneys were summed for each frame. The rectangular shape is idealised for three reasons; it assumes that the injected bolus is what is termed an 'impulse input' and takes zero time to inject; also that all the radiopharmaceutical is taken up by the kidney — in practice, with hippuran, only about 66 per cent is; and finally, that there is a single transit time—in reality there is a spread.

In clinical practice this procedure is not practical and the normal method of studying kidney function is to administer the radiopharmaceutical intravenously. A more complex time-activity curve is then obtained because:

1. By the time the activity arrives it will have smeared out and will no longer be a sharply defined bolus.

2. Only a fraction of the activity will enter the renal arteries; some of the remainder will contribute counts to the image as it will be in tissue above and below the kidneys (background activity).

3. Recirculation will take place before the initial activity has passed through the kidney. There will therefore be a continuous input of activity, not a single pulse.

The first of these complications can only be reduced by good injection technique, the second by using the procedure of background subtraction and the third by a mathematical technique called deconvolution. Before considering deconvolution we shall further consider the renogram, how it is obtained in practice and how background subtraction is carried out.

The renogram

Images are typically collected for 20 seconds over a period of 10 or 20 minutes. With the latter time, often required when there is abnormal function, a total of 60 frames are accumulated. With some computer programs it is possible to alter the frame rate during the study and set it, for example, to be 6 per minute (i.e. every 10 seconds) for the first 5 minutes and then 1 per minute for 15 minutes. This both allows the initial part of the study, when the radionuclide is arriving at the kidney and activity in it is changing rapidly, to be followed in detail, yet saves computer storage (in these examples 45 frames compared with 60).

The region of interest is normally chosen to include all of the kidney — though the pelvis is sometimes excluded — and the computer will automatically plot out the total counts in each kidney ROI for each frame. A background area is also usually selected, for subtraction purposes, and it is normal to monitor the activity in the bladder and so another ROI is set over that organ. A typical set of curves is shown in Figure 28.2.

The renogram shows three phases (Fig. 28.3), nowadays called the first, second and third. The first phase is due to the arrival of activity underneath the camera, it will be steeper the more 'impulse-like' the injection and the height will be determined by the vascular supply. The more gradual slope of the second phase reflects uptake of the radiopharmaceutical in the kidney and the transition to the third phase indicates the onset of excretion of the radiopharmaceutical. It must be appreciated that during the third phase all the following are happening — activity arriving, activity passing through the kidney

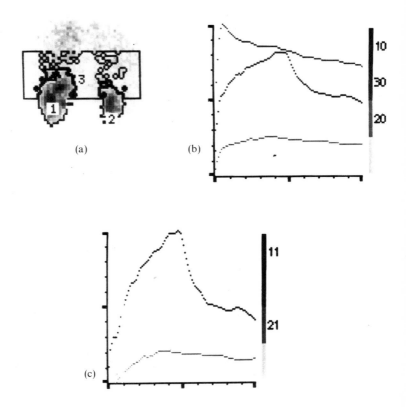

(a)

(b)

(c)

Fig. 28.2 Renogram using ^{99}Tc^m-DTPA. Normal left kidney (LK) but small right kidney (RK) showing poor function due to polyneuritis. (a) Regions of interest: 1. LK; 2. RK; 3. Background. (b) Unsubtracted curves: top, background; middle, LK; bottom, RK. (c) Subtracted curves: top,.LK; bottom, RK. (Courtesy of Dr G. M. Murray, Maelor General Hospital, Clwyd).

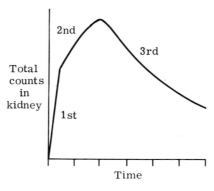

Fig. 28.3 Phases of the classical renogram.

and activity leaving the kidney. The slope and shape of the second and third phases and the transition between the two depend on the relative magnitude of these three processes. This is why the use of the terms vascular, secretory and excretory for the three phases has gone out of favour — they convey too simplistic a view.

The shape of the renogram will not only depend on the renal function of the patient but also on the radiopharmaceutical used. There are two groups, those whose uptake by the kidney is primarily by tubular secretion (e.g. ^{123}I-hippuran) and those where the only mechanism is glomerular filtration (e.g. ^{99}Tc^m-DTPA). The advantage of the former is that the clearance rate is much higher than the latter, thus the blood level will fall more rapidly, leading to a more steeply descending third phase. Also there will be a more pronounced second phase as a higher percentage of the   activity is in the kidney. However, the radionuclide characteristics of ^{99}Tc^m allow high activities of ^{99}Tc^m-DTPA to be administered, leading to less statistical fluctuations.

Background subtraction
The curves generated from the ROIs set so as to encompass the kidneys will also include counts from extra-renal tissue. By subtracting counts from a similar region the interface can be minimised. The background area is usually taken either above or between the kidneys. Figure 28.2 shows the effect of subtraction. It should be noted that the use of the term blood background subtraction is slightly misleading as the activity is both extravascular as well as intravascular. A further point is that the background we wish to subtract also includes the intravascular activity within the kidney.

Quantification of the renogram

Valuable information can be obtained by visual inspection of the subtracted renogram. However, it is often helpful to quantitate the following parameters:

Time to peak. This is the time from arrival of activity at the kidney to the peak of the renogram curve. It is related to the mean transit time.

Ratio of heights of peaks. This is a comparison of the relative function of the two kidneys. Some centres prefer, in order to minimise the effect of statistical functions, other parameters, such as the area underneath the curves between two time limits.

$$\text{Individual percentage function} = \frac{\text{Individual kidney counts}}{\text{Left + right kidney counts}} \times 100$$

Comparing the two kidneys assumes that both are at equal depth and that the skin to collimator distance is the same over both organs.

Effective renal plasma flow (ERPF) and glomerular filtration rate (GFR). The basic principles of determining these parameters have been discussed in Section 12.5, with the determination of GFR being used as an example. No substance is completely removed from the blood with 100 per cent efficiency and the flow rate determined from substances such as hippuran is known as the ERPF. The use of external counting avoids multiple blood samples but at least one sample is required to obtain a measurement of the activity per unit volume of blood; the slope can then be determined from the renogram.

Deconvolution

The purpose of deconvolution is to transform the renogram into an 'impulse retention function' or 'impulse response function', which is the time–activity curve which would be obtained if a bolus injection were given directly into the renal artery, as discussed at the beginning of this section. Let this time–activity curve be denoted by $H(t)$.

In a conventional renal study the activity entering the kidney will be proportional to the ERPF and the concentration (C) of the radiopharmaceutical in the blood. Thus the input rate will be given by:

$$\text{ERPF} \times C(t)$$

The t in brackets after the C indicates that it alters as a function of time. Let the time-activity curve (i.e. the renogram) resulting from this input be denoted by $R(t)$. The input to the kidney during a renogram can be considered a series of impulse inputs, and thus the renogram itself can be considered as the total effect of a whole series of impulse inputs. The magnitude of these impulses will vary with time and reflect the actual input rate. The mathematical procedure for combining a series of impulse inputs $[I(t)]$ with the resulting impulse retention function $[H(t)]$ to obtain a conventional renogram $[R(t)]$ is called convolution (Fig. 28.4). We say that the impulse inputs $I(t)$ are convolved with the impulse retention function $H(t)$ to obtain the conventional renogram $R(t)$.

$$R(t) = I(t) * H(t) \qquad * \text{ means convolved with.}$$

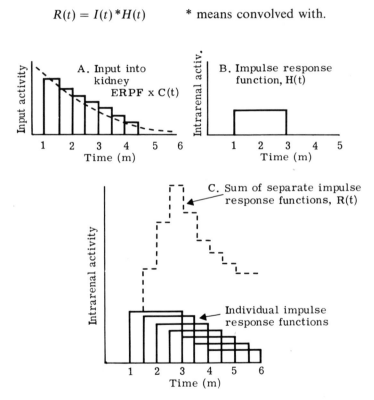

Fig. 28.4 Convolution. Derivation of the renogram (C) from the input rate of the radiopharmaceutical to the kidney (A) and the impulse retention function (B). In this schematic illustration the impulse input are represented by square wave inputs. A true impulse is a square wave of zero width!

The reverse of this process, obtaining $H(t)$ from $I(t)$ and $R(t)$, is known as deconvolution. There are a number of mathematical methods used to carry out deconvolution. A major limitation to these techniques is the statistical fluctuations involved and various smoothing procedures (in space and time) are invoked to minimise the effect of these fluctuations.

In order to obtain $I(t)$ a separate monitor over the head or heart is sometimes used, whilst other procedures use an ROI within the field of view of the camera.

Some deconvolution procedures are carried out on the unsubtracted renogram; this results in an impulse retention function which incorporates the vascular phase of the study.

The initial height of the impulse retention function is proportional to the ERPF; if the impulse retention function is differentiated (i.e. the slope at each point is plotted out) then the width of the resulting curve is a measure of the distribution of transit times (Fig. 28.5).

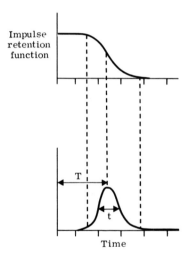

Fig. 28.5 Derivation of distribution of transit times from impulse retention function. T is the mean transit time and t is a measure of the spread of the transit times about the mean.

Functional imaging

The renal studies discussed so far give information about the function of the kidney as a whole. At some centres the pelvis of the kidney is usually excluded and this can help in distinguishing abnormal nephron function from obstruction.

More limited ROIs, with only a part of the kidney being used — such as the superior pole—can be selected. However, processing a number of ROIs can obviously become tedious. Furthermore, visual inspection of individual image frames may not be sufficiently discriminating to show regions where function is different from that of the kidney as a whole.

In functional imaging each pixel is effectively an ROI and time-activity curves are generated for each pixel. One particular parameter (hence parametric imaging as an alternative term for functional imaging) is selected, such as time to peak, and an image formed in which the 'counts' in each display pixel are proportional to the magnitude of the parameter. Thus, in this example, the following might be the grey or colour scale.

Parameter Time to Peak (minutes)	Scale	
	Grey	Colour
<2	1	Red
2–4	2	Orange
4–6	3	Green
6–8	4	Blue
>8	5	Mauve

The amount of computation involved is considerable but the major limitation of this procedure is the statistical fluctuation resulting from the limited number of photons associated with each pixel. To limit the effects of these fluctuations a 32×32 or 64×64 matrix is usually selected and a considerable amount, both spatial and temporal, of smoothing is applied.

38.3. Dynamic cardiac imaging

There have been considerable developments in nuclear cardiology in the last decade and it is now a major branch of nuclear medicine. Earlier development of this subject was limited by the technology available but developments in gamma cameras and associated computers have enabled a number of procedures to be introduced which give information which is either not otherwise available or can only be obtained by invasive techniques.

One heart beat takes about a second—we are therefore dealing with an organ whose functional cycle is between a hundred and a thousand times faster than that of the kidney. The frame length of the images needs to be less than 0·05 seconds to capture the different phases of the cardiac cycle. The fundamental requirement is to collect sufficient counts per frame to obtain adequate images. There are two approaches; the direct one which images a bolus of radioactivity as it passes through the heart (first pass studies) and equilibrium gated studies where information from many cycles are accumulated in such a way that a set of images of an average cardiac cycle is obtained.

First pass studies

Up to a gigabecquerel of a suitable high specific activity radiopharmaceutical (usually $^{99}Tc^m$ as sodium pertechnetate, labelled red cells or human serum albumin) is injected intravenously as a discrete bolus. Data is then collected for the next 20 to 45 seconds. This can be done frame by frame (serial mode) with each frame collecting counts for, typically, 0·05 seconds, or, more commonly, by storing information (time of detection and x-y coordinates) about each scintillation detected. This latter method is known as list mode and has the advantage that it allows complete freedom during subsequent processing to create images with any desired pixel size and of any accumulation period. However, it uses an enormous amount of magnetic disc space in the computer and therefore limits the total length of any study. Not all gamma camera and computer systems are suitable for first pass studies. In the case of cameras, some are not able to cope with the high count rates — typically 50 to 200 000 counts per second — without significant distortion of the image and loss of counts. Multicrystal cameras are especially suited to this type of study (Section 24.5). Computers may be limited by either hardware or software factors.

The advantage of first pass studies is that they allow clear temporal delineation of the cardiac chambers as the radionuclide progresses from the superior vena cava, through the right heart, lungs and left heart. The physician is able to derive considerable information from visual inspection of the images but nuclear cardiography has the advantage, compared with conventional X-ray angiocardiography, that quantitative information can be extracted by processing and analysis of the digital images. However, digital radiology now makes it possible to extract quantitative information from X-ray images.

The detection of shunts can be helped by selection of suitable ROIs and production of time-activity curves. The basic principles of determining cardiac output have been described in Chapter 13.

Left ventricular ejection fraction (LVEF). A widely used index of ventricular performance is the left ventricular ejection fraction, which is computed from the total counts within the left ventricle (defined by an appropriate ROI) at two phases of the heart cycle — end-diastolic and end-systolic (see Fig. 28.6).

$$LVEF = \frac{\text{end-diastolic counts} - \text{end-systolic counts}}{\text{end-diastolic counts} - \text{background counts}}$$

The stroke volume is proportional to the difference between end-diastolic and end-systolic counts.

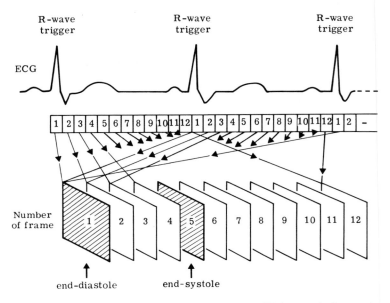

Fig. 28.6 Schematic illustration of a 12-frame gated equilibrium study. In practice at least 20 frames are used and counts from about 100 cycles are collected.

Equilibrium gated studies

Gated studies require a radiopharmaceutical that will remain within the vascular space throughout the study. If human serum albumin or red cells (labelled either *in-vitro* or, more commonly, *in vivo*) are used for a first pass study then gated studies can be carried out at the same session — after the tracer has reached equilibrium in the patient's blood pool (the very opposite of the conditions necessary for first pass studies).

The patient is monitored by ECG and the signal fed to the computer, where the R-wave is detected and used to synchronize the collection of the incoming counts (R-wave trigger). The cardiac cycle is divided into twenty or more phases and an image built up for each phase. Counts from the same phase of successive cardiac cycles are accumulated in the same frame (Fig. 28.6). Thus the total counts per frame steadily increase with time. About a hundred cycles are normally required to produce a sufficient count density in each frame to obtain good images and to minimise statistical fluctuations from pixel to pixel. Some computer programs will detect atopics and reject the information collected during these extra cycles.

The advantage of this type of study is that the high activities required by first pass studies are not necessary and images with good resolution and information density are obtained. Furthermore several views can be obtained and the patient can be studied not only at rest but also after physiological or pharmacological intervention. However, a major disadvantage is the high background activity and the difficulty in separating and outlining the chambers of the heart. The LVEF can be calculated in a similar manner to that discussed under first pass studies and the two procedures have similar accuracy.

Phase analysis. One of the main uses of gated cardiac procedures is to study wall motion. Major defects can be detected by visual inspection of the images but a more sophisticated technique is to use phase analysis. Phase describes the relation between two regular and cyclical motions having the same frequency. If they move exactly together they are in phase, whilst they are described as out of phase if they are moving in opposite directions at a particular point in time (Fig. 28.7). Therefore, when the walls of a cardiac chamber move in and out together they are described as in-phase.

Visual inspection allows assessment of wall motion only along the edges visible in a particular view. Phase analysis circumvents this difficulty by measuring the change in the counts of small areas of the ventricle—that is, time-activity curves for each pixel within the ventricle are generated. The phase difference between the time-activity curves of the pixels are then displayed as an image. This is another example of functional imaging, with phase being displayed rather than time to peak as in the previous discussion of renal studies.

Boundary detection

The normal method of selecting ROIs is to use a light pen or joystick, or some other means of controlling a marker on the screen, and to delineate the organ or area of interest by eye. In cardiac studies the accurate outlining of the various chambers is particularly important and can significantly effect the determination of parameters such as LVEF.

Various automated techniques have been evolved, not only to improve accuracy, but also to make processing of studies faster. There are normally two steps, the first involves background subtraction (if appropriate), smoothing and sometimes sophisticated filtering techniques. This is followed by edge detection, either by determining the contour of a particular count gradient or by threshold detection. In the latter method the contour at which counts are above a certain

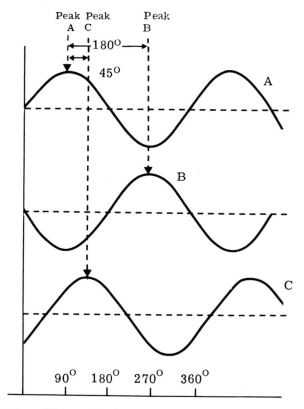

Fig. 28.7 Phase difference. A and B waves are 180° out of phase whilst A and C have a phase difference of 45°.

value — often defined in terms of percentage of the maximum counts per pixel within the ROI — is outlined.

28.4.   Fourier analysis

Nuclear medicine data are usually presented as images (two dimensional [x-y] spatial representations of activity distributions) or as time-activity curves (temporal representations). The term 'object domain' is sometimes used to describe these types of representation of the data. However, using a mathematical procedure called Fourier analysis the data can be 'transformed' and described ('frequency domain representation') in terms of a Fourier series.

The terms 'Fourier analysis', 'Fourier transform' and 'Fourier series', are frequently encountered in descriptions of methods used to process and analyse digital images. The term Fourier analysis has already been briefly encountered when discussing the concept of modulation transfer function in Section 23.4.

Any periodic function (spatial or temporal) can be represented exactly as the sum of a series of cosine waves of different frequencies, amplitudes and phases. This is illustrated in Figure 28.8 where a square wave is represented by a series of cosine waves. The

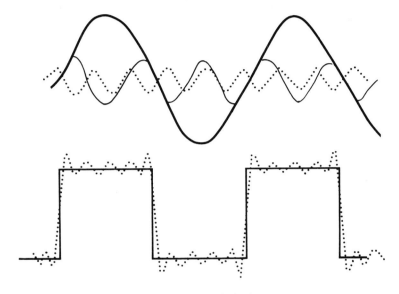

Fig. 28.8 Fourier analysis of a square wave. Only three separate waves are shown in the upper part. In order to obtain the approximation to the square wave shown in the lower part a further two waves have been added. Closer representation could be obtained by adding further cosine waves of higher frequency.

representation is only approximate, if more waves were used then the square wave would be represented with increasing faithfulness. The mathematical expression of a Fourier series is given in Appendix 2 (A2.5).

Fourier analysis can be applied in many situations. Static images can be processed and enhanced to bring out special features of the image or to minimise the effect of statistical fluctuations (the term digital filtering is often applied to this group of techniques). Some methods of deconvolution involve Fourier analysis. In many gated cardiac studies the various analyses also rely extensively on this approach.

28.5.   Modelling

Models are a help in interpreting physical measurements in terms of physiology and pathophysiology. Some models are purely a mathematical concept and bear little relationship to any physical system; more useful are ones which relate directly to the organ or system under study.

The most common type used in nuclear medicine is the compartmental model. The basic elements have been described in Chapter 13. A simple three compartmental model of the renal system is shown in Figure 28.9 . The first compartment is referred to as the

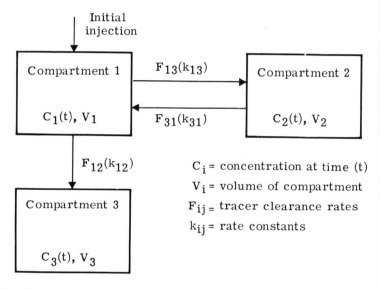

C_i = concentration at time (t)

V_i = volume of compartment

F_{ij} = tracer clearance rates

k_{ij} = rate constants

Fig. 28.9 A three compartmental model for renal tracer studies. See Chapter 13 for a discussion of some of the basic principles involved.

blood or intravascular compartment and a tracer which is injected into this compartment can leave (via the kidneys) and enter the end compartment. There is, of course, no movement of tracer from compartment 3 to compartment 2. There is also exchange between the first compartment and the third compartment. This latter mainly represents extravascular space but also includes tracer in red cells or tracer bound to protein molecules. The quantity of tracer in compartment 2 will rise to a maximum and then fall and eventually all tracer will end up in the end compartment (Fig. 28.10). It must be emphasised that compartments do not necessarily correspond to actual physical spaces. For example, when hippuran is used as tracer,

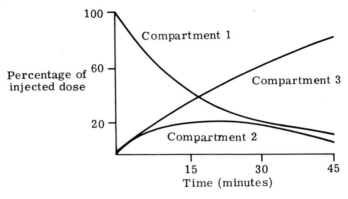

Fig. 28.10 Schematic variation with time of percentage of injected dose of tracer cleared from the blood by the kidneys. Based on model shown in Fig. 28.10.

it is found that the volume of the first compartment is measured to be more than twice the actual blood plasma volume.

Compartmental models assume that there is always instant and uniform mixing of the tracer in all compartments. It is therefore unable to handle the initial effects of bolus injections. Nor do they easily handle transit times. Other models are more appropriate to these situations.

28.6. Conclusion

The bases for a number of techniques used in dynamic imaging have been described by reference to specific examples. However, many of the techniques are used in a wide range of clinical studies. Deconvolution and Fourier analysis techniques will be found, not only in cardiac and kidney studies, but also in the processing of dynamic liver, cerebral and lung investigations.

The processing of digital images and the extraction of quantitative information is only possible using a computer. Details of analytical techniques used and of the computer programs involved have not been described as they are not essential for making clinical use of the various procedures. Nevertheless, an understanding of the principles is important in order to derive the maximum clinical benefit and, conversely, to appreciate the limitations of any particular mode of analysis.

PART FOUR

Basic chemistry

29

What is chemistry?

29.1. Introduction

Much of the discussion in the earlier chapters has been concerned with the properties and interactions of atomic nuclei and sub-atomic particles. However, in nuclear medicine it is not sufficient to understand the elements of radiation physics and to be able to measure the quantity and spatial distribution of radioactive events occurring in the human body. We must also be able to select the appropriate chemical form in which to administer a radionuclide so that it will show a useful degree of localisation in the organ, or region of the body, we wish to examine. Thus it is important that those who are engaged in the practice of nuclear medicine should have sufficient basic knowledge of chemistry to enable them to understand the properties, and methods of preparation of, the radioactive materials currently used in clinical investigation.

It is not easy to define chemistry in a few simple words which adequately describe the full scope of this very large subject. However, a useful working definition is that chemistry is the study of the reactions between *atoms* of two or more *elements* to form *molecules* of a new substance, or *compound*, and the interactions of the molecules of different compounds with each other.

29.2. Law of constant composition

When elements react together to form a new chemical compound the new compound, in a pure state, will always contain the same elements combined together in the same proportions by weight. This statement is known as the *law of constant composition*. Since chemical compounds are formed only by the combination of whole atoms the weights, or masses, of the elements which react together to form a compound will always be directly related to the relative atomic masses of the constituent elements.

29.3. Atomic and molecular mass

The *relative atomic mass* of an element, formerly called the atomic weight, is defined as the number of times by which the mass of one atom of the element exceeds the mass of one twelfth of one atom of the carbon-12 isotope. The *relative molecular mass*, previously called the molecular weight, is defined similarly as the number of times by which the mass of one molecule of a chemical compound exceeds one twelfth the mass of one atom of carbon-12. The relative atomic masses of some important elements are shown in Table 29.1.

Table 29.1 Chemical symbols and relative atomic masses of some elements

Element	Symbol	Relative atomic mass
Hydrogen	H	1·008
Carbon	C	12·000
Nitrogen	N	14·008
Oxygen	O	15·999
Neon	Ne	20·179
Sodium	Na	22·990
Phosphorus	P	30·974
Chlorine	Cl	35·453
Technetium	Tc	99·00
Iodine	I	126·904
Mercury	Hg	200·59
Radium	Ra	226·0

As we saw in Section 29.2, the amounts of the elements which react together to form a chemical compound are always related to the relative atomic masses of the elements. Thus for quantitative work in chemistry it is useful to have a unit for the amount of any substance which is based on the number of atoms or molecules which it contains. This unit is called the *mole* and is defined as the amount of a substance which contains the same number of elementary units as are contained in 12 grammes of carbon-12. The elementary units mentioned in this definition may be atoms of an element, molecules of a compound or, as we shall see in Chapter 30, ions. Thus

1 mole of sodium will have a mass of 22·99 grams
1 mole of chlorine will have a mass of 35·45 grams

and these two will react together to form

1 mole of sodium chloride weighing 58·44 grams.

One mole of any substance always contains the same number of atoms or molecules and this number has been found to be very large, $6·02 \times 10^{23}$. This number is known as *Avogadro's number* or the *Avogadro constant*. The mole is a very large amount of substance and frequently it is necessary to work in decimal fractions of a mole and these are designated by the names and symbols shown in Table A3.2 (Appendix 3).

29.4. Chemical formulae

In order to have a simple and convenient way of describing the atomic composition of chemical compounds chemists have, by international agreement, designated each element by its own unique symbol. These symbols consist of either a single initial letter, for example C for carbon, or two letters, for example Zn for zinc. The symbol represents a single atom of the element. The symbols for some common elements are listed in Table 29.1. Compounds or molecules are designated by the symbols for each of the elements they contain with subscript numbers to indicate the numbers of each atom which are present in the compound. Thus sodium chloride which contains one atom each of sodium and chlorine is written NaCl, water with two hydrogen atoms and one atom of oxygen as H_2O and sucrose, or cane sugar, as $C_{12}H_{22}O_{11}$.

Chemical compounds containing carbon were originally believed to be formed only by or from living organisms and consequently the study of carbon containing compounds is known as organic chemistry and that of all other compounds as inorganic chemistry. Today, these divisions are artificial although still convenient, since an enormous number of man made carbon compounds have been prepared. Many of these such as nylon, polyethylene and the synthetic detergents are now commonplace in our everyday lives.

29.5. The periodic table

It is mentioned in Chapters 3 and 30 that the chemical properties of an element are determined by its electronic structure. Thus it would seem logical to suggest that if there are regularities, or periodicity, in electronic structure there should also be regularities or periodicity in chemical properties. This is in fact correct and we may arrange the elements in a systematic way which demonstrates this. The elements can be arranged in order of ascending atomic number (Z) with elements having similar chemical properties and electronic structures being placed at regular intervals. This arrangement which is called the *periodic table* is illustrated in Figure 29.1. The horizontal rows of elements are called *periods* and the vertical columns of elements are called *groups*. Within a group, or family the elements have a similar electron configuration and therefore marked chemical similarities with a gradation of properties down the group. Within the horizontal periods the elements generally, but not always have dissimilar chemical properties and the number of electrons in the outer electron shells increases regularly across the period. The group of elements on the extreme right of the periodic table have their outermost electron shell completely filled and these elements undergo virtually no chemical reactions. The elements in this group are all gases and are known as the *inert* or *noble gases*.

THE PERIODIC TABLE

Period \\ Group	IA	IIA	IIIA	IVA	VA	VIA	VIIA	VIII			IB	IIB	IIIB	IVB	VB	VIB	VIIB	VIIIB
1	1 H																	2 He
2	3 Li	4 Be											5 B	6 C	7 N	8 O	9 F	10 Ne
3	11 Na	12 Mg											13 Al	14 Si	15 P	16 S	17 Cl	18 Ar
4	19 K	20 Ca	21 Sc	22 Ti	23 V	24 Cr	25 Mn	26 Fe	27 Co	28 Ni	29 Cu	30 Zn	31 Ga	32 Ge	33 As	34 Se	35 Br	36 Kr
5	37 Rb	38 Sr	39 Y	40 Zr	41 Nb	42 Mo	43 Tc	44 Ru	45 Rh	46 Pd	47 Ag	48 Cd	49 In	50 Sn	51 Sb	52 Te	53 I	54 Xe
6	55 Cs	56 Ba	57 La *	72 Hf	73 Ta	74 W	75 Re	76 Os	77 Ir	78 Pt	79 Au	80 Hg	81 Tl	82 Pb	83 Bi	84 Po	85 At	86 Rn
7	87 Fr	88 Ra	89 Ac †															

Main Groups — Transition Elements — Main Groups

* Lanthanide Series	58 Ce	59 Pr	60 Nd	61 Pm	62 Sm	63 Eu	64 Gd	65 Tb	66 Dy	67 Ho	68 Er	69 Tm	70 Yb	71 Lu
† Actinide Series	90 Th	91 Pa	92 U	93 Np	94 Pu	95 Am	96 Cm	97 Bk	98 Cf	99 Es	100 Fm	101 Md	102 No	103 Lr

Fig. 29.1 The Periodic Table.

30

Chemical bonds

30.1. The nature of the chemical bond

The chemical properties of any element are determined by the number and arrangement of the electrons in the outer electron shells or orbitals. In çhemical compounds the atoms are held together by forces called *bonds* which are formed by the transfer, or sharing, of electrons between the atoms. The strength of these bonds varies considerably, some requiring the input of much energy to break them while others are comparatively weak. In the formation of bonds the reacting atoms seek to re-arrange their outer, or *valency*, electrons into the most stable configuration. The most stable electronic configuration is that in which the outer electron shell is completely full and this situation is found in the inert gases, He, Ne, Ar, Kr, Xe and Rn.

Four different types of chemical bond may be formed by electron sharing or electron transfer.

30.2. Ionic bonds

An *ionic*, or electrovalent, bond is formed by the complete transfer of an electron from one atom to another so that one atom achieves the electronic structure of the preceding inert gas and the other the structure of the succeeding inert gas. Let us consider the sodium atom and the chlorine atom reacting together to form sodium chloride. The sodium atom contains one electron in its outer shell and the chlorine atom contains seven electrons in the outer shell. When these two atoms react together one electron is transferred from the sodium atom to the chlorine atom so that both atoms now have completely filled outer electron shells. This can be represented as follows:

$$Na - e^- \rightarrow Na^+$$

(2:8:1)   (2:8)—Neon electron structure

$$Cl + e^- \rightarrow Cl^-$$

(2:8:7)   (2:8:8)—Argon electron structure

The loss of an electron from the sodium atom, leaves a new species of sodium atom with a positive electrical charge, which we write Na^+, and similarly the transfer of an electron to the chlorine atom produces a new negatively charged species which we designate Cl^-. These charged species are called *ions*; positively charged ions are called *cations* and negatively charged ions are called *anions*.

Between any pair of electrical charges of opposite sign there is an *electrostatic force* of attraction and in the molecule of sodium chloride the Na^+ and the Cl^- ions will be held together by electrostatic attraction. Thus the ionic bond may be defined as the electrostatic attraction which occurs between oppositely charged ions which have been produced by the complete transfer of electrons from the outer electron shell of one atom to that of the other.

30.3. Covalent bonds

The removal of one valency electron from an atom requires energy and the removal of further valency electrons from the resulting ion requires very much larger amounts of energy. The carbon atom contains four electrons in its outer electron shell and the energy which would be required to transfer all four of these atoms to other atoms to enable carbon to form ionic bonds is so very large that this process is unlikely to occur. Instead, in forming bonds with other atoms carbon achieves the electronic structure of the inert gas neon by sharing pairs of electrons with other atoms. This sharing of electron pairs requires much less energy than electron transfer and each *shared pair* of electrons forms a *covalent bond* between two atoms. This can be illustrated by reference to two carbon compounds, methane (CH_4) and tetrachloromethane (Carbon tetrachloride) (CCl_4):

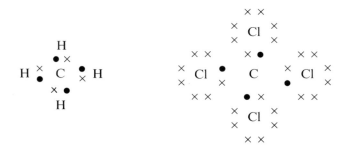

In this diagram the dots represent the four electrons in the outer shell of carbon and the crosses the electrons of hydrogen or chlorine; as can be seen, by sharing electrons each atom achieves the electronic structure of its nearest inert gas, helium for hydrogen, neon for carbon and argon for chlorine.

The covalent bond is of great importance in organic chemistry. In some compounds, in order to achieve an inert gas electronic structure atoms may share more than one pair of electrons to form a bond. This occurs in the gas carbon dioxide (CO_2) where two pairs of electrons are shared with each oxygen atom.

$$\overset{\times\ \times}{\underset{\times\ \times}{\times\ O\ {\overset{\bullet}{\underset{\bullet}{\times}}}\ C\ {\overset{\times}{\underset{\bullet}{\times}}}\ O\ \times}}$$

this type of covalent bond is called a *double bond*.

30.4. Co-ordinate bonds

Some molecules may have pairs of electrons which are not involved in bonding, these pairs of electrons are known as *lone pairs*. Molecules containing such lone pairs may form a bond with another atom by donating both these electrons to form a shared-pair bond, this type of bond is called a *co-ordinate bond*. Ammonia (NH_3) contains one lone pair of electrons and the water molecule has two lone pairs.

Ammonia will react with hydrogen (H^+) ions by donating its lone pair to the H^+ to form the ammonium ion (NH_4^+).

The co-ordinate bond differs from the covalent bond only in that one atom supplies both electrons to form a shared-pair bond.

30.5. Hydrogen bonds

The water molecule contains two lone pairs of electrons which are not involved in the bonding of the two hydrogen atoms to the oxygen.

$$\overset{\bullet\ \ \bullet}{\underset{H\ \ \ \ H}{\times\ {\overset{\bullet\ \bullet}{O}}\ \times}}$$

These lone pairs cause unevenness of the electrical charge over the molecule with the result that the oxygen shows a slight negative charge and the hydrogens a slight positive charge, molecules which show that property are called *polar* molecules. In the ice crystal there is an attractive force between the positive charge on the hydrogen of one water molecule and the negative charge on the oxygen of another. Thus the two water molecules are held together by a weak, but important, bond which is called the *hydrogen bond*. Hydrogen bonding occurs with elements other than oxygen, including fluorine, chlorine and nitrogen.

30.6.   Acids, bases and salts

When a solid compound containing ionic bonds dissolves in water the electrostatic forces which hold the ions together are weakened; as a result the molecules are broken up, or *dissociated*, leaving the individual ions free in the solution. Thus when sodium chloride (NaCl) is dissolved in water the resultant solution will contain sodium ions (Na^+) and chloride ions (Cl^-). Similarly a solution of hydrochloric acid (HCl) will contain hydrogen ions (H^+) and chloride ions (Cl^-).

A substance which yields hydrogen ions (H^+) in solution is called an acid. Since the hydrogen ion is in fact a bare proton, acids may also be defined as any substance which can donate protons, acids may be said therefore to be *proton donors*.

A substance which can yield hydroxide (hydroxyl) (OH^-) ions in aqueous solution is called a base. Sodium hydroxide (NaOH) when dissolved in water yields hydroxide ions as follows:

$$NaOH \rightarrow Na^+ + OH^-$$

Since hydroxide ions react readily with hydrogen ions (protons) to yield water

$$H^+ + OH^- \rightarrow H_2O$$

bases may also be defined as substances which are *proton acceptors*.

When an acid and a base react together in solution the H^+ ions react with the OH^- ions to form water and the anion of the acid reacts with the cation of the base to form a new compound which we call by the general name of a salt; this reaction is known as *neutralisation* of the acid by the base. For example hydrochloric acid and sodium hydroxide react together to form sodium chloride by the following reactions

$$HCl \rightarrow H^+ + Cl^-$$

$$NaOH \rightarrow Na^+ + OH^-$$

$$Na^+ + Cl^- \rightarrow NaCl$$

$$H^+ + OH^- \rightarrow H_2O$$

the overall reaction may be written as:

$$HCl + NaOH \rightarrow NaCl + H_2O$$

The number of hydrogen ions in one molecule of an acid is called the basicity of the acid. Hydrochloric acid contains one hydrogen ion and is a *monobasic acid*, sulphuric acid (H_2SO_4) contains two hydrogen ions and is *dibasic* while phosphoric acid (H_3PO_4) is *tribasic*.

When all the hydrogen ions in an acid are replaced by other cations the resulting salt is called a *normal* salt, but if only part of the hydrogen ions in the acid molecule are replaced the product is called an *acid salt*. An acid salt may not necessarily behave as an acid in solution. Sulphuric acid can react with sodium hydroxide to form both normal and acid salts, thus:

$$H_2SO_4 + NaOH \rightarrow NaHSO_4 + H_2O$$
Sodium acid sulphate

$$H_2SO_4 + 2NaOH \rightarrow Na_2SO_4 + 2H_2O$$
Sodium sulphate

Phosphoric acid can undergo reaction with one, two or three molecules of potassium hydroxide (KOH) to form three salts

KH_2PO_4—Potassium dihydrogen phosphate

K_2HPO_4—Dipotassium hydrogen phosphate

K_3PO_4—Potassium phosphate—the normal salt.

30.7. Strength of acids

Not all ionic compounds dissociate completely into ions on dissolution in water and the degree of dissociation which occurs may vary widely. Substances which are wholly or very extensively ionised in solution are called *strong electrolytes* and those which ionise to only a small extent are termed *weak electrolytes*. An electrolyte is a substance whose solutions can conduct electricity; all acids bases and salts are electrolytes.

Acids ionise to different extents in water. For example, nitric acid (HNO_3) is a strong acid because it is completely dissociated into hydrogen and nitrate ions (NO_3^-) in aqueous solution, thus a solution containing 0·1 mole HNO_3 per litre of solution (a 0·1 molar, or 0·1 M, solution) will contain 0·1 moles H^+ per litre. In contrast acetic acid (ethanoic acid) ionises to a much lesser extent in solution and is a weak acid, a 0·1 M solution of ethanoic acid contains only about 10^{-3} moles H^+ per litre.

The ionisation of any acid can be regarded as a *reversible* reaction

$$HA \rightleftharpoons H^+ + A^-$$

If this reaction is allowed to proceed unhindered by other chemical reactions an equilibrium will be established when the rate at which HA is dissociating into H^+ and A^- ions is exactly equal to the rate at which the ions are recombining to form HA. The proportions of HA and of H^+ and A^- which are present at equilibrium will vary according to the strength of the acid HA, the proportions of unionised acid and the ions are related by the equation:

$$K_a = \frac{[H^+].[A^-]}{[HA]}$$

Table 30.1 Dissociation constants (relative strengths) of some acids in aqueous solution at 25°C

Acid	Reaction	$K_a(mol/dm^3)$
Hydrochloric	$HCl \rightarrow H^+ + Cl^-$	very large
Formic (methanoic)	$HCOOH \rightarrow HCOO^- + H^+$	$1\cdot8 \times 10^{-4}$
Acetic (ethanoic)	$CH_3COOH \rightarrow CH_3COO^- + H^+$	$1\cdot8 \times 10^{-5}$
Carbonic	$H_2CO_3 \rightarrow H^+ + HCO_3$	$4\cdot4 \times 10^{-7}$
Water	$H_2O \rightarrow H^+ + OH^-$	$1\cdot8 \times 10^{-16}$

The square brackets indicate that we are relating concentrations of acids and ions. K_a is a constant for any given acid and is called the *dissociation constant* of the acid. The value of the acid dissociation constant provides a quantitative measure of acid strength which permits comparison of the relative strengths of different acids, since it indicates the extent to which the acid can release hydrogen ions. Strong acids such as hydrochloric acid or nitric acid have very large values for K_a while for weak acids the values are very low. The values of K_a for some acids are given in Table 30.1. The purest water ionises to a very slight extent to produce hydrogen and hydroxyl ions

$$H_2 \rightleftharpoons H^+ + OH^-$$

Thus water can be regarded as an acid and the dissociation constant for water will be given by the expression:

$$K = \frac{[H^+].[OH^-]}{[H_2O]}$$

Measurements of the electrical conductivity of the purest water have shown that at 25°C the concentrations of hydrogen and hydroxyl ions are each 10^{-7} moles per dm^3. Pure water contains 55·5 moles H_2O per dm^3.

Thus

$$K = \frac{[10^{-7}].[10^{-7}]}{55·5}$$

$$= \frac{10^{-14}}{55·5}$$

$$= 1·8 \times 10^{-16}$$

Since the concentration of H^+ and OH^- in pure water is so low compared with the concentration of H_2O the latter can be regarded as constant. The dissociation constant for water can be simplified by incorporating the water concentration into the constants thus

$$[H_2O].K = [H^+].[OH^-] = K_w$$

At 25°C K_w has the value of 1×10^{-14}. K_w is called the *ionic product* for water and, as we shall see in the next Chapter, it can be used to calculate the relationship between the concentrations of hydrogen and hydroxyl ions in any aqueous system at equilibrium.

For weak acids, where the degree of ionisation is small and K_a has a very small value, the hydrogen ion concentration is approximately equal to the square root of the acid dissociation constant multiplied by the concentration of the acid, thus

$$[H^+] \simeq \sqrt{K_a C}$$

where C is the acid concentration in moles per dm^3.

31

pH and buffer solutions

31.1. Hydrogen ions

The concentration of hydrogen ions in a system determines its acid or basic character, and changes in hydrogen ion concentration may affect profoundly the reactions which occur in the system. In living systems the hydrogen ion concentration must be very carefully controlled since quite small increases or decreases may cause severe physiological or biochemical disturbance. Most living systems have a hydrogen ion concentration of about 10^{-7} moles per dm^3, similar to that of pure water.

31.2. The pH scale

The expression of hydrogen ion concentration in moles per dm^3 is inconvenient for general use, and a special scale which permits easy comparison of the acidity of solutions has been developed. This is the *pH scale*. The term pH is defined as the negative logarithm to the base of 10 of the hydrogen ion concentration in moles per litre:

$$pH = -\log_{10}[H^+] \text{ or } \log_{10}\frac{1}{[H^+]}$$

The minimum value on the pH scale is 0 and the maximum is 14, the negative logarithm of K_w the ionic product for water.

Strong acids have a low pH value, for example a 0.1 mole/dm^3 solution of hydrochloric acid has a pH of 1 ($\log_{10}(1/0.1)$).

As we saw in Chapter 30 pure water has a hydrogen ion concentration of 10^{-7} moles/dm^3 thus the pH of water is 7. Since pure water also contains 10^{-7} moles of hydroxyl ions per dm^3 it is neither an acid nor a base and pH 7 is defined as neutral pH.

The ionic product for pure water (K_w) allows the relationship between hydrogen and hydroxyl ions to be calculated simply for an aqueous equilibrium, since

$$pH - \log[OH^-] = 14$$

A solution of sodium hydroxide containing 0·1 moles dm^{-3} contains 0·1 moles of hydroxyl ions dm^{-3} per, thus

$$-\log[OH^-] = 1 \text{ and the pH} = (14 - 1) \text{ or } 13.$$

If we know the values for the acid dissociation constants in a system we can calculate the pH of that system by the use of the expression:

$$pH = pK_a + \log_{10}\frac{[Base]}{[Acid]}$$

pK_a is the negative logarithm to the base of 10 of the dissociation of the acid. At the point where the acid is half dissociated and the concentrations of acid and base are equal $pH = pK_a$.

This expression is known as the *Henderson-Hasselbach equation*. The ratio base to acid can be expressed in terms of the degree of ionisation of the acid (α), that is the proportion of the molecules which are dissociated into ions.

This equation may be used to calculate the pH of solutions of acids or salts. For example: What is the pH of a solution of acetic acid containing 0·01 moles dm^{-3}?

A weak acid, like acetic acid, ionises to only a slight extent in solution and the degree of dissociation is approximately equal to the square root of the acid dissociation constant (K_a) divided by the concentration of the acid (C) in moles dm^{-3}, thus:

$$\alpha = \sqrt{\frac{K_a}{C}}$$

For acetic acid $K_a = 1·85 \times 10^{-5}$ (Table 30.1).
Thus for a 0·01 M solution

$$\alpha = \sqrt{1·85 \times 10^{-5}/0·01}$$

$$= \sqrt{1·85 \times 10^{-3}}$$

$$= 4·301 \times 10^{-2}$$

pK_a for acetic acid is $-\log_{10} 1·85 \times 10^{-5} = 4·733$

$$pH = 4·733 + \log\frac{4·301 \times 10^{-2}}{(1 - (4·301 \times 10^{-2}))}$$

$$= 4·733 + \log\frac{0·04301}{0·95699}$$

$$= 4·733 + \log 0·0449$$

$$= 4·733 + (\bar{2}·6522)$$

$$= 4 \cdot 733 + (-2 + 0 \cdot 6522)$$

$$= 4 \cdot 733 - 1 \cdot 348$$

$$pH = 3 \cdot 385$$

For a weak acid the pH may also be calculated approximately from the expression, see Section 30.7,

or

$$[H^+] \simeq \sqrt{K_a C}$$

$$pH = -\log_{10}\sqrt{K_a . C}.$$

For 0·01 molar acetic acid

$$pH = -\log_{10}\sqrt{1 \cdot 85 \times 10^{-5} \times 0 \cdot 01}$$

$$= 3 \cdot 373$$

31.3.   Measurement of pH

The most accurate way to measure pH is electrometrically using the pH meter. When a glass surface is placed in a solution it gains an electrical potential which is related to the hydrogen ion concentration of the solution. A typical pH meter electrode consists of a thin walled glass bulb containing a standard acid solution of fixed pH in which is inserted a reversible electrode, such as Ag/AgCl. This glass electrode is inserted into the solution whose pH is to be measured, a second reversible electrode, usually a calomel ($Hg/HgCl_2$) electrode, is placed in the solution and the potential difference between the electrodes is measured by means of a sensitive voltmeter. The voltmeter is calibrated in pH units so that a direct reading of pH is obtained.

A simpler, but less accurate method of pH measurement is by the use of *indicators*. In simple terms indicators are weak organic acids or bases in which the unionised molecules have a different colour from the ions into which they dissociate. As these substances ionise in solution the colour of the solution changes over a specific range of pH. Some common indicators are listed in Table 31.1, which also shows the pH range over which the colour changes occur. Indicators may be used as solutions or they may be impregnated on paper to form *indicator papers*. By the use of mixtures of indicators it is possible to produce a *universal indicator* which shows a gradation of colour changes over the whole, or part, of the pH range. Such universal indicators afford a rapid means of making an approximate measurement of the pH of a solution.

Indicators give a much less accurate measurement of pH than the pH meter, but they are simple, cheap and convenient to use. Care

Table 31.1 Some common indicators

Indicator	Acid colour	Alkaline colour	pH range
Methyl orange	Red	Yellow	3·1–4·4
Methyl red	Red	Yellow	4·2–6·3
Bromothymol blue	Yellow	Blue	6·0–7·6
Phenol red	Yellow	Red	6·8–8·4
Phenolphthalein	Colourless	Red	8·3–10.0

must be exercised in their use since the colour changes may be affected by a number of factors including: high temperature, the presence of alcohol or other organic solvents, proteins, soaps, detergents or oxidising and reducing agents in the solution to be measured.

31.4. Buffer solutions

The control of pH is essential for most physiological systems and it is important in the preparation of many medicinal products including radiopharmaceuticals. Some solutions possess the property of being able to maintain their pH at a constant value even when quite large amounts of acid or base are added to the solution. Solutions which have this ability to resist changes in pH are called *buffer solutions.*

If we add successive small amounts of a base, say sodium hydroxide, to a solution of acetic acid and measure the pH after each addition we find, Figure 31.1, that the pH does not increase linearly with each addition of base. Instead the pH changes follow an 'S' shaped curve and there is a region between, about pH 4 and 5, where the pH shows only a small change although a relatively large quantity of base has been added, this is called the *buffer region.* The reason for this is that the acetic acid is only about 1 per cent dissociated into ions

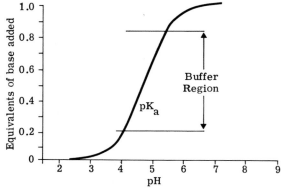

Fig. 31.1 The titration curve of acetic acid

and an equilibrium situation exists between hydrogen ions, acetate ions and unionised acetic acid.

$$CH_3COOH \rightleftharpoons CH_3COO^- + H^+$$

When hydroxyl ions (OH^-) from the base are added these react with the hydrogen ions to produce water. As a result the equilibrium is disturbed and more acetic acid ionises to produce more hydrogen ions to replace those used up by reaction with the hydroxyl ions. The pH does increase, because more acetate (CH_3COO^-) ions have been produced, but the increase is not as large as would have been expected if the acetic acid had not been able to produce more hydrogen ions to neutralise the added hydroxyl ions. If we had been able to keep the concentration of acetate ions constant in the solution the pH would not have been altered at all until a very large amount of base had been added. This can be achieved by ensuring that there is a large excess of acetate ions present in the solution, for example by the addition of the salt sodium acetate. Sodium acetate, unlike acetic acid, is fully dissociated in solution

$$CH_3COONa \rightleftharpoons CH_3COO^- + Na^+$$

If this salt is added to a solution of acetic acid the ionisation of the acetic acid is reduced and the pH of the solution will be greater. However, this mixture will not show any appreciable change in pH even if quite large amounts of acid or base are added.

All buffer solutions are mixtures of strong acids and weak bases, or weak acids and strong bases. In general a weak base mixed with a salt of a strong acid will form a buffer with a pH above 7, while weak acids mixed with salts of strong bases form useful buffer solutions with a pH below 7.

In the blood, pH 7·4, there are a number of buffer systems of which the system carbonic acid H_2CO_3, (a weak acid) — sodium bicarbonate, $NaHCO_3$, is the most important.

Some buffer systems commonly encountered in biology and medicine are listed in Table 31.2.

Solutions of proteins and amino acids also exhibit the properties of buffers.

Table 31.2 Some common buffer systems

Buffer	pH range
Sodium acetate-acetic acid	3·8–5·6
Sodium citrate-citric acid	2·2–5·2
Potassium dihydrogen phosphate- disodium hydrogen phosphate	5·0–8·0
Sodium borate-boric acid	7·0–8·2
Sodium hydroxide-glycine	8·6–12·8

32

Hydrolysis and complex formation

32.1. Hydrolysis

Water is the most abundant component of all radiopharmaceuticals, and of all biological systems, and chemical reactions with water may be of considerable importance in the preparation of radiopharmaceuticals and in determining their biological behaviour.

When a substance dissolved in water and ionises there is a tendency for the ions produced to associate with molecules of water. Thus the simplest ion of all — the hydrogen ion (H^+) — does not exist in solution as a single 'bare' proton but is bound to one molecule of water to form the *hydronium ion* — H_3O^+. Other ions may associate with more than one molecule of water, for example the trivalent ions Cr^{3+} and In^{3+} each bind 6 molecules of water. The water molecules are usually bound to the ion by co-ordinate bonds and the number of such bonds that may be formed with an ion is called the *co-ordination number*. The most common co-ordination numbers are 4 and 6 but some ions have coordination numbers of 2 or 8.

The association of ions with water is called *hydration* and in some circumstances the hydrated ion may undergo further reactions with water which result in water molecules being split into hydrogen ions and hydroxyl ions with the formation of new chemical species. This type of reaction is called *hydrolysis* and is well illustrated by the reactions which occur when some salts are dissolved in water.

If salts were formed from acids and bases of equal strengths their solutions would be neutral and have a pH of 7. For most salts, however, the acids and bases from which they are formed do not have equal strengths and in solution the ions may react with water to produce hydrogen or hydroxyl ions by hydrolysis. For example ammonium chloride is formed by the reaction of a strong acid, hydrochloric acid, with a weak base, ammonia.

$$NH_3 + HCl \rightleftharpoons NH_4Cl$$

In solution NH_4Cl ionises to form ammonium ions (NH_4^+) and chloride ions (Cl^-):

$$NH_4Cl \rightleftharpoons NH_4^+ + Cl^-$$

However, the NH_4^+ ion reacts with water to form ammonia and a hydrogen ion

$$NH_4^+ + H_2O \rightleftharpoons NH_3 + H_3^+O$$

Thus solutions of ammonium chloride contain H^+ ions and have an acid pH value.

Salts of strong bases and weak acids undergo hydrolysis of the anion to yield hydroxyl ions. Thus sodium acetate, a salt of the weak acid acetic acid, ionises in solution to give sodium ions and acetate ions

$$CH_3COONa \rightleftharpoons CH_3COO^- + Na^+$$

The acetate ion then reacts with water to yield acetic acid and hydroxyl ions thus giving the solution an alkaline pH

$$CH_3COO^- + H_2O \rightleftharpoons CH_3COOH + OH^-$$

Such hydrolytic reactions account for the ability of buffer solutions to absorb considerable quantities of H^+ or OH^- ions without causing an appreciable change in the pH of the solution.

32.2. Complex formation

In addition to water, ions may associate with molecules of other substances to form *complex ions*. These other substances, which may be called *complexing agents* or *ligands*, are bound to the ion by co-ordinate bonds and frequently show a much greater tendency than water to react with the ion. Hydrolysis and complex formation are closely related, and often competing, phenomena.

Many substances may function as complexing agents including inorganic ions such as Cl^- or NO_3^-, simple organic acids such as acetic or tartaric and larger molecules such as citric acid, ethylenediaminetetraacetic acid (EDTA) or diethylenetriamine-pentaacetic acid (DTPA) (Fig. 32.1).

When each molecule of complexing agent forms only one co-ordinate bond with the ion the resulting compound molecule is called a *complex*. However, single molecules of some complexing agents such as citric acid or EDTA may form more than one co-ordinate bond with the ion producing a complex with a ring structure which is called a *chelate*. The basic structures of a chelate and a simple complex are shown in Figure 32.2.

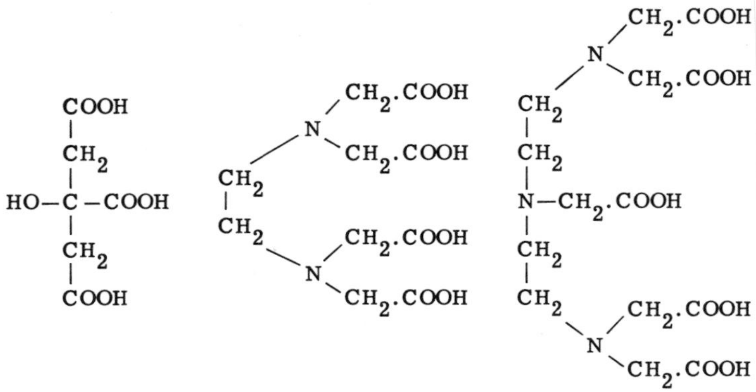

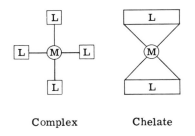

Citric Acid   Ethylenediaminetetra-   Diethylene-Triamine-
                      acetic Acid (EDTA)   Pentaacetic Acid
                                                          (DTPA)

Fig. 32.1

Complex   Chelate

Fig. 32.2

The chemical stability of a complex, that is the tendency for the ligand to be displaced from the ion, depends on the chemical properties of the complexing agent and the complexed ion. Complexes of the same ion with different ligands, or vice versa, may show a very wide range of stabilities. Chelates in general have very great stability and in some instances the normal chemical reactivity of a metal ion may be completely suppressed as a result of chelate formation.

It is frequently desirable to have a numerical value for the stability of a metal ion complex or chelate and this is given by the *stability constant,* which is in fact the equilibrium constant for the overall reaction between the metal and the ligand.

The combination of a single metal atom (M) with several molecules of a ligand (L) can be represented by the following equations:

$$M + L \rightleftharpoons ML$$

$$ML + L \rightleftharpoons ML_2$$

$$ML_2 + L \rightleftharpoons ML_3$$

and so on to

$$ML_{n-1} + L \rightleftharpoons ML_n$$

Since at each step the combination of metal and ligand follows the *law of mass action* the equilibrium constant for each step will be given by the expression

$$K_n = \frac{[ML_n]}{[ML_{n-1}] \cdot [L]}$$

where the symbols in square brackets represent the activities of each component present at equilibrium. The overall stability constant (β_n) for the reaction of the metal ion M with n molecules of ligand is given by the product of the individual constants for each step of the reaction:

$$\beta_n = K_1 \times K_2 \times K_3 \ldots K_n.$$

Stability constants can be determined by various methods including potentiometric titration, spectrophotometry and ion exchange, but their measurement is frequently difficult. For convenience stability constants are often expressed as the logarithm of β_n.

32.3. Interactions of metal ions with water

Another aspect of hydrolysis which is important in relation to the preparation and biological behaviour of some radiopharmaceuticals is the reaction of metal ions with water. As we have already learned (Section 32.1), in solution all ions become associated with one or more water molecules and in certain circumstances the hydrated ions may undergo hydrolysis.

The tendency of solvated ions to hydrolyse depends on the general chemical properties of the ion but hydrolysis occurs most readily with ions of high charge and small size. Thus Fe^{3+}, In^{3+}, Ga^{3+}, Tc^{4+} which are small ions with relatively high ionic charge show a marked tendency to undergo hydrolysis.

The hydrolytic reactions which occur can be illustrated by considering the trivalent indium ion (In^{3+}). In aqueous solution the

In^{3+} ion associates with six water molecules to form the complex ion $[In(H_2O)_6]^{3+}$; this ion is stable in acid solutions but as soon as the pH rises above pH 2·7 hydrolysis begins and the following reactions occur:

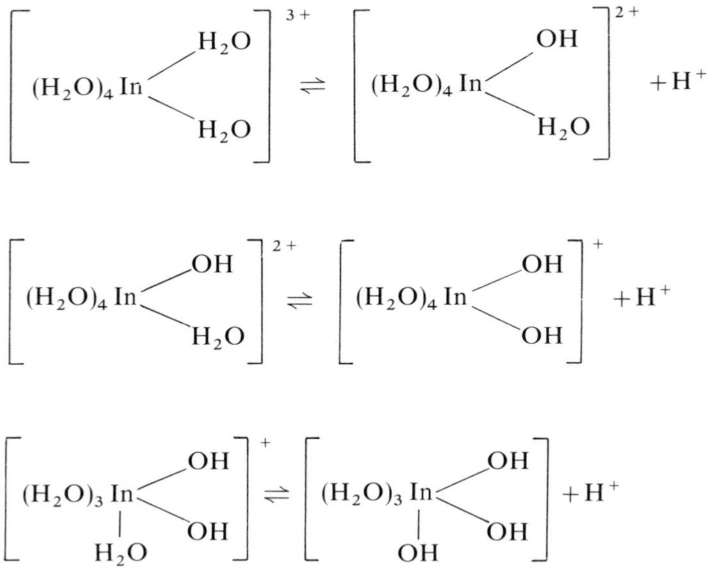

$$\left[(H_2O)_4\,In \diagup_{H_2O}^{H_2O}\right]^{3+} \rightleftharpoons \left[(H_2O)_4\,In\diagup_{H_2O}^{OH}\right]^{2+} + H^+$$

$$\left[(H_2O)_4\,In\diagup_{H_2O}^{OH}\right]^{2+} \rightleftharpoons \left[(H_2O)_4\,In\diagup_{OH}^{OH}\right]^{+} + H^+$$

$$\left[(H_2O)_3\,In\diagup_{\substack{|\\H_2O}}^{OH}\diagdown OH\right]^{+} \rightleftharpoons \left[(H_2O)_3\,In\diagup_{\substack{|\\OH}}^{OH}\diagdown OH\right] + H^+$$

Some of the complex ions produced by hydrolysis may react together in the following manner:

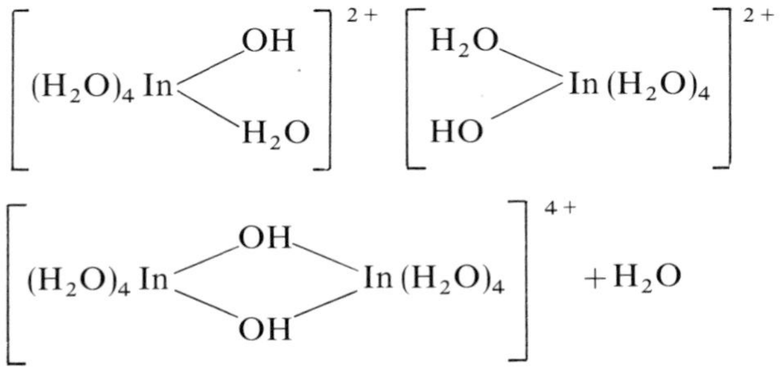

$$\left[(H_2O)_4\,In\diagup_{H_2O}^{OH}\right]^{2+}\left[\begin{array}{c}H_2O\\HO\end{array}\diagup In\,(H_2O)_4\right]^{2+}$$

$$\left[(H_2O)_4\,In\diagup_{OH}^{OH}\diagdown In\,(H_2O)_4\right]^{4+} + H_2O$$

Further hydrolysis and aggregation leads to the formation of aggregates or *polymers* of indium ions linked together by *hydroxyl* bridges (Fig. 32.3). Such aggregates may grow until they contain many thousands or even millions of indium atoms and if the concentration of indium in the solution is large enough precipitation

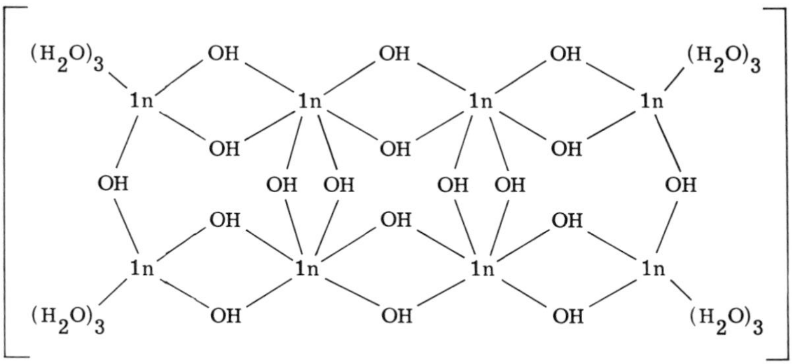

$$
\left[
\begin{array}{c}
(H_2O)_3 \diagdown \quad \diagup OH \qquad \diagup OH \qquad \diagup OH \qquad (H_2O)_3 \\
\quad In \qquad\qquad In \qquad\qquad In \qquad\qquad In \\
\diagup \quad OH \qquad\qquad OH \qquad\qquad OH \\
OH \qquad\qquad OH \quad OH \qquad OH \quad OH \qquad\qquad OH \\
\diagdown \quad \diagup OH \qquad \diagup OH \qquad \diagup OH \\
\quad In \qquad\qquad In \qquad\qquad In \qquad\qquad In \\
(H_2O)_3 \diagup \quad OH \qquad\qquad OH \qquad\qquad OH \qquad (H_2O)_3
\end{array}
\right]
$$

Fig. 32.3

will occur. However, in very dilute solutions, and in radiopharmaceuticals we are generally working with very dilute solutions of the radionuclide, aggregation of ions will still occur to yield particles which are too small to be seen but which will exhibit colloidal properties (see Ch. 33) or show anomalous chemical properties.

32.4. Factors affecting hydrolysis

The extent to which hydrolysis will occur is dependent on a number of factors of which the following are the most important:

1. The pH of the solution.
2. Temperature.
3. The concentration of the metal ion in the solution.
4. The presence of complexing agents in the solution.

Increases in pH, temperature and concentration all favour hydrolysis, thus hydrolysis is *least* likely to occur in strongly acid solutions containing low concentrations of metal ions and held at low temperatures.

Most complexing agents react more strongly than water with metal ions. Thus if a complexing agent is present in a solution containing a hydrolysable ion there will be competition between hydrolysis and complex formation and, if the concentration of the complexing agent is sufficiently high, hydrolysis may be completely prevented.

Hydrolysis and complex formation in relation to radiopharmaceuticals

Hydrolysis, complex, and chelate formation play important roles in determining the biological behaviour of metallic elements and they are important also in the preparation of some radiopharmaceuticals.

The problems which hydrolytic reactions may cause in radiopharmaceutical preparation may be illustrated by reference to the formation of the $^{113}In^m$-DTPA chelate which is sometimes used for brain or kidney scanning. The basic steps in the preparation of this radiopharmaceutical consist of mixing the eluate from the ^{113}Sn-$^{113}In^m$ generator, which contains the $^{113}In^m$ in 0·05 M hydrochloric acid, with a solution of DTPA and raising the pH to about 7. Indium begins to hydrolyse above pH 2·7 and the reaction of indium with DTPA does not occur readily below about pH 4, thus between these two pH values extensive hydrolysis of indium will occur and, as the hydrolysed aggregates of indium react only very slowly with DTPA, the final product is likely to consist of a mixture of hydrolysed aggregates of $^{113}In^m$ and $^{113}In^m$-DTPA. This is undesirable as the $^{113}In^m$ aggregates will not be excreted through the kidneys, like the $^{113}In^m$ DTPA, but will be taken up by reticuloendothelial cells in the liver and spleen. This problem can be avoided by adding a small quantity of sodium acetate to the $^{113}In^m$ solution before adding the DTPA. This prevents the hydrolysis of the In^{3+} ion, by formation of the acetate complex, but does not interfere with the reaction of the $^{113}In^m$ with the very strong chelating agent DTPA with the result that in the final solution the nuclide is present almost exclusively as the $^{113}In^m$-DTPA chelate.

32.6.   Radiocolloids

A phenomenon closely related to hydrolysis and which is of considerable importance in work with radionuclides is *radiocolloid* formation.

This phenomenon was first reported in 1913 by Paneth who found that when he dialysed very dilute solutions of ^{210}Po or ^{210}Bi the nuclides did not pass through a semi-permeable membrane, as ionic polonium or bismuth should have done, suggesting that the solutions were behaving like colloids. (see Ch.'33).

Subsequent work has shown that in very dilute solutions (less than 10^{-9} M) many radionuclides form radiocolloids. The tendency towards radiocolloid formation occurs most frequently with radionuclides of those elements which hydrolyse readily, for example Fe, Ga, In, Tc, Sn, Y, Bi.

Radiocolloids, like colloids in general, do not diffuse through membranes which are normally permeable to ions; they may show anomalous chemical behaviour, such as the slow reaction with DTPA discussed in Section 32.5.

In the human or animal body radiocolloids may show a very different distribution pattern to that of the ionic, or weakly complexed, radionuclide. Radiocolloids may also adsorb onto the surfaces of containers, stoppers and syringes resulting in a loss of radioactivity from the solution.

The formation of radiocolloids is influenced by the same factors which influence hydrolysis, namely, pH, temperature, and the concentration of complexing agents in the solution. In order to minimise the risks of radiocolloid formation, stock solutions of many metallic radionuclides are maintained in fairly strongly acid solutions.

In most work radiocolloid formation is a nuisance rather than an asset. However, occasionally, radiocolloid formation may be turned to advantage in the preparation of radiocolloids for clinical use. Two examples of this are the formation of a $^{99}Tc^m$-technetium dioxide colloid for liver scanning by simple reduction of $^{99}Tc^m$-pertechnetate with sodium borohydride; and the preparation of a colloid suitable for bone marrow scanning by adding an acid solution of $^{113}In^m$ to a phosphate buffer containing gelatin.

33

Colloids

33.1. Introduction

Colloidal preparations are used widely in nuclear medicine, especially for liver, spleen and bone marrow scanning.

A colloid may be defined, in simple terms, as a solution which contains *particles* of one substance *permanently dispersed* in a continuous phase of another substance. The particles are larger than the small molecules ordinarily encountered in chemistry but too small to be seen easily under a light microscope. The word colloid, which was originally invented by Thomas Graham in 1861, generally refers to dispersions in which the particles are between 1 and 500 nm in diameter. In the colloid preparations used in nuclear medicine the particles are invariably dispersed in an aqueous medium.

33.2. Properties of colloids

Colloids show no distinctive chemical properties *per se* and their chemical reactions will be related to the chemical nature of the substance of which the particles are composed. However, the chemical properties of a colloidal dispersion may show some differences from those of a simple solution of the same substance. This anomalous chemical behaviour of colloids, compared with non-colloidal solutions of the same substance, is most commonly manifested in differences in the rates at which particular chemical reactions occur.

Colloids do show certain common physical properties of which the three most important are: a slow rate of diffusion, the power to remain almost completely dispersed in the solvent and certain electrical properties.

The rate of diffusion of colloidal substances is very much slower than that of simple solutions of small molecules and colloidal particles will not pass through a cellophane or other membrane which is freely permeable to ions or small molecules. In the body colloidal particles do not diffuse through the membranes lining the pleural and peritoneal cavities and this property has been utilised in the treatment of pleural or peritoneal effusions with radioactive colloids, such as ^{198}Au-colloid.

In colloidal preparations the particles remain permanently suspended in the solvent and do not sediment even after standing for long periods of time. This power of remaining permanently dispersed is due largely to the electrical charges which occur at the boundary between the particle and the solvent. All colloids are two phase systems consisting of a solid and a liquid, or a liquid and a gas; preparations containing colloidal size droplets of liquid, or solid particles, dispersed in a gas are called *aerosols*. At any phase boundary there exists an *electrical double layer* consisting of positive and negative charges. The positive charges are attached to one of the phases and the negative charges to the other, consequently in a colloid the particles all carry an electrical charge of the same sign and tend to repel each other. In a stable colloid these repulsive charges are sufficiently strong to prevent the individual particles coming close enough together for the short range, attractive, *van der Waals forces* to cause adhesion and aggregation into larger particles which would fall out of solution.

Since all colloidal particles carry an electric charge they will migrate in an electric field; this migration is called *electrophoresis* and has important applications in the analysis of colloidal preparations and especially of protein solutions.

33.3.   Types of colloid
There are two types of colloidal solution the *lyophilic*, or 'solvent-loving' colloid and the *lyophobic* or 'solvent-hating' colloid.

Lyophilic colloids are solutions of naturally soluble substances whose molecules are large enough to be in the colloidal size range. These include proteins and starches which are soluble in water. Solutions of lyophobic colloids are often viscous and if the concentration of colloid particles is high enough the solution may set to form a plastic solid or gel. The ordinary table jelly, which is an aqueous solution of the protein gelatin, is a good example of a gel.

Lyophobic colloids are dispersions of naturally insoluble particles of colloidal dimensions and may be regarded as consisting essentially of very fine particles in suspension in the solvent.

33.4.   Stability of colloids
All lyophilic colloids form stable solutions in which the molecules remain permanently dispersed in the solvent. This stability is due largely to the size of the electric charges at the particle-solvent

boundary. If the electrical status of the colloidal solution is altered by the addition of small quantities of salts, especially those with a polyvalent ion having a charge of opposite sign to that of the colloid particles, the molecules may aggregate and precipitate out of solution, this process is called *salting out*. In some instances the precipitate may be redissolved by simply diluting the solution but in other circumstances the precipitate may be very difficult to re-dissolve.

Lyophobic colloids are less stable than lyophilic colloids since the electrical charges on the particles are frequently weaker and consequently the particles may show a much greater tendency to aggregate to form larger particles, greater than 400 to 500 nm, which settle out of solution. The stability of a lyophobic colloid may often be increased by the addition of a lyophilic colloid to the solution. The molecules of the lyophilic colloid, which may be called the *protective colloid*, adsorb onto the insoluble particles and render the latter less hydrophobic and less likely to aggregate into larger particles. The protein gelatin and the glucose polymer dextran are often used as protective colloids in the preparation of radioactive colloids for clinical use. In the absence of a protective colloid, colloidal gold is quite unstable and the gold particles tend to precipitate out, however the addition of a small quantity of gelatin to the solution results in a gold colloid which remains stable for years.

33.5. Types of colloid used in nuclear medicine

Radioactive colloids have many important applications in nuclear medicine. Labelled proteins such as ^{125}I-labelled human serum albumin, ^{99}Tc^m-labelled human serum albumin and ^{113}In^m-transferrin which are used for vascular and other studies are lyophilic colloids.

However, the colloids used for organ visualisation are all lyophobic. Gold-198 colloid, which is one of the oldest colloidal radiopharmaceuticals, is a suspension of particles of metallic gold, 10 to 20 nm in diameter, in an aqueous solution stabilised by gelatin. The very commonly used ^{99}Tc^m sulphur colloid is another lyophobic colloid consisting of ^{99}Tc^m, probably as technetium heptasulphide adsorbed onto colloidal sulphur and stabilised with gelatin, or dextran. The labelled macroaggregates of human serum albumin used for lung scanning and the albumin microspheres used for circulation studies are not true colloids, since the sizes of the albumin particles, 10 to 70 μm, are considerably greater than 400 nm which is the upper limit of the colloidal size range.

The preparation of radioactive colloids for organ visualisation is generally achieved by a controlled precipitation procedure. The individual preparation methods have been worked out very carefully to yield a stable colloid having particles in the size range required for the particular clinical investigation to be carried out. In preparing colloidal radiopharmaceuticals great care must be exercised in following exactly the recommended procedure, and in ensuring that the reagents are of the required quality, since small variations in salt concentration or pH may result in a product which is unsuitable for the required purpose.

34

The chemistry of some elements of importance in nuclear medicine

34.1. Introduction

Some of the more important radionuclides used in nuclear medicine today, e.g. $^{99}Tc^m$, ^{67}Ga, $^{113}In^m$, are isotopes of relatively rare elements the chemical properties of which are not usually discussed in school or pre-clinical chemistry courses. A sound knowledge of the principal chemical properties of the radionuclides used is essential to the understanding of the principles and practice of radiopharmaceutical production. The purpose of this Chapter is to present brief reviews of the chemical properties of technetium, gallium and indium with special reference to their use in radiopharmaceuticals. Some aspects of the chemistry of iodine are also reviewed with particular emphasis on the labelling of proteins and other molecules.

34.2. The chemistry of technetium

The nuclear properties of technetium-99m make it an almost ideal radionuclide for imaging and other investigations, and $^{99}Tc^m$ is probably the most widely used nuclide in contemporary nuclear medicine. However, despite very wide interest in $^{99}Tc^m$ preparations for clinical investigation the chemistry of technetium compounds, especially in aqueous systems, is still incompletely understood.

All the known isotopes of technetium are radioactive. The element was first isolated by Perrier and Segre in 1937 by the bombardment of molybdenum with deuterons in the cyclotron at Berkeley in California.

Technetium-99, the decay product of $^{99}Tc^m$, has a half life of $2 \cdot 12 \times 10^5$ years and its specific activity of $1 \cdot 6$ g/GBq is sufficiently low to permit chemical studies using weighable amounts of the element.

Technetium, atomic number 43, is assigned to Group VII A of the Periodic Table (Fig. 29.1) together with manganese and rhenium. In broad terms the chemistry of technetium resembles that of rhenium more closely than that of manganese.

Oxidation states of technetium

Technetium has the electronic configuration (Kr) $4d^6 5s^1$, indicating that it has the electronic structure of the inert gas krypton plus six electrons in the 4d energy shell and one electron in the 5s shell. These two valency shells contain seven electrons and compounds of technetium are known with oxidation (or valency) states ranging from $+7$ to -1. In aqueous solution the most stable oxidation states of technetium are the pertechnetate ion TcO_4^- ($+7$) and the insoluble oxide TcO_2 ($+4$).

Oxidation state, or number, is related to the valency of the atom and represents the charge which the atom would have in a given compound if the electron-transfer tendency were carried to completion. Atoms in an elementary state have an oxidation state of zero, thus the oxidation state of technetium metal is zero. The oxidation state of an ion is the same as the ionic charge number, thus oxygen normally has an oxidation state of -2 and hydrogen has an oxidation state of $+1$ in most of its compounds. The algebraic sum of the oxidation states of the atoms in a compound is always zero, thus the oxidation state of any atom can be calculated from the oxidation states of the other atoms in the compound. For example in sodium pertechnetate, which may be written as $Na^+ Tc(O^{-2})_4$, the oxidation state of the technetium atom is $(4 \times -2) + 1$ or $+7$. Oxidation numbers may also be indicated by roman numerals, thus $Tc(+7) \equiv Tc(VII)$. An *oxidation* reaction is one in which the oxidation state is increased and a *reduction* reaction results in a decrease in oxidation state.

Technetium-99m is eluted from a ^{99}Mo-$^{99}Tc^m$ generator as the TcO_4^- ion but this chemical form is suitable for use in only a limited number of clinical investigations and for the preparation of many $^{99}Tc^m$ radiopharmaceuticals it is necessary to reduce the TcO_4^- to a lower oxidation state. This reduction may be achieved by the use of *reducing agents*, such as stannous chloride ($SnCl_2$), ferrous chloride ($FeCl_2$), or ascorbic acid, or by electrolytic reduction. The oxidation states which are present in most radiopharmaceuticals containing $^{99}Tc^m$ are not known precisely because contemporary methods of measurement are not sufficiently sensitive to permit the determination of oxidation state at the very low technetium concentrations, less than 10^{-9} M, contained in these preparations. More precise chemical studies are possible using ^{99}Tc at concentrations of 10^{-4} to 10^{-5} M, but the oxidation states observed at these concentrations may not be identical with those existing at very much lower concentrations.

The chemical forms of technetium which are probably present in some commonly used ^{99}Tc^m radiopharmaceuticals are discussed in the next section.

The chemical form of technetium in some radiopharmaceuticals

Pertechnetate. The product obtained by the elution of a ^{99}Mo-^{99}Tc^m generator with physiological saline, Na^{99}Tc^{m}O$_4$, may be used for brain or thyroid scanning without any chemical treatment. The TcO$_4^-$ ion, which has a similar ionic radius and charge to the iodide (I$^-$) ion, shows a similar biological distribution to iodide with concentration in the thyroid, salivary gland, choroid plexus and stomach. However, unlike iodide, TcO$_4^-$ is not converted into organic compounds *in vivo* and, apart from possible weak binding to albumin and other proteins, the ion is virtually unreactive in biological systems.

Technetium-99-human serum albumin. The labelling of human serum albumin with ^{99}Tc^m necessitates the reduction of TcO$_4^-$ to a lower oxidation state. This labelling may be achieved by mixing ^{99}Tc^{m}O$_4^-$ with human serum albumin solution in the presence of a reducing agent such as stannous chloride or ascorbic acid. Alternatively a mixture of human serum albumin and ^{99}Tc^{m}O$_4^-$ may be electrolysed with zirconium electrodes. It is not yet clear whether the radionuclide is bound to the albumin in the Tc($+5$) or Tc($+4$) state.

Other radiopharmaceuticals, containing reduced technetium. A large number of radiopharmaceuticals containing reduced ^{99}Tc^m have been described and a number, such as the ^{99}Tc^m-diphosphonate, ^{99}Tc^m-polyphosphate, ^{99}Tc^m-DTPA, or ^{99}Tc^m-glucoheptonate complexes have found extensive clinical use. However, in most cases the nature of the reduced ^{99}Tc^m species present in these complexes is unknown. The preparation of the ^{99}Tc^m-DTPA complex by treating ^{99}Tc^{m}O$_4^-$ with an excess of both SnCl$_2$ and DTPA is believed to result in the formation of a ^{99}Tc^m($+3$) DTPA complex. Intuitive guesswork suggests that in the pyrophosphate complex used for bone scanning the ^{99}Tc^m is present in the ($+4$) state.

Quality control of technetium radiopharmaceuticals

For any radiopharmaceutical _preparation which involves the chemical manipulation of ^{99}Tc^{m}O$_4^-$ it is necessary to have rapid and reliable methods of analysis to ensure that the radionuclide is present predominantly in the required chemical form. These techniques are additional to the analytical procedures needed to monitor the eluate from any radionuclide generator for breakthrough of the parent radionuclide or of column material (see Ch. 37) and for the presence of other unacceptable contaminants.

Some form of chromatography, paper, thin-layer, ion-exchange or gel-permeation, is the usual method of choice for the analysis of $^{99}Tc^m$ radiopharmaceuticals. However, the method, or preferably methods, of analysis used for a particular radiopharmaceutical must be carefully selected and tested if the results of the analyses are not to be misleading.

When TcO_4^- is reduced in an aqueous medium in the absence of any complexing agent the reduced technetium undergoes hydrolysis to form polymerised, hydrolysed species of what is probably $Tc(+4)$ (Ch. 32). These hydrolytic reactions may also occur to some extent even in the presence of complexing agents and the presence of hydrolysed $^{99}Tc^m$ species in a radiopharmaceutical preparation may be missed unless the analytical procedures are well chosen. These hydrolysed technetium species are bound by the cellulose of chromatographic paper or by Sephadex gels and they pass through a column of anion exchange resin in the same way as complexed technetium. If a preparation of $^{99}Tc^m$- albumin is analysed by paper chromatography, using 85 per cent methanol as the developing agent, any unreacted $^{99}Tc^mO_4^-$ will move on the paper with an R_f of 0·5 to 0·6 but the $^{99}Tc^m$-albumin will be denatured and remain behind at the point of application (the origin), together with any hydrolysed reduced technetium. Thus, this method of analysis will indicate the amount of free unreacted $^{99}Tc^mO_4^-$ which may be present but will not distinguish between hydrolysed reduced technetium and the albumin complex. A more satisfactory method of analysis is to use isotonic saline as the developing agent since in this solvent the hydrolysed material does not move, the $^{99}Tc^m$-albumin complex moves with the solvent front and free $^{99}Tc^mO_4^-$ moves with an intermediate Rf value, thus all three $^{99}Tc^m$ species may be clearly distinguished on the chromatogram. Reduced technetium compounds may be oxidised by atmospheric oxygen and to avoid misleading results it is necessary to carry out chromatographic analyses in an inert (nitrogen) atmosphere. Further problems in the analysis of $^{99}Tc^m$ complexes may arise from dissociation of the complex due to reaction with the chromatographic support or as a result of dilution of the complex during the analysis. These problems are discussed in more detail in the references cited in Appendix 8.

34.3. The chemistry of gallium

Gallium is placed together with boron, aluminium, indium and thallium in Group III B of the Period Table, Figure 29.1. The electronic configuration of gallium is (Kr) $4s^2 4p^1$ and compounds of oxidation state $+1$, $+2$ and $+3$ are known, however only the $+3$ state is stable in aqueous solution.

The Ga^{3+} ion has a small ionic radius (0·062 nm) and the combination of high ionic charge and small size results in a tendency to undergo extensive hydrolysis in solution. Insoluble or colloidal hydrolysed species of gallium are produced when an acid solution is raised to pH 1·5 to 2·3 in the absence of complexing agents. Gallium is an amphoteric element thus it exhibits both acidic and basic behaviour, and gallium hydroxide, or hydrolysed gallium species, dissolve in ammonia or alkali metal hydroxides to form gallates.

At the present time only a very limited range of gallium radiopharmaceuticals are in use and of these the most important are the ^{67}Ga citrate and ^{68}Ga-EDTA complexes. With the increasing interest in positron-emitting radionuclides for scanning a wider range of ^{68}Ga radiopharmaceuticals may be expected to be developed. The ^{68}Ge-^{68}Ga generators which are currently available are eluted with EDTA solution producing the ^{68}Ga-EDTA chelate. In order to convert this to other chemical forms it is necessary to separate the ^{68}Ga from the EDTA moiety. This may be achieved by a simple anion exchange procedure which produces a solution of ^{68}Ga in dilute hydrochloric acid. Other complexes may be formed by lowering the pH of this solution to about 2, adding the complexing agent and increasing the pH to about 7. It is unwise to raise the pH of the ^{68}Ga solution to above 2·3 before adding the complexing agent otherwise hydrolysed gallium species or gallates may be formed.

In vivo, following administration of ^{67}Ga citrate the radionuclide is bound to the plasma proteins, principally to transferrin, in the blood and to unidentified proteins in the tissues.

34.4.   The chemistry of indium

Indium has the electronic configuration (Xe) $5s^2 5p^1$ and like gallium compounds exhibits $+1$, $+2$ and $+3$ oxidation states, with the $+3$ state being predominant in aqueous solution.

Having a larger ionic radius, 0·081 nm, the In^{3+} ion shows a slightly lesser tendency to hydrolyse than Ga^{3+} with insoluble or colloidal species being produced at pH 2·7 to 3·4. This tendency to hydrolyse to produce colloidal species has been utilised for clinical application and colloidal preparations of $^{113}In^m$ hydroxide or phosphate have been used for liver, spleen and bone marrow scanning.

A considerable number of $^{113}In^m$ or ^{111}In radiopharmaceuticals have been used in clinical investigation either as colloidal or aggregate forms or as soluble complexes. The generator produced nuclide $^{113}In^m$ is usually eluted from the ^{113}Sn-$^{113}In^m$ generator with 0·05 M hydrochloric acid to yield an indium chloride solution which is a convenient starting point for the preparation of all types of radiopharmaceutical. The $^{113}In^m$ solution eluted from the generator in 0·05 M hydrochloric acid is a mixture of hydrated In^{3+} ions and chloro complexes, the principal species being:

$$In(H_2O)_6^{3+} \qquad 5·85\%$$

$$In(H_2O)_5Cl^{2+} \qquad 80·5\%$$

$$In(H_2O)_4Cl_2^+ \qquad 11·65\%$$

$$In(H_2O)_3Cl_3 \qquad 2·00\%$$

The preparation of the $^{113}In^m$ DTPA complex has been discussed in Chapter 32 and other complexes may be formed in the same general manner.

In vivo, indium radionuclides appear to bind strongly to the plasma protein transferrin and following injection most indium complexes appear to dissociate releasing the metal to form the indium transferrin complex.

Lipid-soluble complexes of ^{111}In with 8-hydroxyquinoline (oxine), acetylacetone or tropolone are now used for the high efficiency labelling of platelets, neutrophils and lymphocytes *in vitro*. The labelled cells, which appear to retain the ^{111}In label strongly *in vivo* , are used for various types of scintigraphic study such as thrombus localisation, lymphocyte circulation and the localisation of inflammatory lesions.

34.5.   The chemistry of iodine

Iodine is one of the group of elements, fluorine, chlorine, bromine, iodine and astatine, called 'halogens' which occupy Group VIIB of the Periodic Table. The chemical properties of iodine are well described in general chemistry textbooks and only those aspects of its chemistry which are of special relevance to radiopharmaceuticals will be discussed here.

Iodine has the electronic configuration $(Kr)4d^{10}5s^25p^5$. Compounds of iodine are known with oxidation states of -1, $+1$, $+3$, $+5$ and $+7$, but from the radiopharmaceutical point of view the -1 and $+1$ oxidation states are probably the most important.

The -1 oxidation state, the iodide ion, I^-, is itself an important radiopharmaceutical for thyroid studies and as the starting material for the preparation of most iodinated compounds.

The iodination of proteins

The iodide ion cannot form a stable linkage with proteins and the formation of a stable carbon–iodine bond requires iodide to be oxidised to a higher oxidation state. The nature of the iodine species which is involved in protein iodination is uncertain, it is usually considered to be the I^+ oxidation state but this species is so reactive in solution that it has not yet been possible to prove that it plays a role in protein iodination.

The first step in the iodination of a protein is the oxidation of an iodide to form the reactive iodine species, this is assumed to be I^+ in the following discussion. When a solution of a protein is mixed with a solution containing the reactive iodine species the first reaction to occur will be the oxidation of any sulphydryl (—SH) groups which may be present.

$$I^+ + R-SH \quad \rightarrow R-SI + H^+$$

$$R-SH + R-SI \rightarrow R-S-S-R + H^+ + I^-$$

This reaction does not result in any iodination of the protein and the formation of the disulphide bond (R—S—S—R) may destroy or alter the biological function of the protein.

From the point of view of labelling proteins with radioactive iodine the most important reaction is the iodination of tyrosine in the protein, to form the mono- or di-iodo tyrosyl residues.

This reaction is rapid and is catalysed by bases. The rate of the reaction is dependent on the hydroxyl ion concentration and is inversely proportional to the square of the concentration of iodide in the reaction mixture.

At higher iodine concentrations histidine residues in the protein may be iodinated

This latter reaction is undesirable from the point of view of protein labelling as it may cause deleterious changes in the protein.

If the structural and biological integrity of the protein is to be preserved after iodination it is important to avoid over-iodination as the latter may lead to iodination of histidine residues and the destruction of other amino acids such as methionine and tryptophane. The usual working rule is that if the biological integrity of the labelled protein is to be preserved an average of not more than one iodine atom should be incorporated into each protein molecule.

For some radiopharmaceutical applications complete retention of biological integrity is not necessary, for example in macro-aggregated albumin, and in such cases a higher level of iodination may be acceptable. Indeed, a higher degree of iodination may in some cases improve the properties of the radiopharmaceutical. It has been suggested that fibrinogen labelled with up to 100 atoms of iodine per protein molecule may be superior to a less highly labelled fibrinogen for thrombus localisation since the highly iodinated protein retains its major biological activity but is cleared more rapidly from the plasma thus allowing a higher thrombus to background radioactivity ratio to be achieved.

The most important step in the iodination of proteins is the generation of the reactive iodine species; this must be carried out under mild conditions and in such a way that high local concentrations of iodine in the solution are avoided in order to minimise the risks of damaging the protein. A number of methods have been developed to achieve these conditions and these are described briefly below.

The *iodine monochloride* (ICl) method was one of the earliest procedures used for the radioiodination of proteins. Iodine monochloride was generated by the oxidation of sodium iodide with sodium iodate and hydrochloric acid, and the ICl and protein solutions were carefully mixed together in stoichiometric proportions by a jet mixing method which produced rapid and complete mixing. This method gives a theoretical maximum utilization of I^+ of 100 per cent for tyrosine iodination but any iodine used to oxidise sulphydryl groups in the protein will be lost from the system as I^-, thus reducing the yield.

This latter problem and the need for careful and rapid mixing of the ICl and protein solutions were avoided by the development of the chloramine-T process which permitted the continuous oxidation of iodide in the protein solution thus permitting 100 per cent of the iodine present to be used for protein iodination. Chloramine-T is the sodium salt of N-monochloro-p-toluene sulphonamide

$$\left[CH_3 \,\langle\bigcirc\rangle\, SO_2NCl \right]^{-} Na^{+}$$

and is a mild oxidising agent. In this method solutions of the protein, iodide and chloramine-T were mixed together, the I^- was oxidised *in situ* to I^+ and after a short interval the iodination was stopped by addition of the reducing agent sodium metabisulphite. This method of protein iodination has been in widespread use for many years but for some applications it has now been superseded by the more gentle methods discussed below. One problem encountered in protein iodination with chloramine-T has been the tendency of some proteins, for example fibrinogen, to form macromolecular aggregates which may adversely affect the biological behaviour of the labelled protein.

In all protein iodination work it is important that the radioactive iodide solution used should be free from reducing agents and a solution supplied specifically for protein iodination should be used. Most commercial solutions of radioiodide which are intended for use in investigations of thyroid function etc. contain reducing agents as 'stabilisers' in order to reduce the risk of spontaneous oxidation of the iodide and the resultant risk of release of volatile radioiodine species into the atmosphere.

In recent years the need to prepare radioiodinated proteins with high specific activities which retain the biological properties for use in radioimmunoassay and other investigations has led to the development of other iodination procedures.

One of these procedures is the electrolytic method in which the protein is dissolved in physiological saline containing radioiodide and placed in an electrolytic cell. The electrolytic cell consists of a platinum vessel with a large surface area, which forms the anode (+ve), and a platinum cathode which is separated from the protein + iodide solution in the vessel by a cellophane membrane. The rate of oxidation of iodide depends on the current flowing through the cell, thus the rate of protein iodination can be closely controlled by regulating the electric current. This method also permits 100 per cent utilisation of the radioiodine for protein labelling.

Another procedure is the enzymatic iodination method in which the oxidation of radioiodide is catalysed by the enzyme lacto-peroxidase. In this method the protein is mixed with radioiodide, hydrogen peroxide and the enzyme in a suitable buffer. The lactoperoxidase may be insolubilised on a suitable support medium to permit easy separation from the reaction mixture by centrifugation. This method has been used to iodinate immunoglobulins, fibrinogen, transferrin and other proteins yielding a high specific activity product which retains a high degree of biological activity.

Recently a new indirect method of labelling proteins with ^{125}I has been described. In this method an ^{125}I-labelled reagent, iodinated 3-(4-hydroxyphenyl)propionic acid-N-hydroxysuccinamide ester, reacts with free amino groups in the protein to produce a conjugate which has a high specific activity and appears to cause minimum interference with biological activity. This reagent, the so-called *Bolton-Hunter Reagent*, has been used to prepare labelled human growth hormone with a specific activity of $6 \cdot 3$ MBq/μg protein which showed the same immunoreactivity as the unlabelled compound.

The iodination of other compounds

Iodine radioisotopes have been used for many years to label a wide variety of compounds for clinical studies. The recent introduction of ^{123}I into clinical use on a fairly large scale has re-aroused interest in the development of radioiodine containing radiopharmaceuticals and many interesting new compounds are being developed. Examples of the non-protein, iodinated radiopharmaceuticals are [123]I- or ^{131}I-labelled Hippuran for renal function studies, [131]I-19-iodocholesterol for adrenal imaging and [123]I- or ^{131}I-labelled fatty acids for cardiac studies.

The methods of iodination used in the preparation of these non-protein radiopharmaceuticals vary widely and may range from a simple addition of iodine to a convenient double bond $\left(\begin{array}{c} \diagdown \\ \diagup \end{array} C = C \begin{array}{c} \diagup \\ \diagdown \end{array} \right)$ in a compound to a complex multi-stage synthesis. With ^{123}I the technique of excitation labelling has been introduced for the preparation of some iodinated compounds. In this method the compound to be labelled is mixed with the radioactive precursor of ^{123}I, [123]Xe, and the resultant radioactive decay produces an *excited* [123]I species which reacts readily with the substrate. Exchange reactions in which a radioactive iodine atom is exchanged for an inactive iodine atom, or another atom such as hydrogen, in a compound may be used to prepare some iodinated radiopharmaceuticals. Such exchange reactions may be carried out in solution or, if the parent compound is stable at its melting point, in the molten state. This method may be used to prepare ^{123}I-labelled oestradiol by reacting Na[123]I with molten oestradiol.

34.6.   Other halogens

The increasing availability of dedicated cyclotrons in nuclear medicine centres and the development of positron emission tomography has awakened considerable interest in the use of compounds containing ^{18}F ($T_{1/2} = 110$ min) or ^{77}Br ($T_{1/2} = 56$ h) as radiopharmaceuticals. The bromination of proteins and other compounds may often be carried out using techniques similar to those used for iodination, including direct bromination, enzymatic, exchange and excitation labelling.

Although ^{18}F appears to be a very good label for radiopharmaceuticals in view of the very wide variety of compounds which can be fluorinated and the great strength of the $C - F$ bond, the preparation of fluorinated radiopharmaceuticals at an acceptable degree of purity and at high specific activity presents many problems and in general their production involves relatively complicated synthetic pathways. Further problems are created by the short half-life of ^{18}F and the consequent requirement that the synthetic and purification procedures must be completed within about 1 to 3 hours. A detailed discussion of fluorine chemistry is beyond the scope of this book but substances containing aromatic (ring) systems may be relatively easily fluorinated via the Balz-Schiemann reaction using a diazonium fluoro-^{18}F-borate, while some other compounds may be labelled by ^{18}F^{-} exchange reactions or by direct fluorination with elemental fluorine.

34.7.   Other elements

Recent developments in nuclear medicine have focussed attention on the use, or potential use, of a number of other less common elements for clinical investigation. For example ^{81}Rb, ^{129}Cs and ^{201}Tl for cardiac imaging, ^{81}Kr^{m} for lung function studies and ^{167}Tm or ^{169}Yb for bone scanning or for tumour or abscess imaging. In general these nuclides are used as simple soluble inorganic salts or as complexes with citrate or other anions and their formulation into radiopharmaceuticals does not present sufficient chemical problems to justify discussion of their chemical properties in this work.

Another result of the development of medical cyclotrons and positron imaging systems has been a wide interest in the use of the very short lived, positron emitting nuclides of carbon and nitrogen, ^{11}C ($T_{1/2} = 20\cdot40$ min), ^{13}N ($T_{1/2} = 9\cdot96$ min), in radiopharmaceuticals. For example ^{11}C- and ^{13}N-labelled amino acids have been developed for pancreas imaging and ^{11}C-2-deoxyglucose has been used to demonstrate differences in metabolic activity in different regions of the brain during various activities or in disease. The development of such radiopharmaceuticals, which may include a very wide variety of metabolic substrates as well as drugs, offers enormous potential for the quantitative investigation of metabolic activity in localised areas of the human body in both health and disease. The preparation of such compounds imposes special problems since the half-lives of the nuclides requires that the synthetic and purification procedures should normally be completed in 10 to 30 minutes. However the, often very elegant, techniques which have been developed utilise standard synthetic organic chemical, or biosynthetic, reactions.

35

Proteins

35.1. What are proteins?

Proteins are large complicated organic molecules which are essential components of all animals, plants and micro-organisms. In animal systems, including man, proteins perform many vital functions which may be classified under four main headings. The *structural proteins* which are important contributors to the strength and physical properties of tissues, for example collagen in bone and tendon. The large group of *enzymes*, or biological catalysts, which facilitate the very large numbers of complex chemical reactions which occur in the body. The *carrier proteins* which transport essential substances round the body, for example haemoglobin which carries oxygen or transferrin which transports iron and some other metals. The *regulatory proteins* which control many biological functions, for example the antibodies which are responsible for the immune reactions and some of the hormones, for example insulin, which regulate critical chemical processes in the body.

Proteins are polymers built up from hundreds of simpler molecules called *amino acids*. The large protein molecules, which are often described as *macromolecules*, have relative molecular masses ranging from about 5000 to 500 000. Hydrolysis of proteins by enzymes or by heating in acid releases about twenty different amino acids.

35.2. Amino acids

Amino acids are organic compounds characterised by the presence of a primary amino ($-NH_2$) group and a carboxylic acid group ($-COOH$) in the molecule. The general formula for amino acids is

$$NH_2$$
$$|$$
$$R-CH-COOH$$

where R may be hydrogen, or a carbon skeleton. Some examples of amino acids are shown in Figure 35.1. Some amino acids contain two

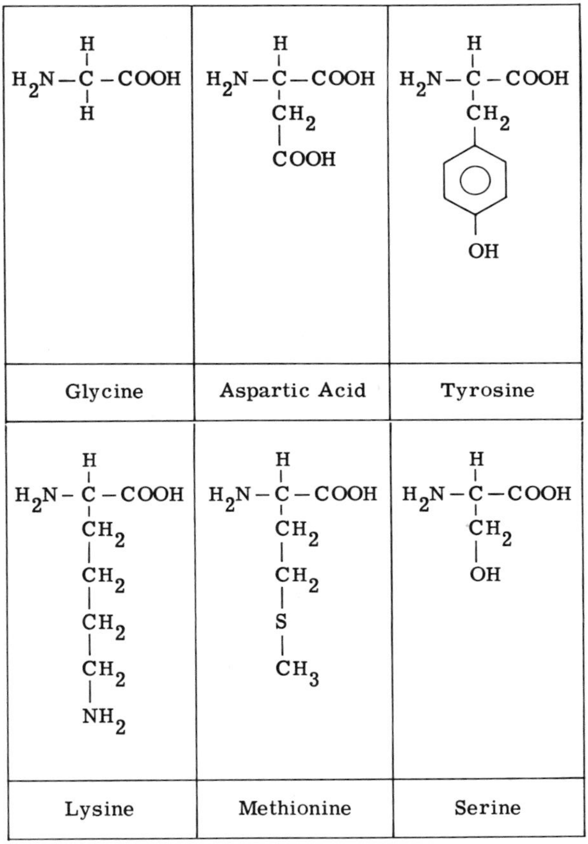

H | $H_2N-C-COOH$ | H	H | $H_2N-C-COOH$ | CH_2 | $COOH$	H | $H_2N-C-COOH$ | CH_2 (benzene ring) OH
Glycine	Aspartic Acid	Tyrosine
H | $H_2N-C-COOH$ | CH_2 | CH_2 | CH_2 | CH_2 | NH_2	H | $H_2N-C-COOH$ | CH_2 | CH_2 | S | CH_3	H | $H_2N-C-COOH$ | CH_2 | OH
Lysine	Methionine	Serine

Fig. 35.1 Structures of some amino acids.

carboxylic acid groups in the molecule and these are described as *dicarboxylic* amino acids. The amino group is capable of acting as a proton acceptor and is, therefore, a base (Ch. 30.6); some amino acids contain two amino groups in the molecule and these are described as basic amino acids. Three amino acids, cysteine, cystine and methionine, contain sulphur, as well as carbon hydrogen and oxygen, in the molecule.

The carboxyl groups of amino acids ionise in a similar way to those of simple acids; for most amino acids the pK_a lies in the region of 2 to 3. The basic amino groups also ionise with a pK_a of about 10. One special property of amino acids is that the carboxylic acid group can donate its proton (H^+) to the amino group of the same molecule, thus forming a salt within the molecule. In the solid state, or in solutions at pH values between 4 and 9, amino acids exist with two ionised groups—one anion, one cation—forming a *dipolar ion* or *zwitterion*. For example glycine may be written as

$$^+H_3N—CH_2—COO^-.$$

Over this pH range the molecule carries little net electrical charge and there is one point, the *isoelectric point*, at which the net charge is zero.

This zwitterion behaviour of amino acids is important in conferring buffering capacity to their solutions. Proteins also have similar buffering capacity due to their constituent amino acids.

35.3.   The peptide bond

In all proteins the amino acids are linked together by a bond which is formed by the reaction of the carboxyl group of one amino acid and the amino group of another with the elimination of a molecule of water:

The linkage $-\overset{O}{\overset{\|}{C}}-\overset{H}{\overset{|}{N}}-$ is called a *peptide bond*, the compound formed in the reaction shown above contains two amino acids and is called a *dipeptide*. Since dipeptides still contain reactive carboxylic and amino groups they can react with other amino acids to form polymers with many peptide linkages called *polypeptides*. All proteins are polypeptides.

35.4.   Protein structure

There are about twenty naturally occurring amino acids which are present in most proteins. In any protein the number and sequence of the amino acids is not a random arrangement but follows a highly organised pattern, which is under genetic control.

The number and sequence of the amino acids in a protein chain is known as the *primary structure* of the protein. The formation of hydrogen bonds (Ch. 30.5) between the oxygen of the carboxyl groups and the nitrogen of the amide groups in the protein may produce a regular, or fairly regular, folding of the protein backbone to give a *secondary structure*. Other reactions between amino acid side chains may result in further folding of the molecule to give a *tertiary structure*. Finally some protein molecules, for example insulin or haemoglobin, may consist of two or more distinct polypeptide chains linked together, this aggregation of sub-units is the *quaternary structure* of the protein.

Some proteins may contain other types of molecule in addition to amino acids. Proteins containing carbohydrate (sugar) residues are called *glycoproteins* and *mucoproteins*, other proteins may contain fatty acids, cholesterol or phospholipids and are called *lipoproteins*. These proteins which also contain non-amino acid residues are called *conjugated proteins*. Haemoglobin is a conjugated protein which contains a complex iron-containing substance called *haem*. These non-amino acid components of conjugated proteins are frequently important in relation to both the biological activity of the protein and its structure.

The overall structure, or conformation, of a protein is often of critical importance in relation to its biological function. An irreversible change in the structure of a protein, *denaturation*, frequently results in complete loss of biological activity, but even slight alterations in protein conformation may have a profound effect on the biological activity or metabolism of a protein. This latter point is important in the preparation of radioactively labelled proteins for clinical investigations and labelling techniques must be carefully chosen to minimise the risks of damage to the protein structure.

35.5. General properties of proteins

Most proteins dissolve in water or dilute salt solutions to yield colloidal dispersions. At higher salt concentrations some proteins may be insoluble.

All protein solutions exhibit colloidal behaviour (Ch. 33). Each protein molecule carries a net electrical charge and consequently the protein molecules will migrate in an electric field. Since the electric charge on the molecule varies in different types of protein, the distance the different protein molecules will migrate in a given electric field will vary and thus electrophoresis is a very important and useful method of analysis for protein mixtures.

When protein solutions are subjected to heat or to the addition of acids, metallic salts, alcohols, organic solvents, or a number of other substances the proteins precipitate, usually as a result of irreversible denaturation. However, under certain carefully controlled conditions salts, such as ammonium sulphate, or organic solvents, such as acetone, may be used to precipitate certain types of protein from solution in an undamaged form. These controlled precipitation reactions are important in the separation and purification of individual proteins.

35.6. Protein synthesis

It was mentioned in Section 35.4 that the number and sequence of amino acids is under genetic control, this control is exercised by a complex mechanism which can be described only very briefly here. The deoxyribonucleic acid (DNA) of the cell nucleus contains four main building blocks, the purine and pyrimidine bases adenine, guanine, thymine and cytosine. The arrangement of these bases in certain sections of the very large DNA molecule determines the order in which the amino acids will be assembled in any given protein.

When a protein is to be synthesised a section of the DNA molecule is transcribed into a special form of ribonucleic acid (RNA), called 'messenger RNA' or m-RNA. This m-RNA migrates from the cell nucleus into the cytoplasm and becomes attached to a structure called a *ribosome*. In association with the ribosome the m-RNA acts as a template for the assembly of the new protein molecule, Fig. 35.2. The amino acids used for the assembly of the new protein molecule are themselves associated with specific small pieces of RNA, called 'transfer-RNA' or t-RNA which enable them to find their correct place in the newly forming protein molecule. Protein synthesis occurs in all animal cells but certain organs, or groups of cells within an organ, synthesise proteins for export to other parts of the body. For example some cells in the pancreas produce a number of digestive enzymes which are secreted into the duodenum, while the cells of the Islets of Langerhans produce the protein hormone insulin which is secreted into the blood and assists in the control of carbohydrate metabolism.

The amino acids used for protein synthesis may be derived from the diet or synthesised *de novo* in the body. In man, and many animals, not all amino acids can be synthesised *de novo* and two classes of amino acid are recognised, the essential amino acids, which cannot be synthesised *de novo* but must be derived from the diet, and the non-essential amino acids which can be synthesised in the body.

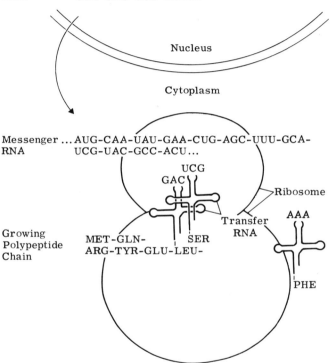

DNA   ...ATG-CAA-CGT-TAT-GAA-CTG-AGC-TTT-GCA-
TCG-TAC-GCC-ACT-GTT-TCT-ATT-GCA...

...TAC-GTT-GCA-ATA-CTT-GAC-TCG-AAA-CGT-
AGC-ATG-CGG-TGA-CAA-AGA-TAA-CGT...

Messenger ...AUG-CAA-CGU-UAU-GAA-CUG-AGC-UUU-GCA-
RNA   UCG-UAC-GCC-ACU...

Nucleus

Cytoplasm

Messenger ...AUG-CAA-UAU-GAA-CUG-AGC-UUU-GCA-
RNA   UCG-UAC-GCC-ACU...

UCG
GAC

Ribosome

Transfer   AAA
RNA

Growing   MET-GLN-   SER
Polypeptide   ARG-TYR-GLU-LEU-
Chain

PHE

Fig. 35.2 Diagrammatic representation of protein synthesis.

35.7. Protein breakdown

In the body proteins may be degraded to their constituent amino acids by the action of a number of different *proteolytic* enzymes.

In the gastrointestinal tract the dietary proteins are hydrolysed first to small polypeptides and finally to individual amino acids. The released amino acids are absorbed from the small intestine and utilised for the synthesis of new protein in the body or metabolised.

Protein digestion begins in the stomach by the action of the enzyme *pepsin*. Pepsin is called an *endopeptidase* and it attacks peptide linkages within the protein chain, especially those containing an aromatic amino acid such as tyrosine or tryptophane. Pepsin acts preferentially in the acid conditions of the stomach at pH 1 to 2. The enzyme is secreted in an inactive form as *pepsinogen* and under the influence of hydrogen ions part of the molecule is split off leaving the active enzyme pepsin.

The digestion of dietary protein continues in the duodenum by the action of three major groups of proteolytic enzymes which are secreted by the pancreas. The first of these is another endopeptidase *chymotrypsin*. This enzyme is secreted into the duodenum in two inactive forms *chymotrypsinogen* A and B which are activated by the action of trypsin or chymotrypsin. The second pancreatic enzyme is *trypsin*, another endopeptidase which preferentially attacks peptide linkages containing basic amino acids such as lysine. Trypsin is secreted as *trypsinogen* which is activated by the action of trypsin itself. The final group are the *carboxypeptidases* which are *exopeptidases* and attack the peptide linkages at the carboxyl end of the protein chain. All these enzymes show maximal (optimal) activity at pH 7 to 8.

The enzymes in the stomach and duodenum break down proteins to polypeptides of varying sizes. The hydrolysis of these peptides to the individual amino acids is completed in the small intestine by a number of *peptidases*, for example *leucine aminopeptidase* which is an exopeptidase which attacks the terminal linkages at the amino end of the protein chain.

Most tissues of the body contain proteolytic enzymes which are capable of carrying out the intracellular digestion of proteins. These enzymes include the *cathepsins*, which are endopeptidases, as well as leucine aminopeptidase and various di- and tri-peptidases.

35.8. Protein turnover

All proteins in the body are constantly being broken down and resynthesised. In any tissue the concentration of a specific protein at any time reflects the balance between the rates of protein synthesis and degradation.

The plasma contains a number of proteins which occur in fairly closely defined concentrations in normal individuals. The normal concentrations of the principal serum proteins are shown in Table 35.1.

The plasma proteins are synthesised mainly in the liver. The synthetic capacity of the liver is sufficient to replace about nine per cent of the liver protein and 25 per cent of the plasma proteins each day. This represents a capacity to synthesise about 55 g of new protein per day.

Table 35.1 The protein concentrations in normal human serum

Protein	Concentration (g/l)
Albumin	36·6
α_1-Globulins	3·1
α_2-Globulins	6·8
α_2-Macroglobulin	2·9
α_2-Haptoglobin	0·8
α_2-Caeruloplasmin	0·4
β-Globulins	8·7
β_1-Lipoprotein	3·6
β_1-Transferrin	3·0
γM-Globulins	0·7
γG-Globulins	13·1
Total protein	79·7

Adapted from *Documenta Geigy Scientific Tables*, 7th Ed. 1970.

The daily turnover rates for some plasma proteins in normal individuals, as determined by radioactively labelled proteins, are shown in Table 35.2.

In the plasma the concentrations of the albumins, globulins and fibrinogen are closely related to each other and a major factor controlling the plasma protein concentration is probably the colloid-osmotic pressure. The albumins play a principal role in this regulation and in disease the albumin concentration may fall but rarely rises.

In healthy individuals the total plasma protein concentration may be rather variable and only major fluctuations are of clinical significance. The total plasma protein concentration may rise in diseases such as cholera where there is severe salt and water loss due to diarrhoea and vomiting, but the albumin/globulin ratio does not alter. In infectious diseases and in plasmacytoma the globulin fractions may increase markedly. The total protein content may fall in kidney disease, cancer and some forms of diabetes. The fall may reflect

Table 35.2 Daily turnover rates of some serum proteins in normal individuals

Protein	Turnover Rate	
	g/d	%/d
Albumin	8·9	8·0
Transferrin	1·7	17·0
γG-Globulin	2·9	6·6

Adapted from *Radioisotopes in Medical Diagnosis*, Eds. Belcher and Vetter, Butterworth 1971.

a general loss of protein or decreases in the concentration of specific proteins.

35.9.   The labelling of proteins with radionuclides

Proteins labelled with a suitable radionuclide can yield clinically useful information in a number of situations.

The ideal labels for studies of the metabolic behaviour of proteins *in vivo* would be radionuclides of carbon, nitrogen, hydrogen or sulphur which could be incorporated into the proteins by biosynthesis following administration of an appropriately labelled amino acid. Unfortunately the available nuclides are not suitable for this approach to be feasible for most human studies. Consequently it is necessary to label proteins *in vitro* by the attachment of a suitable radioactive atom or group to a purified protein preparation.

Although in principle a number of radionuclides can be used to label proteins, in practice only ^{131}I, ^{125}I, ^{99}Tc^m and ^{51}Cr^{3+} have been used widely in clinical practice. The radionuclides of iodine, ^{131}I and ^{125}I, have proved to be most useful up to the present time since they form a stable linkage to the protein, by iodination of tyrosine residues, (see Ch. 34) and their relatively long half-lives permit studies to be carried out over a period of several days or weeks.

If labelled proteins are to be useful indicators of the behaviour of the native protein *in vivo*, the labelling procedure must be carried out in such a way that any significant change in the protein conformation is avoided. This means that heating or exposure to highly acid or alkaline conditions must be avoided and in the case of iodine labelling the amount of iodine bound should not exceed one atom per molecule of protein.

Recently a new and potentially valuable approach to protein labelling has been developed. This involves the binding to the protein of a so-called *bifunctional chelating agent* which can also bind a metallic radionuclide such as ^{111}In. One example of this type of compound is shown in Figure 35.3; in this substance a *p*-benzenediazonium group has been bound to one of the methylene groups of the powerful chelating agent ethylenediaminetetraacetic acid (EDTA see Ch. 32.2). Attachment to a protein occurs through reaction of the diazonium ($-N{=}N-$) group with an amino group on the protein, subsequently a suitable metallic radionuclide may be chelated by the EDTA moiety. This approach has been used to label fibrinogen and albumin with ^{111}In without any apparent significant change in the biological properties of the proteins.

General labelling of plasma proteins *in vivo* may be achieved by the intravenous administration of ^{51}Cr as chromic chloride. The ^{51}Cr^{3+}

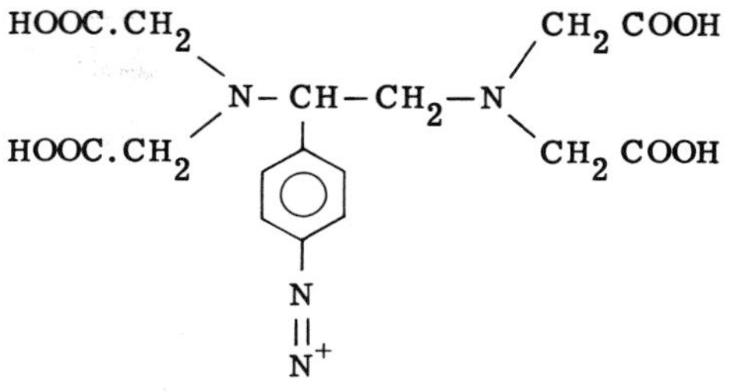

1 - (p - Benzediazonium) - Ethylenediamine -
N.N.N^1.N^1 - Tetraacetic Acid

Fig. 35.3

ion binds almost instantaneously and firmly to the plasma proteins. This type of labelling is valuable for certain types of study which will be discussed in the next section.

35.10.   Labelled proteins in nuclear medicine

Labelled proteins are now used widely in clinical investigation. Studies of the metabolism of plasma proteins can yield the following information:

1. The intravascular protein mass and the total protein mass in the body.

2. The rate of protein transfer between the intra- and extravascular pools.

3. The rate of protein synthesis.

4. The rate of protein turnover, that is the fraction of the intravascular protein which is broken down and replaced per day.

This type of study involves the intravenous administration of a suitably labelled protein and measurement of the changes in the plasma levels and the excretion of the label over a period of up to about four weeks. For such studies it is essential, if meaningful results are to be obtained, that the labelled protein retains as closely as possible the conformation and biological properties of the native (unlabelled) protein. At the present time ^{125}I- or ^{131}I-labelled proteins are used for this type of study.

Human serum albumin labelled with ^{125}I or ^{131}I is also commonly used for the measurement of plasma volume.

Radiolabelled proteins are also used for the study of abnormal protein loss, for example through the gastro-intestinal tract. A labelled protein is administered intravenously and the rate of excretion of the label in the faeces and urine is measured. A number of labelled proteins can be used for this type of study, including ^{125}I- or ^{131}I-human serum albumin and ^{51}Cr-labelled plasma proteins. Labelled polymers of high molecular weights such as ^{131}I-polyvinyl pyrolidone (^{131}I-PVP) or ^{59}Fe-dextran can be used in place of labelled protein for the measurement of gastro-intestinal protein loss. None of these protein or non-protein test substances meets the full criteria needed for accurate measurement of the rate of abnormal protein loss and the information they provide is only semiquantitative.

A number of labelled human serum albumin preparations are used for organ visualisation. Iodine-131-labelled human serum albumin has been used for brain scanning and for tumour localisation, and macroaggregates of albumin labelled with ^{99}Tc^{m}, or ^{131}I, are used for lung scanning.

Fibrin labelled with ^{131}I or ^{125}I is used for the detection of thrombi, and a number of labelled antibodies are being evaluated as tumour localising agents.

An increasingly important use of radiolabelled proteins is in radioimmunoassay procedures for the determination, *in vitro*, of very small quantities of hormones and other biologically important molecules in blood and other body fluids (Ch. 14).

PART FIVE

Radiopharmaceuticals

36

Production of radioactive nuclides

A knowledge of the various methods of production is important in understanding why certain nuclides are cheap, others expensive; some readily available, others in limited supply; some have a low specific activity, others high; and some contain only the radionuclide desired, others have radionuclide impurities. There are also certain general rules which are useful, for example nuclides produced in a reactor are normally beta emitters, which can be readily appreciated when the mechanism of production is understood.

Table 36.1 summarises the main sources of radionuclides and these will be discussed in turn. Radionuclide generators play such an important role in nuclear medicine that they are dealt with in the next

Table 36.1 The principal sources of radionuclides

1. Naturally Occurring Radionuclides
2. The Nuclear Reactor
   (a) Neutron Bombardment
   (b) Fission Products
3. The Cyclotron
   Charged particle bombardment

chapter. The parent nuclides of generators are produced by the methods described in this chapter and generators should therefore be considered as a secondary source of radionuclides.

36.1. Naturally occurring radionuclides

The most famous of the naturally occurring radionuclides is ^{226}Ra; this was first used for treatment in 1901. It is still used in many places but is being steadily replaced by artificially produced nuclides, such as ^{137}Cs. Radium-226 has a half-life of 1620 years and is one member of a series named after its first member, ^{238}U. Each radionuclide of the series decays into the next member, which is itself radioactive until the chain finishes in stable lead (Fig. 36.1). There are two other series or families, the Actinium and Thorium chains, both also finishing in

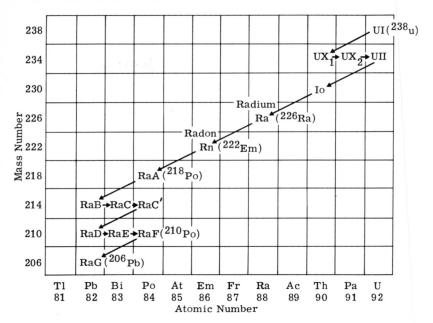

Fig. 36.1 The uranium series of naturally occurring radionuclides.

stable isotopes of lead. The first members of the series, along with other nuclides, were created by fusion reactions occurring in a star (probably our own sun) and if the earth had existed for much longer than the lifetime of the first members of the series (4.5×10^9, 7.1×10^8 and 1.4×10^9 y) then no activity could be detected today as it would have decayed to a negligible level.

The naturally occurring radionuclides discussed above all have high atomic numbers ($Z > 82$). The only other significant naturally occurring radionuclides are potassium-40 (^{40}K) and carbon-14 (^{14}C). 0.012% of natural potassium is ^{40}K, and as the human body contains about 190 g of potassium this represents an activity of approximately a kilobecquerel. Measurement of this activity can be used to determine the mass of potassium present in a human and to follow its change with treatment (Section 21.6). Carbon-14 is produced in the upper atmosphere due to the effect of cosmic radiation and becomes incorporated into plants and animals, including man. The levels of activity are extremely low but can be used in archaeology to date objects containing organic material.

The naturally occurring radionuclides are not used as unsealed sources in medicine and the major importance is their contribution to background radiation (Ch. 10). Some naturally occurring radio-nuclides, for example ^{226}Ra, are still used as sealed sources, and reactor-produced ^{14}C is used as an unsealed source in some clinical investigations.

36.2. Radionuclides produced by neutron bombardment

This is the most important method of producing artificial radionuclides. A target which is composed wholly or partly of the nuclide to be transformed is bombarded by neutrons. A neutron enters the nucleus of one of the atoms of the target, the nucleus re-arranges and a new nuclide is formed. The re-arrangement is accompanied by the expulsion of a particle (proton or alpha) or a gamma ray.

The nomenclature used for this process is

$$A(n, x)B$$

where

A is the initial nucleus
B is the final nucleus
n is the bombarding particle, a neutron in this case, and
x is the emitted particle (p or α) or gamma ray (γ).

The source of neutrons is usually a nuclear reactor and the target to be irradiated is placed inside the core (Ch. 8).

Carrier-free radionuclides

If the material produced by a particular production process contains only radioactive atoms of the element of interest, then it is termed 'carrier-free'. This will occur if the radionuclide is not an isotope of the target element.

A radioactive solution which is carrier-free is likely to have a very high specific activity (Section 4.4) and the concentration may well be of the order of $10^{-9}\,\text{mol}\,\text{dm}^{-3}$. This has advantages and disadvantages; some of the disadvantages are discussed in Chapters 37 and 38. The advantages of dealing with very low masses of the element are that the question of chemical toxicity rarely arises and the radionuclide can be used as a tracer without disturbing the system being studied. If necessary carrier can always be added to a carrier-free solution.

(n, γ) reactions

This type of reaction accounts for the majority of radionuclides produced. An example is the production of phosphorus-32. If stable phosphorus is placed in a nuclear reactor and irradiated with neutrons, the nucleus captures a neutron, re-arranges and emits a gamma ray:

$$^{31}_{15}P + ^{1}_{0}n \rightarrow ^{32}_{15}P + \gamma.$$

This reaction may be abbreviated to:

$$^{31}P(n, \gamma)^{32}P.$$

The nuclide produced is an isotope of the target material and therefore chemical separation is not possible; thus the ^{32}P produced will contain stable carrier phosphorus, and the specific activity will usually be relatively low.

Only low energy neutrons are required to give high yields and so the target is placed in a part of the reactor core where the neutrons have been slowed down by the moderator. Table 36.2 lists some of the radionuclides produced using this reaction.

(n, p) reaction
This is a less common reaction and requires high energy (fast) neutrons. The target is placed in the reactor near to a uranium rod and is therefore exposed to unmoderated fission neutrons. An important reaction of this type is the production of ^{14}C, extensively used for labelling organic molecules required in biological and medical research.

$$^{14}_{7}N + ^{1}_{0}n \rightarrow ^{14}_{6}C + ^{1}_{1}p$$

$$^{14}N(n, p)^{14}C.$$

Notice that the equation must always balance, both as regards atomic mass and number.

$$\text{Atomic Mass:} \quad 14 + 1 \rightarrow 14 + 1$$

$$\text{Atomic Number:} \quad 7 + 0 \rightarrow 6 + 1$$

The nuclide produced in this case is a different element from that of the target and therefore can be chemically separated, producing carrier-free ^{14}C.

(n, α) reaction
The only example of importance in medicine is the production of tritium, an isotope of hydrogen, by the irradiation of lithium with fast neutrons

$$^{6}_{3}Li + ^{1}_{0}n \rightarrow ^{3}_{1}H + ^{4}_{2}He$$

$$^{6}Li(n, \alpha)^{3}H.$$

Table 36.2 Some common radionuclides used in medicine which are produced by the (n, γ) reaction

$^{31}P(n, \gamma)^{32}P$	
$^{58}Fe(n, \gamma)^{59}Fe$	
$^{59}(Co(n, \gamma)^{60}Co$	
$^{74}Se(n, \gamma)^{75}Se$	
$^{98}Mo(n, \gamma)^{99}Mo \xrightarrow{\beta} {}^{99}Tc^m$	(1)
$^{112}Sn(n, \gamma)^{113}Sn \xrightarrow{\beta} {}^{113}In^m$	(1)
$^{124}Xe(n, \gamma)^{125}Xe \xrightarrow{\beta} {}^{125}I$	(2)
$^{130}Te(n, \gamma)^{131}Te \xrightarrow{\beta} {}^{131}I$	(2)

Notes:
(1) Generator systems. See Chapter 37.
(2) The iodine is obtained by allowing the parent to decay

All these mechanisms involve the addition of a neutron to the nucleus with the emission of either a γ-ray or charged particles (p or α). Therefore the product nucleus will have an enhanced neutron to proton ratio and is likely to decay by β^- emission.

Calculation of activity produced by neutron bombardment
Whilst a target is being bombarded by neutrons the atoms in the target are being steadily changed into radioactive atoms. However these radioactive atoms are in turn transforming and so the total number of radioactive atoms present depends both on the rate of production and the rate of decay. The rate of production itself will depend on the neutron flux (F) and the activation cross-section (σ) (see Ch. 8). If there are N target atoms per unit volume the number of activations per unit volume per unit time will be $NF\sigma$.

The rate of decay will depend on the transformation constant (λ), and the activity of the product will depend on the relative rates of the two processes. The water level in a washbasin is an analogous situation; the total amount of water in the basin (radioactivity of product) depends on the rate of flow of water from the tap (activation) and the rate of flow down the drain (decay) (Fig. 36.2). Initially there is no water in the basin but the level builds up till the rate of addition equals the rate of loss; thereafter the level will stay constant.

When the rate of activation of the target equals the rate of decay saturation has been achieved and equilibrium exists. The number of radioactive atoms decaying per second (the activity) will equal the activation rate $(NF\sigma)$. The activity at saturation (A_s) is thus:

$$A_s = NF\sigma \text{ Bq m}^{-3} \qquad \text{Units:} \, F \, \text{ m}^{-2}$$
$$N \, \text{ m}^{-3}$$
$$\sigma \, \text{ m}^2$$

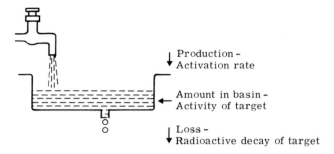

Fig. 36.2 Analogy of water flowing in and out of basin for the build up of activity in a target bombarded by neutrons.

The maximum activity is therefore independent of λ, but the rate at which saturation is reached is dependent on λ. The activity at time t (see Fig. 36.3) is given by

$$A_t = A_s(1 - e^{-\lambda t})$$

which is derived in Appendix 2.3. Writing this in terms of the half-life of the product:

$$A_t = A_s(1 - \exp[-0.693t/T_{1/2}])$$

If $t = T_{1/2}$ $A_t = 0.5\, A_s$ $(e^{-0693} = 0.5)$

If $t = 2 \times T_{1/2}$ $A_t = 0.75\, A_s$ $(e^{-0.693 \times 2} = 0.25)$.

It can be seen that there is no point in irradiating a target for longer than 3–4 half-lives as the increase in yield is not commensurate with cost. Often a considerably shorter irradiation time is used to minimise radionuclide impurities (Section 36.5).

When the target material is composed of several nuclides care has to be exercised as to whether the cross-section refers to all the nuclides or just the nuclide involved in the reaction.

36.3. Fission products

The basic process of fission and the wide range of resulting radionuclides have been discussed in Chapter 8. The principal radionuclides of interest are listed in Table 36.3. Long lived radionuclides can be extracted from spent fuel rods and are available in very large amounts whilst short lived radionuclides are normally obtained by neutron bombardment of a uranium target (normally enriched in ^{235}U) in a reactor. The uranium target is withdrawn at the optimum time, depending mainly on the half life of the radionuclide required, and the nuclides are separated by chemical methods. The

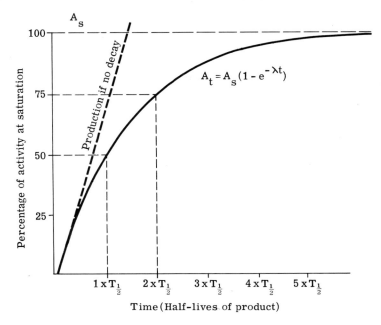

Fig. 36.3 Activation by neutron bombardment. Graph of activity in the target as a function of time. The neutron flux is constant.

products are normally carrier free and beta emitters. This latter property arises as ^{235}U has a large excess of neutrons to protons (143 to 92) and when split by fission into two medium mass nuclides each will be unstable due to a larger neutron to proton ratio than is required for stability.

36.4.   Radionuclides produced by charged particle bombardment

For positively charged particles to transmutate a nuclide they must overcome the electrostatic repulsion of the nucleus and supply it with enough energy to bring about the reaction. This normally requires a minimum energy of several MeV and the most common machine used for accelerating particles to this energy is the cyclotron (Ch. 8).

The same nomenclature as in neutron bombardment is employed to specify the reaction involved. In all cases the product is a different element and can therefore be chemically separated. This results in one general feature of cyclotron produced radionuclides — they are carrier-free. Another very important characteristic is that they are neutron deficient and therefore decay by positron emission, electron capture, or both.

Table 36.3 Radionuclides used in medicine which can be produced by fission of uranium

Long lived: $\qquad U(n, f) \rightarrow {}^{137}Cs$ $\qquad U(n, f) \rightarrow {}^{90}Sr$	
Shorter lived: $\qquad U(n, f) \rightarrow {}^{99}Mo \xrightarrow{\beta} {}^{99}Tc^m$ $\qquad U(n, f) \rightarrow {}^{131}Te \xrightarrow{\beta} {}^{131}I$ $\qquad U(n, f) \rightarrow {}^{132}Te \xrightarrow{\beta} {}^{132}I$ $\qquad U(n, f) \rightarrow {}^{133}Xe$	(1) (1)

Notes:
(1) Generator system. See Chapter 37.

(d, n) reaction

The bombarding particle is a deuteron and a neutron is released. It is unfortunate that the only γ-emitting isotopes of the three major elements of the body, carbon, nitrogen and oxygen, have short half lives in the range 2–30 minutes. However, they can all be produced in a cyclotron and for ^{15}O the reaction is

$$^{17}_{7}N + {}^{2}_{1}H \rightarrow {}^{15}_{8}O + {}^{1}_{0}n.$$

Checking the balance of this equation:

Atomic mass: $\qquad 14 + 2 \rightarrow 15 + 1$

Atomic number,: $\qquad 7 + 1 \rightarrow \;\; 8 + 0$

This equation is written in the abbreviated form as $^{14}N(d, n)^{15}O$, the equations for the other two radionuclides being: $^{12}C(d, n)^{13}N$ and $^{10}B(d, n)^{11}C$.

(α, np) reaction

Here an α-particle is used to bombard the nucleus and two particles are released, a neutron and a proton. An important radionuclide produced using this reaction is ^{18}F:

$$^{16}_{8}O + {}^{4}_{2}He \rightarrow {}^{18}_{9}F + {}^{1}_{1}p + {}^{1}_{0}n$$

or

$$^{16}O(\alpha, pn)^{18}F.$$

(α, 2n) reaction

An example of this reaction is provided by the production of ^{123}I from ^{121}Sb (antimony):

$$^{121}Sb + {}^{4}_{2}He \rightarrow {}^{123}I + {}^{1}_{0}n + {}^{1}_{0}n$$

or

$$^{121}\text{Sb}(\alpha, 2n)^{123}\text{I}.$$

There are several side reactions which create radionuclide impurities as discussed below.

Other important examples of this method are $^{65}\text{Cu}(\alpha, 2n)^{67}\text{Ga}$ and $^{109}\text{Ag}(\alpha, 2n)^{111}\text{In}$.

Other processes

Although most radionuclides for medical applications are produced using alpha particle or deuteron beams some are prepared with a beam of protons. An example is the production of ^{34}Cl by the reaction $^{34}\text{S}(p, n)^{34}\text{Cl}$. Other examples of production processes will be found in Appendix 6.

Calculation and specification of yield

The same considerations regarding the activity of the product are applicable both to charged particle bombardment and neutron bombardment. However as a charged particle beam is narrow and it is the total number of particles per second striking the target which is important the unit of flux is not generally used. The beam current, in units of microamperes, is normally stated and when the product has a half-life long compared to the irradiation time the yield is usually expressed in terms of megabecquerels per microampere-hour or similar units. With short lived products the activity at the end of irradiation is stated for a given current.

36.5. Radionuclide impurities

There is often a choice of production method for a particular radionuclide and contamination by other radionuclides produced in the same target is often an important factor. The general aim in choosing a reaction, target and operating conditions is to maximise the yield of the desired radionuclide and to minimise radionuclidic impurities.

If the unwanted radionuclide has a short life compared with that of the main product then by storing the irradiated material the impurity can decay to an acceptable level before use. An example is the production of ^{67}Ga by alpha bombardment of copper. Natural copper is composed of 31 per cent ^{65}Cu and 69 per cent ^{63}Cu. The reaction used is $^{65}\text{Cu}\,(\alpha, 2n)\,^{67}\text{Ga}$ but the alpha beam also interacts with the ^{63}Cu leading to contamination by ^{66}Ga. However, ^{66}Ga has a half-life of 9·3 h compared with the 78 h half-life of ^{67}Ga and so the level of ^{66}Ga will fall to an acceptable level after storage for 1–2 days.

A more serious problem arises when the impurity has a longer half-life than the main radionuclide. An example is the contamination of ^{123}I by ^{124}I and ^{125}I due to the reactions ^{123}Sb(α, 2n) ^{125}I and ^{121}Sb(α, n)^{124}I. There are three possible solutions. The first is to use an enriched target containing a higher percentage of the required isotope, in this case ^{121}Sb. This is expensive and will only minimise the ^{125}I. A second possibility is to alter the energy of the beam to reduce the yield of the impurity, but this will inevitably also lower the amount of the required product. The third solution is to use another reaction. In the above example the only suitable one involves high energy particles (see Section 36.7).

A technique sometimes employed in the production of radionuclides in a reactor is to irradiate the target for less than the optimum time. This can reduce the proportion of impurities by taking advantage of the different rates of production (see Section 36.2). The production of ^{198}Au is an example. ^{198}Au(n, γ)^{199}Au is a secondary reaction and to minimise the production of ^{199}Au the irradiation time is limited to 2–3 hours rather than the days one would expect from consideration of the half-life of ^{198}Au.

36.6. Szilard-Chalmers processes

When a nucleus undergoes a nuclear transformation considerable energy is imparted to the atom and the chemical bonds binding it to other atoms within a molecule may be broken. This effect can be used to obtain radionuclides of high specific activity even when they are produced by reactions in which the product nucleus is an isotope of the target material, for example in a (n, γ) reaction. The nucleus which has been transformed, although still of the same element, will be part of a different chemical species and so can be chemically separated from the target molecules.

The preparation of high specific activity ^{51}Cr provides an example. A target of potassium chromate (^{50}NaCrO$_4$) is irradiated with neutrons, ^{50}Cr(n, γ)^{51}Cr. On formation of the ^{51}Cr sufficient energy is imparted to the atom that it breaks the bonds linking it to the oxygen atoms. The target is dissolved forming a solution of unaltered potassium chromate and the hydroxide ^{51}Cr(OH)$_3$. The ^{51}Cr can therefore be separated from the ^{50}Cr, usually by simply filtering the solution since the hydroxide is insoluble.

36.7. High energy reactions

Certain reactions can be carried out only by using high energy particles, more energetic than those obtainable in most cyclotrons used in the production of medical radionuclides. Several facilities are now available for preparation of radionuclides using these reactions. They are either high energy cyclotrons or linear accelerators and were built primarily for high energy nuclear physics. The Linear Accelerator at Brookhaven National Laboratory, U.S.A. accelerates protons up to an energy of 200 MeV. With energies of this magnitude pure ^{123}I can be prepared using the reaction

$$^{127}I(p,5n)^{123}Xe \overset{EC}{\to} {}^{123}I$$

In the U.K. pure ^{123}I is produced at the Harwell centre of the U.K. Atomic Energy Authority. Certain nuclides can only be obtained with a large yield by using a high energy reaction, for example $^{133}Cs(p, 2p5n)^{127}Xe$.

36.8.   Summary and comparison of different methods of radionuclide production

The main bulk of radionuclides used in medicine today are produced in nuclear reactors even though this method does, in general, only produce beta emitting radionuclides. Many of the products of medical interest have comparatively long half-lives, in the range days to months, allowing a wide geographical distribution. Furthermore they are relatively cheap.

Since cyclotrons are expensive to run, and usually only a single target can be irradiated at one time, the cost of cyclotron produced radionuclides is high. The products decay either by positron emission or electron capture, or by a combination of these processes. Positron emission allows the use of coincidence counting techniques (Section 26.5) whilst radionuclides decaying by electron capture give comparatively low absorbed doses per unit activity administered (Ch. 11). Many cyclotron produced radionuclides of interest are comparatively short-lived (minutes to days) limiting their application to institutions close to the machine. However cyclotron produced radionuclides are playing an increasingly important part in nuclear medicine and several hospitals have installed cyclotrons wholly or partly for radionuclide production. Most of these cyclotrons are of limited capability but can produce adequate quantities of radionuclides such as ^{11}C or ^{18}F.

Table 36.4 summarises some of the characteristics of radionuclides produced in nuclear reactors and by cyclotrons.

Table 36.4 The nuclear reactor and the cyclotron. Summary of some of the characteristics of the radionuclides produced. These statements should only be taken as a general guide

	Nuclear reactor	Cyclotron
Mode of operation	Neutron bombardment Fission	Bombardment by protons, deutrons and alpha particles
Major reactions	(n, γ), (n, p) (n, α) $U(n, f)$	(d, n), (α, d) (α, np) (p, n) and others
Neutron-proton ratio	Neutron excess	Neutron deficient
Mode of decay	β^-	β^+, EC
If carrier-free	(n, γ) No $\left.\begin{array}{l}(n, p) \\ (n, \alpha) \\ U(n, f)\end{array}\right\}$ Yes	Yes
Cost	Comparatively low	Comparatively high

37

Generators

The introduction of $^{99}Tc^m$ in the middle 1960's made a major impact on nuclear medicine and it is now the most important radionuclide used in organ visualisation. Whilst the physical characteristics of $^{99}Tc^m$ make it almost an ideal nuclide for many procedures (Ch. 11) it could never have attained such widespread use unless it was readily available in hospitals located far from reactors and cyclotrons. This availability was made possible by the development of simple and reliable generator systems, often colloquially referred to as 'cows' as they are 'milked' to obtain the radionuclide.

The generator concept was developed in the early years of this century in order to provide a supply of radon gas from ^{226}Ra (Fig. 37.1). The requirement of any generator system is that the radionuclide of interest should be a short-lived daughter of a relatively longer-lived radionuclide from which it can be separated. Either physical or chemical methods can be used to separate the two radionuclides and this is done either continuously or, more usually, when required.

A number of generator systems have been developed and Table 37.1 lists those of most importance in nuclear medicine. Systems in

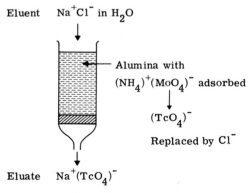

Eluent Na^+Cl^- in H_2O

Alumina with $(NH_4)^+(MoO_4)^-$ adsorbed

$(TcO_4)^-$

Replaced by Cl^-

Eluate $Na^+(TcO_4)^-$

Fig. 37.1 Basic principles of a ^{99}Mo-$^{99}Tc^m$ generator.

Table 37.1 Radionuclide generator systems

Parent		Daughter		Decay product
^{68}Ge	$\xrightarrow[280d]{EC}$	^{68}Ga	$\xrightarrow[68\,m]{\beta^+ EC}$	^{68}Zn
^{81}Rb	$\xrightarrow[4\cdot5\,h]{EC\beta^+}$	^{81}Kr^m	$\xrightarrow[13\cdot5s]{IT}$	^{81}Kr*
^{99}Mo	$\xrightarrow[67\,h]{\beta^-}$	^{99}Tc^m	$\xrightarrow[6h]{IT}$	^{99}Tc*
^{113}Sn	$\xrightarrow[118d]{EC}$	^{113}In^m	$\xrightarrow[1\cdot7h]{IT}$	^{113}In
^{132}Te	$\xrightarrow[78h]{\beta^-}$	^{132}I	$\xrightarrow[2\cdot3h]{\beta^-}$	^{132}Xe

* Products are radioactive but have half-lives of more than 10^5 years.

which the daughter decays by isomeric transition (IT) have advantages (Ch. 11) but this is not a basic requirement. The only limitation to the use of generators, as regards location of the hospital, is the half-life of the parent. Whilst the ^{99}Mo-^{99}Tc^m generator will be discussed in some detail many of the points raised are applicable to other systems.

37.1.   The ^{99}Mo-^{99}Tc^m generator

The parent molybdenum is obtained from a nuclear reactor, either by an (n, γ) reaction or by fission of uranium. The most common method employed to separate the daughter technetium is ion exchange. The molybdenum is prepared as ammonium molybdate $(NH_4)^+(MoO_4)^-$ and adsorbed on alumina contained in a glass or plastic column. The ^{99}Mo decays and ^{99}Tc^m is formed as the pertechnetate ion $(TcO_4)^-$. When a saline solution is passed through the column the chloride ions exchange with the $(TcO_4)^-$ but not the $(MoO_4)^-$ ions. After passing through the column the saline solution contains sodium pertechnetate $Na^+(^{99}Tc^mO_4)^-$. (See Fig. 37.1).

The column is said to be *eluted* by the *eluent* (saline) to give the *eluate* (sodium pertechnetate in saline). After elution the ^{99}Tc^m activity on the column builds up and the column can be re-eluted.

There are various commercial systems available with slightly different methods of mounting the column and eluting (Figs. 37.2 and 37.3). Two separate techniques are used for passing the saline over the

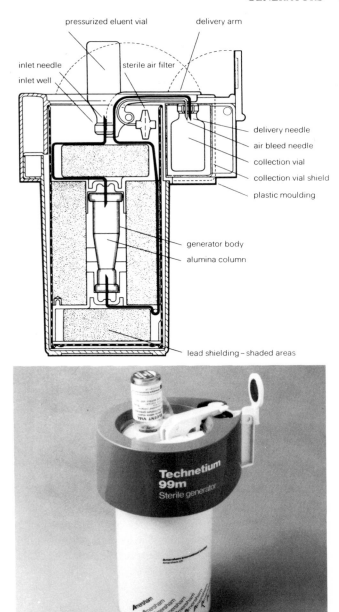

Fig. 37.2 A commercial ^{99}Mo-^{99}Tc^m generator system. (*Courtesy of Amersham International Ltd*)

alumina. Positive pressure systems operate either by using pressure to pass the saline through the column or by allowing the saline to flow through by gravity. Negative pressure systems use vacuum vials to suck the saline through from a reservoir. The columns are enclosed in lead for radiation protection. Most have been sterilized by autoclaving and will produce a sterile eluate if eluted according to the manufacturers instructions.

The volume of eluate obtained varies from 5 to 25 ml according to the manufacturer. Physiological (0·9 per cent w/v) saline is now universally used as the eluent as it can be injected intravenously without modification.

Build-up and yield are discussed in detail in the next section but Figure 37.4 shows the activity-time curves for the ^{99}Mo-^{99}Tc^{m} system. The ^{99}Tc^{m} in the eluate is essentially carrier-free, as are all radionuclides derived using generator systems, and for the radioactive element concentrations of the order of 10^{-9} mol dm^{-3} are typical (Appendix 7.4, problem 1). These very low levels can give rise to difficulties in the radiochemistry (Ch. 38). The decay product ^{99}Tc is also radioactive but as its half-life is $2\cdot1 \times 10^5$y, about 10 becquerels of ^{99}Tc are produced from the decay of 3 gigabecquerels of ^{99}Tc^{m}.

37.2. Build-up and yield
The activity of the daughter radionuclide on a column depends on the activity of the parent, the percentage conversion of the parent to the daughter, and the time since the previous elution.

Activity of parent
The activity on a column is normally referred to in terms of the activity of the parent. For example, a ^{99}Mo-^{99}Tc^{m} generator will have an activity of 5 gigabecquerels of ^{99}Mo at a stated time on a specified date (the calibration date and time).

Percentage conversion
Conversion of the parent to the daughter of interest is not always complete, for example 8·6 per cent of ^{99}Mo decays to ^{99}Tc without passing through the 142 keV metastable level (Section 5.5). This effect is illustrated in Figure 37.4.

Time since previous elution
To understand the build-up of activity after elution it is helpful to study the equations governing the activity of the parent and daughter. A full derivation, which involves simple calculus, is given in Appendix 2.4. Consider a general case where the parent, with initial activity A_1^0,

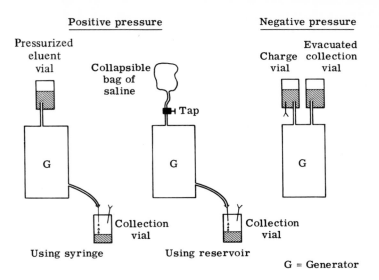

Fig. 37.3 Various methods used to elute generators.

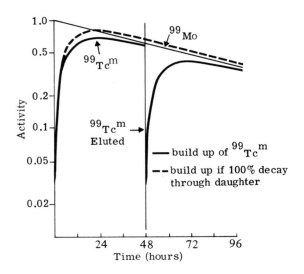

Fig. 37.4 Activity-time curves for a ^{99}Mo-^{99}Tc^m generator. Also shown (dashed line) is the relative activity of the daughter if all the ^{99}Mo decayed to the metastable state (Section 32.2).

decays into the daughter which has an activity A_2 at time t after elution. The transformation constants are λ_1 and λ_2, see Figure 37.5. The activity of the parent is governed by the basic radioactive decay equation

$$A_1 = A_1^0 e^{-\lambda_1 t} \qquad (37.1)$$

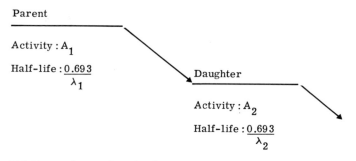

Parent

Activity : A_1

Half-life : $\dfrac{0.693}{\lambda_1}$

Daughter

Activity : A_2

Half-life : $\dfrac{0.693}{\lambda_2}$

Fig. 37.5 Decay of parent into daughter.

The activity of the daughter is not governed by such a simple equation but will depend on:

1. Rate of formation of daughter. This is equal to the rate of decay of the parent ($A_1^0 e^{-\lambda_1 t}$).
2. Rate of decay of daughter (propor$^{\cdot}$ λ_2).
3. Time since elution, t.

The activity of the daughter is given by

$$A_2 = \frac{\lambda_2}{\lambda_2 - \lambda_1} A_1^0 (e^{-\lambda_1 t} - e^{-} \qquad (37.2)$$

This equation can be simplified in special situations.

If $\lambda_1 \ll \lambda_2$. Here the daughter has a very much shorter half-life than the parent. An example is the ^{113}Sn-^{113}In^m generator system. The decay of the parent can be ignored relative to that of the daughter, so $e^{-\lambda_1 t} = 1$. Also ($\lambda_2 - \lambda_1$) compared to λ_2. Therefore (37.2) becomes

$$A_2 = A_1^0 (1 - e^{-\lambda_2 t}) \qquad (37.3)$$

This equation is plotted in Figure 37.6. After a time which is long compared with the half-life of the daughter, $e^{-\lambda_2 t}$ will tend to zero and thus

$$A_2 = A_1^0 \qquad (37.4)$$

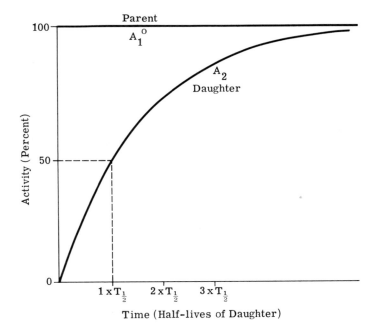

Fig. 37.6 Build-up of daughter when parent has a long half-life compared to the daugher.

The build-up is exactly analogous to the production of a radionuclide by neutron bombardment in a reactor (Ch. 36). In the one case the neutron flux is constant and in the other the rate of decay is virtually constant.

If $\lambda_1 < \lambda_2$. In this case the half-life of the daughter is shorter than the parent but not to the extent of the previous case, so we are unable to assume that $e^{-\lambda_1 t} = 1$. This situation is encountered with the ^{99}Mo-^{99}Tc^m system. No approximation can be made during build-up and equation (37.2) has to be used in full. Figure 37.4 shows the build-up and decay for ^{99}Tc^m.

The time when there is maximum daughter activity after elution is given by:

$$t = \frac{1}{\lambda_2 - \lambda_1} \ln \frac{\lambda_2}{\lambda_1}$$

(see Appendix 2.4 for derivation).

After t becomes sufficiently large (about five half-lives of the daughter) $e^{-\lambda_2 t}$ becomes small compared with $e^{-\lambda_1 t}$. Equation (37.2) then simplifies to

$$A_2 = \frac{\lambda_2}{\lambda_2 - \lambda_1} A_1^0 e^{-\lambda_1 t}. \qquad (37.5)$$

The daughter thus decays with the half-life of the parent. This is known as Transient Equilibrium.

Now $A_1 = A_1^0 e^{-\lambda_1 t}$ (Equation 37.1) and substituting into equation (37.5)

$$A_2 = \frac{\lambda_2}{\lambda_2 - \lambda_1} A_1$$

The daughter activity is therefore greater than that of the parent by a factor

$$\frac{\lambda_2}{\lambda_2 - \lambda_1}$$

Continuous elution

An example of a generator which is continuously eluted is the ^{81}Rb-^{81}Kr^m generator where air can be continuously passed over the column, thereby removing the ^{81}Kr^m. The number of atoms of the daughter being produced per unit time is equal to the decay rate of the parent.

Decay rate of parent $= \lambda_1 N_1 =$ Rate of formation of daughter.

The activity of the daughter formed per second will be the number of atoms formed ($\lambda_1 N_1$) times the transformation constant (λ_2).

Activity of daughter formed per second $= \lambda_1 \lambda_2 N_1$.

Now $\lambda_1 N_1 = A_1$ activity of parent.

$\therefore$ Activity formed per second $= \lambda_2 A_1$.

Nomograms

The calculation of the activity of the daughter on the column is very simple if a nomogram is available. Figure 37.7 is a nomogram for a ^{99}Mo-^{99}Tc^m generator. If a ruler is laid across the nomogram so that it intersects the left hand scale at the appropriate time and similarly the right hand scale then the centre scale gives the ^{99}Tc^m on the generator as a percentage of the nominal ^{99}Mo activity at reference time.

Yield

Using the nomogram or the appropriate equations the activity of the daughter on the column can be obtained. However when the column

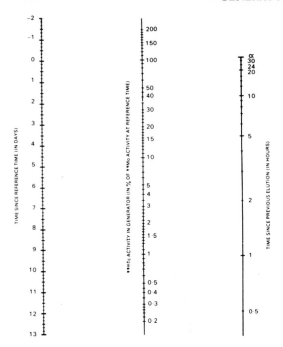

Fig. 37.7 ^{99}Mo-^{99}Tc^m generator system nomogram. (*Courtesy of Amersham International Ltd*)

is eluted not all this activity can be removed. One of the reasons for this is radiolysis due to the radiation arising from the activity on the column. Free radicals are formed which are extremely reactive and can cause reduction of the daughter to a lower oxidation state. Some manufacturers add oxidising agents either to the eluent or to the column itself to improve the yield. A typical value for elution efficiency would be eighty per cent yield of the activity present on the column. Table 37.2 summarises the factors involved in a calculation of the final yield.

Table 37.2 Factors affecting the elution yield of a generator

---

Activity of eluate depends on—

    1. Activity of daughter on column. This is governed by
             Activity of parent
             Percentage of conversion
             Time since previous elution
   Calculated using nomogram or equation (37.2)

    2. Elution efficiency

37.3.   Methods of separating the daughter from the parent

Chromatographic columns

This is the principal method and has been discussed briefly in connection with the ^{99}Mo-^{99}Tc^m generator.

The method consists of fixing the parent on a mineral or organic adsorbent, the daughter being separated by the use of a suitable solution. Two types of adsorbent are suitable:

1. Organic ion exchange. Anionic, cationic or complexing resins can be used.

2. Mineral adsorbents. The use of these is more widespread due to their stability under irradiation. Alumina is used as the adsorbent for the ^{99}Mo-^{99}Tc^m, ^{68}Ge-^{68}Ga and ^{132}Te-^{32}I systems and hydrated zirconium oxide for the ^{113}Sn-^{113}In^m system.

Solvent extraction

This makes use of the different partition of the parent and daughter between two immiscible solvents. An example is the extraction of ^{99}Tc^m using methyl ethyl ketone (MEK) from a solution of ^{99}Mo. This system of extraction has not found favour for commercial generators.

Gas elution

If the daughter product is a gas, such as ^{81}Kr^m, then if the parent is adsorbed on a suitable column the daughter can be separated by passing air over the column.

Volatilisation

This method is based on the different volatilities of the parent and daughter. It can be used for large scale separation of the oxides of molybdenum and technetium; however it is not employed very much because of the complexity and the low yield of about twenty-five percent.

37.4.   Quality control

Siting, assembly and elution

Most commercial generators are designed to provide a sterile eluate. It is essential therefore that they are sited in a suitable environment. If the eluate will not be subsequently sterilized then the elution must be carried out under aseptic conditions. This will normally require the generator to be kept in a laminar flow cabinet or in an appropriate clean area (see Section 39.1). Additional lead shielding may be required for higher activity generators in order to reduce the radiation exposure of the operator. It need only be sited in a fume cupboard if the eluate is, or could easily become, volatile as with the ^{132}Te-^{132}I generator. The manufacturer's instructions must always be carefully followed when assembling and eluting to ensure that the eluate is sterile.

Physical and chemical control
The activity of the eluate must always be measured, reliance on calculation of yield being insufficient.

Radionuclide impurities can be measured using gamma ray spectroscopy, semiconductor detectors being especially useful due to their excellent energy resolution (see Fig. 18.6). A simpler way of detecting any clinically significant breakthrough of ^{99}Mo is to use a re-entrant ionization chamber to measure the eluate both with and without a suitable lead pot. The 140 keV gamma rays of ^{99}Tc^m will be highly attenuated whilst the higher energy rays of ^{99}Mo will only be moderately attenuated. The maximum permitted breakthrough of ^{99}Mo is 0·1 per cent of total eluate activity.

Routine testing of commercial generators to ascertain the level of contamination by column adsorbent is not normally necessary. However there are simple chemical tests available and the concentration of column material contamination can affect the preparation of certain radiopharmaceuticals. The filter located on the outflow side of most generators is valuable in trapping small particles of the column material.

Pharmaceutical control
It is not possible to carry out a test for sterility prior to administration but regular tests should be carried out to maintain surveillance of procedures and techniques.

37.5. Specific generator systems
The main systems are listed in Table 37.1.

^{68}*Ge-*^{68}*Ga.* This system has the advantage that the parent has a long half-life but the physical characteristics of ^{68}Ga are not well matched to modern imaging systems, except those specifically designed for use with positrons.

^{81}*Rb-*^{81}*Kr^m.* The half-life of the parent (only 4·5 h) requires that the user be within a reasonable distance of a cyclotron. The system can be eluted either by passing air over the column, thus allowing direct inhalation of ^{81}Kr^m, or by running sterile physiological saline through it and thus permitting 'on-line' intravenous administration.

^{99}*Mo-*^{99}*Tc^m.* This has been discussed in some detail previously in this chapter. At present several systems use ^{99}Mo produced by neutron irradiation of molybdenum, but fission produced ^{99}Mo is now increasingly being used, especially for higher activity generators. The advantage of the fission material is that a higher specific activity is possible and therefore columns can be smaller leading to lower elution volumes, which is an advantage in some labelling procedures. A disadvantage is the higher level of radionuclide impurities and the greater processing required.

^{113}Sn-$^{113}In^m$. This has the advantage over the ^{99}Mo-^{99}Tc^m system in that the parent has a much longer half-life. It is therefore suitable for centres very remote from the manufacturer or those with small usage. Although for most procedures the absorbed radiation dose from ^{113}In^m is very similar to that from ^{99}Tc^m the former has a higher γ-ray energy and is therefore less well matched to the Anger γ-camera, the detection efficiency being about twenty-two per cent compared with over ninety per cent for ^{99}Tc^m. Parent breakthrough can be tested by allowing the ^{113}In^m to decay for 48 hours and then measuring the residual activity, which should be less than 0·01 per cent of the activity at time of elution.

^{132}Te-^{132}I. This was the first of the modern radionuclide generator systems. However, the high γ-ray energies of ^{132}I preclude its widespread use for diagnostic investigations.

38

Radiopharmaceuticals

38.1. Introduction

Radiopharmaceuticals are medicinal products, designed for use in the investigation or treatment of human disease, which contain a radionuclide as an integral part of the main ingredient. Apart from their radioactivity, radiopharmaceuticals differ from conventional pharmaceutical products in one important respect, namely that the mass of the principal ingredient which is administered is generally too small to produce a pharmacological response in the patient. However, since radiopharmaceuticals are administered to human subjects, usually by intravenous injection, they must meet the same stringent criteria of quality which are laid down for conventional pharmaceuticals.

Prior to the introduction of short-lived radionuclides into clinical investigation most radiopharmaceuticals were purchased from commercial suppliers who guaranteed that their products were of the required pharmaceutical quality. The advent of the short-lived, generator-produced radionuclide made it necessary for many radiopharmaceuticals to be prepared in hospitals. Further the short half-lives of the radionuclides makes it impossible to carry out full quality control tests before the preparation is administered to the patient. Thus the preparation of radiopharmaceuticals imposes special problems and responsibilities upon the nuclear medicine service of a hospital, these matters will be discussed in more detail in Section 38.4.

38.2. The preparation of radiopharmaceuticals

The preparation of any radiopharmaceutical can be divided into two main parts:

1. The preparation of the primary radionuclide.

2. The conversion of the primary radionuclide into the chemical form required for radiopharmaceutical use.

The production of radioactive nuclides in nuclear reactors or charged particle accelerators has been discussed in Chapter 36. At the end of the bombardment it is generally necessary to separate the radionuclide from the 'target' material and to carry out further purification procedures. In nuclear reactors the targets are usually in solid form, but gases, liquids or solids may be bombarded in charged particle accelerators.

In principle any suitable chemical separation technique can be used to isolate and purify the radionuclide. However, because of the very small scale on which many separations have to be carried out some methods may not be applicable. Further problems arise due to the intense radioactivity of the targets and separations must be carried out in appropriately shielded cells, using remote handling devices if necessary.

Separation methods will not be discussed in detail. Most methods involve dissolution of the target and the isolation and purification of the required radionuclide by one or more of the following procedures: co-precipitation, solvent extraction, ion exchange or liquid chromatography, distillation or volatilization. An example of a typical method is the preparation of ^{131}I. In this case the target material is tellurium dioxide (TeO_2) which is irradiated with neutrons in a nuclear reactor to produce ^{131}I by the reaction

$$^{131}Te(n, \gamma)^{131}Te^m \xrightarrow[30h]{\beta^-} {}^{131}I$$

After the irradiation, which may last from 1 to 4 weeks, the target is removed from the reactor and dissolved in 10 per cent sodium hydroxide. The solution is then acidified with sulphuric acid, a small quantity of ferric sulphate is added as an oxidising agent and the ^{131}I is distilled off and collected in dilute sodium hydroxide. Alternatively, the TeO_2 may be heated to 600–800°C for several hours in a stream of oxygen. The ^{131}I is released from the hot TeO_2 and may be trapped in a dilute solution of sodium hydroxide.

The conversion of the elemental radionuclide into the chemical compounds required for radiopharmaceutical use may involve only very simple chemical steps or may require complicated synthetic procedures. While in theory any convenient chemical procedure may be used, special problems may arise in relation to the synthesis of radiopharmaceuticals containing very short-lived radionuclides, for example compounds containing $^{11}C(T_{1/2}\ 20\cdot4\,m)$, $^{13}N(T_{1/2}\ 10\,m)$ or $^{18}F(T_{1/2}\ 110\,m)$, since the whole procedure must be completed as rapidly as possible, within a period of two half-lives, and on a microchemical scale.

Three general methods of preparation can be used for the preparation of radiopharmaceuticals namely:

1. Chemical synthesis
2. Biosynthesis
3. Exchange reactions.

Chemical synthesis is the most widely used technique for the preparation of radiopharmaceuticals containing either long- or short-lived radionuclides. The procedures may range in complexity from the simple solution of $^{67}GaCl_3$ in pyrogen-free 3·8 % sodium citrate to the complicated synthetic pathways required to produce compounds like ^{131}I-19-iodocholesterol or ^{18}F-p-fluorophenyl-alanine.

Biosynthetic procedures rely on biochemical reactions to synthesise the required compound in a specific stereochemical form. The procedure may involve a complete biological system, for example the production of ^{75}Se-Selenomethionine by yeast cells grown in a medium containing ^{75}Se-Selenite. Alternatively highly purified enzymes may be used as catalysts, for example the preparation of ^{11}C-thymidine from ^{11}C-formaldehyde and deoxyuridine by the crystalline enzyme 'thymidylate synthetase'. Biosynthetic procedures are not widely used for radiopharmaceutical preparations at the present time.

Exchange reactions, which involve the exchange of a non-radioactive atom in a compound with a radioactive atom have not been widely used until recently, but there is now considerable interest in the use of exchange reactions for the preparation of compounds containing radioactive iodine or bromine. The exchange may occur between a non-radioactive and a radioactive atom of the same element, for example ^{3}H for ^{1}H or ^{123}I for ^{127}I, or between atoms of different elements, for example ^{123}I for ^{1}H.

The exchange reactions may take place in the gaseous phase, in solution or, for compounds which do not decompose at their melting point, in the molten state. This latter procedure has been used to prepare ^{123}I-labelled oestradiol.

A detailed discussion of the preparation of individual radiopharmaceuticals is outside the scope of this book but examples of simple preparations using radiopharmaceutical kits will be given in Section 38.5.

38.3.   Pharmaceutical aspects of radiopharmaceuticals

All radiopharmaceuticals must be regarded as medicinal products and consequently all their ingredients must be of appropriate quality for administration to human beings, and the final product must meet all the pharmaceutical and statutory requirements of the country in which they are to be used.

The standard of purity and the quality control testing which must be met by all the different types of pharmaceutical are laid down in a special manual called a *Pharmacopoeia*. The standards prescribed in the pharmacopoeia are determined by a national commission and many countries publish their own pharmacopoeia. In the United Kingdom the pharmaceutical standards which must be met are prescribed in the *British Pharmacopoeia* and other well-known works are the *European Pharmacopoeia* and the *United States Pharmacopoeia*. The conditions under which pharmaceuticals may be prepared or manufactured are also subject to official control. In the United Kingdom pharmaceutical production is licensed by the Department of Health and Social Security under the terms of the Medicines Act, 1968, and strict quality control is required during the manufacturing process in order to ensure that the final product meets the requirements of the *British Pharmacopoeia*. Most other countries exercise some form of official control over the manufacture of pharmaceutical products and the required standards are laid down in an appropriate Pharmacopoeia.

Pharmaceuticals which are to be administered by injection are subject to particularly strict control and, in addition to acceptable chemical purity, injection preparations are required to be sterile and pyrogen-free. Pyrogens are products of microbial metabolism which produce fever when injected into human subjects; they are heat-stable and are not destroyed by normal methods of sterilisation. All conventional injectable pharmaceutical products are required to pass prescribed sterility and pyrogen tests before they are released for administration. This requirement cannot be met for many radiopharmaceuticals due to the fact that the time required for testing is very long compared with the half-life of the radionuclide. This problem is discussed in more detail in Section 38.4.

Methods of sterilization
There are four methods of sterilization which may be used in pharmaceutical practice.

Sterilization by moist heat is the most reliable method for the sterilization of aqueous solutions and of capped bottles or vials which are to be used as final containers for sterile products. A trace of moisture must always be left in a capped container otherwise sterilization is not satisfactory. In this method the items to be sterilized are placed in an *autoclave* in which steam is generated under pressure to produce sterilising temperatures. Temperatures of 115°C for 30 minutes or 121°C for 15 minutes are satisfactory for sterilization. Heat sensitive preparations, such as proteins cannot be sterilised by autoclaving.

Sterilization by dry heat requires that the items to be sterilised are subjected to a temperature of 160° for 1 hour. This method is rarely suitable for radiopharmaceuticals but is a valuable method for the sterilization of glassware.

Sterilization by filtration is applicable only to solutions and is carried out by passing the solution through a sterile membrane filter. These filters, which are usually made from cellulose or polycarbonate, are placed in a special holder and the solution is passed through the filter into a sterile container. Membranes with a pore size of 220 nm are generally advised for sterilization, but a pore size of 450 nm is adequate for most solutions. The solution may be forced through the filter by positive pressure, but for radiopharmaceuticals it is preferable to filter under negative pressure by allowing the fluid to be sucked through the sterile filter into an evacuated sterile container. Sterilization by filtration should be used only when the solution cannot be sterilised by autoclaving. Unless the preparation is to be injected immediately, sterilization by filtration should be carried out under aseptic conditions.

Radiation sterilization which requires exposure to at least 25 to 30 kilograys of gamma radiation is of only very limited value for the sterilization of pharmaceuticals. However, it is of very great value for the sterilization of disposable plastic syringes and other items which may be used in radiopharmaceutical preparation.

Pyrogens

Pyrogens cannot be removed from radiopharmaceutical preparations by any process analogous to sterilization and control of pyrogens must be achieved by using only pyrogen-free reagents and glassware and maintaining very high pharmaceutical standards throughout the preparation.

38.4.   Special problems related to the preparation of radiopharmaceuticals

The presence of the radionuclide in radiopharmaceuticals creates certain additional problems which are not encountered in the preparation of non-radioactive pharmaceuticals. Firstly, the need to protect the operator from any radiation hazard resulting from the radionuclide means that in all radiopharmaceutical preparations good radiochemical practice must be superimposed on good pharmaceutical practice. Secondly, radiopharmaceuticals containing short-lived radionuclides cannot be subjected to all the usual quality control procedures before they are released for administration to patients. This applies especially to tests for sterility and apyrogenicity since these tests take several days to complete.

The quality control checks required for radiopharmaceuticals include the following, in addition to pyrogen and sterility testing:

Chemical purity. This is defined as the fraction of the total mass of the main ingredient which is present in the required chemical form. This is normally not a problem with radiopharmaceuticals although often it may be difficult to measure the chemical purity due to the extremely low mass of the main ingredient which is present in the preparation.

Radiochemical purity. This is defined as the proportion of the radionuclide which is present in the required chemical form. For example in a preparation of ^{131}I-labelled Hippuran to be used for renal function studies at least 98 per cent of the ^{131}I must be present in the form of labelled Hippuran. Determination of radiochemical purity will usually involve the use of paper, thin-layer, gel permeation or ion exchange chromatography to separate the respective chemical forms in which the radionuclide is present. Often such analyses can be completed within a few minutes.

Radionuclide purity. This is defined as the proportion of the total radioactivity in the preparation which is present as the specified radionuclide. Radionuclidic impurities may cause an unnecessarily high radiation dose to the patient or may reduce the accuracy of, or even invalidate, the result of a test. Radionuclidic purity may be assessed by gamma-ray spectroscopy or other suitable means.

A very large number of the radiopharmaceuticals currently in clinical use contain ^{99}Tc^m, or some other short-lived radionuclide, and cannot be subjected to full 'pre-issue quality testing'. Consequently very special care must be used in the preparation of such radiopharmaceuticals since the production method must be so designed that the risks of the product being unsterile or containing pyrogens are remote. This means that the procedures must be rigidly defined and the preparation must be carried out in the appropriate clean or aseptic facilities. Before any preparative procedure is put into routine clinical use, a number of production runs should be carried out and the products subjected to full pyrogen, sterility and other quality control tests. Only if these tests show that the product is consistently of the required quality may the procedure be introduced into clinical use. However, once introduced the procedure should be rigidly adhered to, and where possible a portion of each batch should be set aside for subsequent quality tests. If this latter is not possible, regular test batches of the product should be prepared specifically for quality testing.

38.5. Radiopharmaceutical kits

The need to be able to produce, on a routine basis, high quality radiopharmaceuticals which can be safely administered to patients without prior quality control has led to the development of the radiopharmaceutical 'kit'. These kits contain all the non-radioactive ingredients required for the preparation of an injectable radio-pharmaceutical in a prepackaged, sterile form which has been subjected to full quality control testing prior to use.

The kits are so designed that the preparative procedure is reduced to a few simple operations which can be carried out under suitable aseptic conditions. A large number of 'kits' are now available commercially for the preparation of a wide range of radiopharmaceuticals and many others have been described in the literature.

The principle of the kit will be illustrated by an example involving a single step. The MDP kit (Amersham International Ltd.) for the preparation of ^{99}Tc^m-methylene diphosphonate for bone scanning consists of five individual units, each of these will provide up to five patient doses of the radiopharmaceutical. A unit consists of a 10 ml glass vial containing a freeze-dried mixture of 5 mg methylene diphosphonic acid (as sodium salt) and 0·34 mg of stannous fluoride, sealed under an inert nitrogen atmosphere with a rubber closure. It has been sterilized by exposure to 25 kGy of gamma radiation which causes brown colouration of the glass. To prepare the radiopharmaceutical a suitable volume (3–8 ml) of the sterile eluate from a technetium generator is transferred aseptically to the vial by means of a syringe. Before removing the syringe an equivalent volume of gas from the space above the solution is withdrawn to normalise the pressure in the vial, which is then shaken for 10 seconds to ensure complete dissolution of the vial. The pertechnetate is reduced by the stannous fluoride to a cationic species which is then complexed by the methylene diphosphonate.

From a pharmaceutical point of view a multi-stage kit is less desirable than the single-stage procedure since each additional step increases the small but finite risk of introducing microbial contamination into the preparation.

38.6. Stability and storage of radiopharmaceuticals

Many pharmaceutical preparations, especially when in solution, decompose on storage and in the case of radiopharmaceuticals the decomposition may be accelerated by self-irradiation from the radionuclide.

Three main types of decomposition may occur on storage and each of these processes may be minimised by storing the product under the most appropriate conditions.

Chemical changes may occur due to the inherent thermodynamic instability of one or more of the ingredients of a preparation, or by poor choice of storage environment, for example exposure to strong sunlight or excessive heat.

Primary radiolysis may cause decomposition of one or more ingredients as a result of direct interaction of beta particles or gamma rays with molecules of the compounds.

Secondary radiolysis, the production of reactive species as a result of radiation damage to the solvent may cause decomposition of other components. We saw in Chapter 10 that the radiolysis of water may produce electrons, hydrogen and hydroxyl free radicals and hydrogen peroxide, any of which may produce deleterious chemical changes in sensitive compounds.

Chemical changes may often be minimised by storage under appropriate conditions, for example at low temperature or protected from light. Radiolytic effects may be reduced by dispersal of the radioactive molecules by dilution, by cooling to low temperature or the addition of free radical scavengers. However, these conditions may be inappropriate for some radiopharmaceuticals.

Radiation induced damage to the main ingredient of a radiopharmaceutical may not always be the factor which limits the storage life of a long lived radiopharmaceutical. Radiopharmaceuticals supplied in multi-dose containers frequently contain a bacteriocide to reduce the risk of growth of any bacteria introduced during the withdrawal of individual doses. Some of the bacteriocides used are themselves sensitive to radiation damage which may destroy their bactericidal properties or produce undesirable decomposition products. For example chlorocresol may liberate hydrochloric acid as a result of radiolysis, similarly benzyl alcohol, a widely used bacteriocide may liberate benzoic acid.

For most commercially produced radiopharmaceuticals the recommended storage conditions are stated on the label together with an 'expiry date' giving the last date on which the product is considered to be safe for human use. Non-radioactive pharmaceuticals and radiopharmaceutical kits also frequently have an expiry date. No product should be used for clinical investigations after the expiry date.

Short-lived radiopharmaceutical preparations are not necessarily stable for the whole period over which they contain a useful amount of radioactivity. Some ^{99}Tc^m complexes may show marked decomposition 2–3 hours after preparation.

38.7. Radionuclide-labelled cells and other biological materials

Red blood cells labelled with ^{51}Cr have been used for many years for the determination of red cell mass and red cell survival and, more recently, heat-damaged ^{51}Cr- or ^{99}Tc^m-labelled red cells have been used for spleen imaging. There is now considerable interest in the use of granulocytes, lymphocytes and platelets labelled with ^{111}In, or, to a lesser extent, with ^{99}Tc^m, for various types of investigation including the measurement of leucocyte kinetics and the detection of abscesses, areas of inflammation, tumours and other disease processes. The preparation of labelled cells presents special problems since the biological properties of the cells may be altered by even mild mechanical, chemical or heat damage. Further because they are chemical- and heat-sensitive and larger than bacteria, labelled cells cannot be terminally sterilised by any of the available sterilisation procedures. Consequently the techniques used for cell separation and labelling must be gentle and must be carried out under aseptic conditions (Chapter 39).

The procedures involved may be illustrated by reference to the preparation of ^{51}Cr-labelled red cells for a red cell mass estimation. Twenty cm^3 of blood is withdrawn from the patient into a sterile syringe and transferred aseptically to a bottle containing 5 cm^3 of a sterile acid-citrate dextrose solution. The contents of the bottle are mixed by gentle inversion and the bottle is placed in a laminar-flow cabinet. The top of the bottle is swabbed with an antiseptic solution and 1 cm^3 sterile saline containing 1·8 MBq ^{51}Cr-sodium chromate is introduced from a sterile syringe. The contents of the bottle are mixed and the bottle is left to stand at room temperature for 30 minutes. During the period of incubation with ^{51}Cr the hexavalent chromate, ^{51}CrO$_4^{2+}$, ion passes through the red cell membrane and becomes firmly bound to the protein, principally the globin, chains of the haemoglobin molecules.

After standing the bottle is centrifuged for 10 minutes at 3000 rpm to sediment the red cells. The bottle top is again swabbed with antiseptic and the plasma and any unreacted ^{51}Cr are withdrawn using a sterile syringe fitted with a long, sterile needle. Ten cm^3 of sterile saline for injection are added to the bottle and the contents are mixed by inversion. The bottle is centrifuged again for 10 minutes at 3000 rpm and the saline is removed as before; this saline washing is repeated twice. Finally the red cells are resuspended in 10 ml sterile saline for injection and injected back into the patient.

The labelling of leucocytes, lymphocyte or platelets with the oxine, acetyl-acetone or tropolone complexes of ^{111}In involves similar incubation and washing procedures. However, with these cells the preparation is more complicated because it is necessary first to isolate the individual cell type required from a blood sample, this procedure is usually achieved by a sedimentation technique. In order to reduce the risks of microbial infection of the cells during the labelling procedure it is important that the whole process should be carried out in a suitable laminar flow cabinet or in an appropriate clean facility. In all cell labelling procedures there is a small but finite risk of the operator, or of cells from other patients, becoming contaminated with radioactivity or with a virus such as the Hepatitis virus. The operator should therefore take special precautions to minimise the chances of personal contamination through spillage of the sample or by the generation of aerosols during the manipulations, especially during the washing procedures. So far as is practicable only cells from a single patient should be labelled, or be present, in any facility at any one time.

The preparation of labelled proteins has been discussed in Chapter 30 and we learned that proteins were easily damaged by heat and exposure to certain chemicals. Labelled protein solutions cannot be sterilised by heating but they can be sterilised by filtration through a sterile 220 nm pore diameter membrane filter. However, macro-aggregated albumin or albumin microspheres consist of particles which are too large to pass through a sterilising filter and therefore at least part of the preparation of labelled microspheres or macro-aggregates must be carried out using aseptic procedures.

39

Laboratory facilities and procedures

39.1. Design of laboratory

The design of a laboratory for handling radioactivity will vary enormously, from a designated bench in a normal chemical or pathology laboratory to a purpose designed and built radiation laboratory. In a hospital with a nuclear medicine facility there is an additional requirement of pharmaceutical safety when radiopharmaceuticals are being prepared and dispensed. The facilities required to prepare clean and safe radiopharmaceuticals do not conflict in most cases with those needed to handle safely radioactive substances. However, there are certain situations where a compromise is necessary.

Radiation safety

There are two fundamental principles: to minimise radiation exposure to the persons handling the activity and to prevent the spread of contamination outside the laboratory. Radiation exposure can arise from direct external irradiation from a source, or from contamination of the working area with radioactive materials; internal irradiation may arise from inhalation or ingestion of radionuclides. The methods used to reduce direct irradiation and contamination are dealt with in Section 39.2.

The hazards associated with radionuclides will depend on the procedures being carried out, the toxicity of the radioactive compound and the activity involved. The International Atomic Energy Authority (IAEA) have divided the common radionuclides into various classes of toxicity (Table 39.1) and laid down limits of activity for each class which may be handled in three grades of laboratory, A, B and C. The International Commission on Radiological Protection (ICRP Report Number 25) and various national agencies have adopted a similar approach. The handling of sealed sources is not considered in this text.

The radiotoxicity is only a rough guide to the hazard as the calculations have been carried out assuming a simple form of the

379

Table 39.1 Classification of radionuclides according to relative radiotoxicity per unit activity.

Classification	Examples
High toxicity (Class 1)	Most alpha emitters e.g. Radium-226.
Medium toxicity Upper sub-group A (Class 2)	Iodine-125 Iodine-131
Lower sub-group B (Class 3)	Carbon-14 Phosphorous-32 Chromium-51 Molybdenum-99 Cobalt-57 Selenium-75
Low toxicity (Class 4)	Hydrogen-3 Carbon-11 Technetium-99m Indium-113m Xenon-133

elements whilst the actual chemical form will affect its distribution and retention in the body. Limits given below for the various laboratories are approximate and are quoted for normal chemical operations. Limits are higher for storage or simple dispensing but lower for complex procedures.

Grade A laboratories are for handling high levels of activities not normally encountered in a hospital. The most hazardous operations usually met is dispensing therapy doses (3–8 GBq) of ^{131}I for treatment of carcinoma of the thyroid. Should labelling procedures with ^{123}I and ^{131}I be undertaken they may also involve a gigabecquerel or so of these radionuclides. These can be safely carried out in a Grade B laboratory.

Most hospitals will have at least a Grade C laboratory for handling the low levels such as encountered in *in vitro* tests. Up to a few tens of megabecquerels of a Class 2 radionuclide, e.g. ^{125}I, may be handled in a Grade C laboratory or a hundred times as much of a Class 3 radionuclide. Some hospitals may only require a Grade C laboratory to meet all their requirements.

The main features of a Grade B laboratory are listed in Table 39.2 and these will be discussed later. The requirements for Grade C laboratories are obviously lower and can usually be met with little, if any, modification to a modern chemical or pathology laboratory. Further details of all three Grades can be obtained from the references given in Appendix 8. A Grade B laboratory will normally have parts of it set aside specifically for washing up and storage.

Table 39.2 Some general features of a Grade B laboratory.

Specifically set aside for handling radionuclides.

Protective clothing used. Gowns or overalls, gloves and overshoes.

Negative pressure. Extraction fans to outside of building to prevent spread of contamination inside building.

Fume cupboards.

Floors, walls and benches should be smooth and without cracks. Must have non-absorbent and washable surfaces.

Benches strong enough to support lead shielding.

Wash basin with elbow and/or foot operated taps.

Sink with direct access to main drain for disposal of radioactive liquid waste.

Fume cupboards. Any operation involving a significant possibility of the generation of radioactive vapours or aerosols with the consequent risk of inhalation of activity, such as iodination or dispensing large activities from unsealed containers, should be carried out in a fume cupboard. These must exhaust to the outside of the building, the exact location of the outlet is important, and details of desirable air flow rates and design considerations are given in the reference in Appendix 8.

Pharmaceutical

Most radiopharmaceuticals are administered intravenously and therefore the environment in which they are prepared must be such as to permit the preparation of clean and safe agents. Even more reliance has to be placed on the environment and procedures used in radiopharmacy than in normal pharmacy as in many cases conventional quality control tests, such as the sterility test, cannot be carried out before administration of the radiopharmaceutical (Ch. 38). The quality of environment required will depend on the procedure being carried out and the subsequent method, if any, of sterilization. Any radiopharmaceutical which cannot, or will not, be sterilized in its final container — terminally sterilized — must be prepared under aseptic conditions. Thus the preparation of radiopharmaceuticals from kits should be carried out under aseptic conditions, either in a laminar flow cabinet or in an appropriate clean area.

Aseptic conditions. These can be most easily provided by a unidirectional airflow cabinet, often referred to as a laminar flow cabinet. Many designs are not suitable for use with radiopharmaceuticals as the airflow is ejected into the room. The essential feature of all the cabinets is to provide a working area which is in an airstream which has been highly filtered and is therefore sterile. One design in which ninety per cent of the airflow is recirculated and ten per cent expelled outside the building is shown in Figure 39.1. Any radiopharmaceutical which cannot be terminally sterilized must be prepared under aseptic conditions. The cabinet should be located in a clean area.

Clean area. One of the main features of a clean area is that the air supply should be filtered, although not to the same level as for a unidirectional airflow cabinet. Ideally it should be at positive pressure in order to keep dust out, but this conflicts with the general requirement for radioactive materials to be handled in a negative pressure laboratory. The solution chosen will depend on the procedures involved and activities being handled. The laboratory and work surfaces must be easily cleaned and 'dust traps' avoided. Sources of microbial contamination, such as sinks, are undesirable.

Apart from providing an environment suitable for locating a unidirectional airflow cabinet, a clean area is used for carrying out

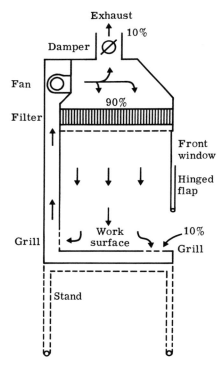

Fig. 39.1 Essential features of one type of laminar flow cabinet.

other pharmaceutical procedures not requiring aseptic conditions. The need to use a special clean area is not always essential for certain procedures, such as the preparation of oral doses. There is some controversy concerning the minimum standards which are necessary in a radiopharmacy in which only short-lived radiopharmaceuticals, e.g. $^{99}Tc^m$ radiopharmaceuticals, will be prepared. Current thought in the United Kingdom and in some other European countries is that the facilities should reach the same standard as those required in any pharmaceutical establishment which prepares injectable products. Discussion and guidance on these matters will be found in the references in Appendix 8.6.

39.2. Handling of radioactive materials

Certain basic rules apply to all work with radiation; in most cases the risks arise from external radiation from either a bottle or syringe containing the radionuclide or the patient himself following injection. There are three cardinal points to remember: *Time, Distance and Shielding.*

Time, because obviously the shorter the time of exposure the less the dose received. Procedures should be practised with inactive materials, and all operations with radioactive sources should be carried out as rapidly as is consistent with the satisfactory and safe performance of the task.

Distance, because the radiation intensity decreases by the square of the distance from the source, i.e. the dose rate at 2 metres from the source is only one quarter of that at 1 metre. Do not handle very active sources directly, and do not stand close to the patient unnecessarily. Remote handling tongs or long forceps should be used whenever possible.

Shielding with some material which will absorb a large proportion of the radiation is necessary when the work cannot be carried out quickly enough or at such a distance that the radiation is reduced to an acceptable level. The amount and type of shielding will depend on the type and intensity of the source, and was considered in chapters 6 and 7. For γ-rays we may need several centimetres of lead, whereas high energy β-particles will be stopped by a few centimetres of transparent plastic. Low energy β-particles will not be transmitted by the walls of a glass container, although bremmstrahlung will be produced with low efficiency. With very active sources of penetrating radiation, such as an isotope generator, it may be necessary to shield the source from all directions including below bench and ceiling levels.

Intelligent use of *Times, Distance* and *Shielding* is required in all work with radiation sources. In addition, if unsealed sources are used care must be taken to contain any accidental contamination. It is good practice to carry out procedures in large shallow dishes, preferably lined with absorbent paper. Any surface on which contamination is likely can be covered with disposable plastic backed absorbent material so as to facilitate decontamination.

Suitable protective clothing must be used whenever radioactive materials are handled (see Section 39.4). Eating, drinking and smoking must not be carried out in any radiochemical laboratory.

39.3. Laboratory instrumentation and equipment

A wide variety of equipment will be required; the major items which might be found in a radiopharmacy are listed in Table 39.3. Some of these are discussed below:

Radiation monitoring. There will normally be several instruments available for measuring the level of radiation and for detecting contamination. Instruments with G.M. tubes are widely used as contamination detectors and radiation monitors. For quantitative gamma measurements and high sensitivity gamma probes scintillation detectors are employed. A selection of instruments is shown in Figure 39.2.

Quality testing instrumentation. Some of these will incorporate radiation detectors such as radiochromatogram scanners, whilst others measure classical physical and chemical quantities, such as pH or particle size. The range and amount of equipment will depend on

Table 39.3 Some of the major items of equipment which might be found in a radiopharmacy suite.

Re-entrant ionization chamber
Radiation monitoring equipment
Refrigerator
Autoclave
Lead shielding
Handling equipment—forceps etc.
Balance
Centrifuge
Quality testing equipment
    Radiochromatogram scanner
    Scintillation detector and multichannel analyser
    pH meter
    Microscope
    Thin layer chromatography (TLC) and/or paper chromatography apparatus

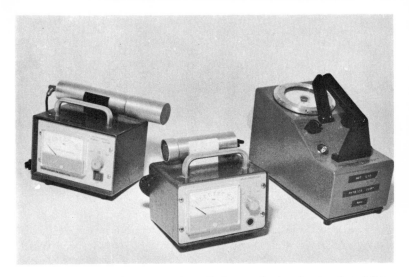

Fig. 39.2 A selection of instruments for radiation monitoring showing, from left to right, a thin window scintillation counter and a Geiger counter for general monitoring, and a scintillation dose-rate meter providing a logarithmic response over a wide range.

the size of the nuclear medicine facility. For measuring radionuclidic purity a detector and multichannel analyser is required. The best energy resolution is obtained using a semiconductor detector (Ch. 18) but sodium iodide scintillators are widely used and are satisfactory for many applications.

Graduated glassware. Work in nuclear medicine necessitates the use of pipettes, volumetric flasks, measuring cylinders, and, occasionally, burettes. All these items are specially calibrated to contain or deliver specified volumes of liquid—they are accurately calibrated and expensive pieces of equipment and must be treated with care.

Volumetric glassware is available in two standards of calibration: *Grade A*—which is generally reserved for work of the highest accuracy, and *Grade B*, which is the grade used in most laboratory work.

All graduated glassware is marked with the volume it contains and the temperature at which is was calibrated—normally 20°C. 'Bulb' pipettes are all calibrated 'to deliver' the specified volume after draining for 15 seconds and removing the last drop from the pipette by touching the side of the vessel or the surface of the liquid; all pipettes drain in a vertical position. Graduated or 'serological' pipettes are graduated in fractions of a ml—1/100, 1/50, 1/10, 1/5 depending on the total volume. Such pipettes calibrated to the tip are either calibrated 'to deliver' or more generally as 'blow out' which means that if the entire volume is required the last drop must be blown out of the pipette. Blow out pipettes are now frequently marked 'blow out'.

All volumetric glassware should be treated with care and should not be exposed to very high temperatures if it is to be used for accurate work.

A wide range of 'disposable' pipettes is now available and although these are relatively expensive they have many advantages in radiopharmaceutical work. In radioisotope laboratories liquids should never be drawn into pipettes by mouth suction—suitable pipetting devices must always be used.

Balances. A good balance for weighing out chemicals or for weighing injection vials before and after injection is an essential in the nuclear medicine laboratory. The most suitable balance is a modern analytical balance which is capable of weighing to 0·0001 g with a high degree of accuracy. The analytical balance is a precision instrument which must be handled with care. The balance must be carefully set up on a vibration-free mounting; its maintenance and adjustment is a skilled job and should be carried out only by an experienced balance technician.

Centrifuges. A centrifuge is required for the separation of blood cells and plasma and for some other operations in nuclear medicine. In general a standard laboratory centrifuge with a maximum speed of 3000 to 4000 r.p.m. and a 4 or 6 × 50 ml capacity is all that is required. Automatic timers are now common and are a very useful accessory.

The essential point in using a centrifuge is to ensure that the buckets diametrically opposite each other contain the same weight and size of tube or bottle. Tubes or bottles should be balanced against each other using a simple balance. For minor differences in weight the buckets may be balanced by placing small quantities of water between the bucket and the tube. If there are major differences in the weights of sample tubes, each sample tube, in its bucket, should be balanced separately against a similar tube filled with approximately the same volume of water or other suitable liquid.

Failure to balance centrifuge buckets and contents will result in 'rough' running of the centrifuge. If the imbalance is small the rate of wear and tear on the machine will be increased, but major imbalance may lead to rotor failure which can cause extensive damage to the machine and laboratory and result in serious injury to staff.

Care must always be taken to ensure that the rubber cushions are in place in the centrifuge buckets. The cover of the centrifuge should always be closed before the machine is started up and not opened again until the machine has run down to a complete stop. Braking should never be assisted by placing the hand on the rotor or windshield—this can result in severe injury!

Regular cleaning of the centrifuge bowl and buckets should be carried out and damaged buckets, rotors, or rubber cushions should be replaced at once.

39.4. Procedures

Protective clothing. This must always be worn when handling radioactivity: at the minimum this involves gloves and gown or laboratory overall. In a Grade B laboratory overshoes should be worn.

Dispensing. A stock solution may be divided either by volume or by weight. The latter is the most accurate but is time consuming and, unless special precautions are taken, the most hazardous, due to direct irradiation of the operator. In most routine dispensing pipettes or syringes are used. Syringes must be shielded and are only accurate to a few per cent. However, they are the only method of carrying out aseptic transfers (to and from sealed containers). Pipettes are more accurate but require open containers. Due to the length of the pipette the radiation dose received by the hands is reduced compared with syringes.

Aseptic procedures. In many radiopharmaceutical procedures it is necessary to maintain sterility throughout the preparation. In such circumstances it is essential to use aseptic conditions and techniques. These techniques involve the use of sterile and pyrogen-free reagents, glassware, syringes and other materials. Usually aseptic operations are carried out with the reagents contained in serum vials, transfer being effected by sterile syringes and needles, and the rubber of each vial being carefully swabbed with a suitable antiseptic solution immediately prior to puncture. In certain circumstances less stringent environmental conditions may be acceptable but, as in all situations relating to aseptic procedures, the advice of a qualified pharmacist should be sought.

Measurement of activity. The activity of all incoming radio-pharmaceuticals and also the eluate from generators must be measured using a re-entrant ionization chamber (Ch. 18). There are a number of commercial instruments available and these can be calibrated using radioactive standards supplied by national laboratories or commercial firms. Ionization chambers are capable of measuring most radionuclides to within one or two per cent. The activity of the final patient vial must be within the limits for that radiopharmaceutical (if listed) laid down in the appropriate Pharmacopoeia; in many cases this is $\pm 10\%$. When dispensing is done from a stock solution of known radioactive concentration it is desirable that the dispensed activity should be checked to ensure that no errors have been made.

39.5. Waste disposal

Radioactive waste arises from a variety of sources, for example the excretion of radioactivity by patients after the injection of a radiopharmaceutical or the contaminated glassware used in the preparation of that radiopharmaceutical. Waste may be solid, liquid or gaseous in form and contain either long-lived or short-lived radionuclides.

The disposal of radioactive waste is covered by government regulations in most countries and these limit the amounts of activity which may be disposed by various means. In the United Kingdom disposal is strictly controlled by the Department of the Environment and each hospital and institution must have a certificate of authorisation for the disposal of waste. The limits laid down in the certificate are legally enforceable under the Radioactive Substance Act 1961.

In general a policy of local disposal by maximum dispersion in non-active material is encouraged. In the case of liquids this means flushing the activity down a drain leading to the main sewer of the institution. In the main sewer the activity is further diluted by all the other non-active liquid waste. The amount of activity which can be disposed by this method is mainly limited by the need to keep the concentration at the outlet of the sewer down to a safe level. In many regulations radionuclides are divided into short and long-lived, with a dividing line of the order of three months. A typical example of a liquid waste disposal regulation might be several gigabecquerels per month of short-lived and a few tens of megabecquerels per month of long-lived nuclides.

Solid waste is dispersed either by incineration or in the normal refuse collection. Limits are usually set in terms of both the activity per unit volume and the maximum activity per article (typically $0 \cdot 04$ MBq). The outlet for gaseous waste must be such that the waste is dispersed to the atmosphere and not drawn into another part of the same building, or into any other building.

In general it is easier to dispose of liquid waste and so empty stock bottles can be washed and the activity flushed down the sink. Waste with an activity which is too large for immediate disposal must be stored. In this case care must be taken not to mix short and long-lived radionuclides as the lengths of time involved before the activity has fallen to a low level are very different. For high activities of long-lived radionuclides local disposal may not be feasible within a reasonable length of time and long storage in a hospital is not desirable. In this case alternative procedures, such as collection and disposal by a government agency should be used. In the United Kingdom this agency is the National Waste Disposal Service operated by the Atomic Energy Authority.

3.9. Records

Records are required for a variety of purposes and in many cases are a legal requirement. Each institution has to devise its own system to suit local arrangements but simplicity should always be aimed at. Complex records are unlikely to be completed, thereby defeating the aim of the system.

Records of radioactive substance should be such that the complete life history of the consignment is available, from delivery to final disposal as waste. This is necessary not only for the efficient running of the department but also for radiation safety reasons and waste disposal requirements. All containers of radioactive material must be clearly labelled with the radionuclide, physical and chemical form and activity.

Pharmaceutical records are essential to ensure that the right radiopharmaceutical is administered to the patient at the correct time. These records can often be combined with radiation records to produce one comprehensive system for a nuclear medicine facility.

3.9. Emergency procedures

In the case of a spill of radioactivity the action will depend on the activity involved and the radiotoxicity of the radionuclide. The procedure discussed in this section apply to all significant spills, which may be defined as those which involve more than about a tenth of a megabecquerel amounts of a medium or low radiotoxicity radionuclide. National regulations or guidance must be studied, as well as any local regulations. Staff involved with ionising radiation in United Kingdom hospitals must read the relevant part of the *Code of Practice* (see Appendix 8).

Equipment should be kept readily available for use in emergency in any department where significant amounts of activity are handled. The essential items will depend on the type of work being carried out but will include protective clothing; decontamination materials; warning signs; equipment for the handling, temporary storage and disposal of contaminated articles; and portable monitoring equipment.

The following sequence of actions should be adhered to when a spill occurs.

When the accident has involved injury to staff or patients, first aid must be administered. At the same time a person qualified in protection, such as a physicist, must be called and the Radiation Safety Officer or equivalent informed.

The next concern is to stop the spread of contamination and clear people from the area of the spill. Care should be taken that people leaving the site are not contaminated, especially that they do not spread activity with their shoes. Before any further action is taken anybody involved must wear adequate protective clothing; this will involve at the minimum, overshoes or boots, gloves and gown. A suitable respirator may be needed.

Decontamination of persons takes priority over clearing up the spill. Protective and, if possible, other outer clothing which is contaminated with radioactive substances should be removed and left in the contaminated area. Activity in the eye should be washed out with copious amounts of saline or water. Contaminated skin must be washed thoroughly with soap and water. If this fails to remove the activity detergent may be used but any further action should only be taken with care as the skin must not become broken or porous. A shower bath may be required but only after the major areas of contamination have been cleaned. When there is any question of ingestion of radioactivity then medical advice must be sought or a whole body count carried out.

In clearing up spills appropriate equipment must be used. For simple spills this only means soap, water and absorbent material. Commercial detergents and decontamination agents can be of great value. Contaminated articles, clothing and waste can be removed from the site of the spill in plastic or non-absorbent bags. For short-lived radionuclides, if activity still remains on a surface after decontamination, the surface should be suitably covered until the radioactivity has decayed to a sufficiently low level.

Safety within the department of nuclear medicine

40.1. General safety

All members of staff are in frequent contact with potentially dangerous equipment and materials, careless or improper use of which can result in serious accident and physical injury to both themselves and others. If, however, they are aware of the risks and behave in a responsible manner, the likelihood of an accident is very small. Safety is a matter of informed commonsense on the part of everyone working in the department or area.

In many countries workers' safety is now covered by legislation; in the United Kingdom this is contained in the Health and Safety at Work Act. The ultimate responsibility for safety lies with the employing organisations and Heads of Departments are responsible for ensuring that a proper safety code is prepared and operating. Notwithstanding any legal requirements every member of staff has a primary responsibility for ensuring that all proper safety procedures are carried out, and potential hazards reported, so that neither the individual nor his or her patients and colleagues come to any harm. Never ignore a potentially dangerous situation and do not be afraid to ask advice, admit a mistake or 'make a fuss'.

This chapter deals briefly with a wide range of possible hazards. Radiation risks are usually widely appreciated and hence well controlled. In practice they are often small compared with other less publicised risks within the department. For all cases certain general rules apply:

1. Always seek expert advice if you are in doubt.

2. Deal with any hazardous situation immediately—don't leave it until a more convenient time!

3. Be well acquainted with the layout of your Department, particularly with regard to emergency exits and evacuation plans, firefighting appliances, radioactive emergency equipment, telephones, first-aid kits and the like.

4. Keep gangways, passages and exits clear at all times.

5. Be acquainted with any specific emergency instructions applicable to your Department.

6. Good records should be kept, including the date of regular safety checks, faults found and when rectified, and details of any accidents.

Various specialist pamphlets are available, a selection of which is listed in Appendix 8.

40.2. Radiation safety

Hazards from radioactive materials create the most obvious potential risk in a nuclear medicine department, and therefore tend to attract the most attention. The biological effects of ionising radiation and the international regulations governing their use have already been discussed in Chapter 10. With proper care it is possible to keep the radiation exposure of staff down to a small fraction of the maximum permissible levels.

In the majority of countries there is legislation requiring the regular monitoring of both staff and of laboratory areas. Personnel monitoring is usually carried out using film badges, or thermo-luminescent dosemeters containing lithium fluoride. Monitors must be worn at all times when the staff-member is likely to be in the neighbourhood of a radiation source.

Apart from the obvious chances of exposure within the radiopharmacy (see Ch. 39) personnel are most exposed by being in proximity to patients who have been injected, or in handling syringes containing radiopharmaceuticals. In the first case distance and time can reduce the exposure considerably, whilst syringe shields constructed from suitable materials significantly reduce the finger dose when injecting.

It is often useful if the dose-rate due to a γ-emitter can be estimated. This can be quickly calculated, provided the nature and amount of radioactivity to be handled is known, by the use of 'exposure rate constant' Γ, formerly known as the k-factor. It is defined as the exposure rate at 1 cm in air from a point source whose activity is 1 GBq, and normally has units of $C\,kg^{-1}\,h^{-1}\,GBq^{-1}$ at 1 cm. It may be calculated from a knowledge of the decay scheme and values for common radionuclides are given in Table 40.1. The exposure rate constant is also given in terms of röntgen per hour for 1 mCi of activity at 1 cm as tables of Γ in these old units are still widely found.

As an example consider a patient containing 2 GBq of ^{131}I who is being measured at a distance of 2 m from the operator. Since the Γ for ^{131}I is $0\cdot015\,C\,kg^{-1}\,h^{-1}$ per GBq at 1 cm the exposure rate at 1 cm from a 2 GBq source will be $0\cdot03\,C\,kg^{-1}\,h^{-1}$. At 2 m (i.e. 200 cm) it

Table 40.1 Exposure rate constants, Γ, for selected γ-ray emitters.

Nuclide	Energies and percentage abundances (in brackets) of principal γ and X-rays. (MeV)				Γ C kg^{-1} GBq^{-1} h^{-1} at 1 cm	R mCi^{-1} h^{-1} at 1 cm
^{24}Na	1·37	(100)	2·75	(100)	0·13	18.4
^{42}K	1·52	(18)			0·010	1·4
^{51}Cr	0·32	(9)			0·0011	0·16
^{59}Fe	1·1	(56)	1·29	(44)	0·045	6·4
^{57}Co	0·12	(87)	0·14	(18)	0·0062	0·88
^{58}Co	0·81	(99)	0·51	(30)	0·038	5·4
^{99}Tc^m	0·14	(90)	0·019	(8)	0·0054	0·77
^{123}I	0·028	(89)	0·16	(83)	0·010	1·46
^{125}I	0·027–0·032	(140)	0·035	(7)	0·0042	0·6
^{131}I	0·36	(83)	0·64	(7)	0·015	2·2
^{137}Cs	0·66	(85)	0·03	(7)	0·022	3·1

will have dropped to 0.75×10^{-6} C kg^{-1} h^{-1} according to the inverse square law. If we wish to reduce to $<0.1\,\mu$C kg^{-1} h^{-1} then lead shielding will be required. From Table 7.1 the half value thickness of ^{131}I γ rays in lead is 6 mm. Thus 3 HVTs ($=1.8$ cm) will reduce the dose by 2^3 ($=8$), that is to $0.09\,\mu$C kg^{-1} h^{-1}. Should the operator remain in this position for 15 minutes he will receive a total exposure of $0.02\,\mu$C kg^{-1}.

The exposure rate constant can also be used for quick dosimetry calculations—if the radioactive content of one organ is known, then the exposure rate at another part of the body can be estimated. It may also be of assistance in rough estimates of total body retention of therapy doses of ^{131}I; a measurement of the exposure rate at a known distance from the patient, such as 2 m, is used to calculate the amount of ^{131}I from a knowledge of Γ.

40.3. Mechanical safety
Mechanical safety of equipment should be checked frequently by a senior member of staff, and periodically by a qualified expert. In addition the operator of the equipment should be alert for possible faults. Points to watch include collimator fastenings, rigidity of heavy equipment, particularly that placed over patients (such as γ-cameras), sharp edges, corrosion, worn drives and 'free play'.

40.4. Electrical safety
Again repeated checks are obligatory. Likely sources of hazard are damaged or worn cables and particularly plug connections and cable clamps. Plugs for power sockets may have been wrongly or carelessly wired, and must only be attended to by qualified persons. The earth

connection may not be satisfactory and must be regularly checked. Particular care needs to be taken with any equipment likely to come in contact with patients—it is possible for the EHT supply to a photomultiplier to short onto the housing and the collimator, which may not be properly earthed!

Emergency switches for turning off all equipment should be installed and clearly marked.

40.5. Chemical safety

The two principal causes of accidents within chemical laboratories are exposure to toxic chemicals and carelessness in assembling and using equipment such as centrifuges or glassware. Great care must be taken when using, carrying, storing and disposing of any dangerous chemicals. When handling poisons and corrosive chemicals protective clothing must be worn, including eye shields if there is any possibility of splashing. Eating, drinking and smoking should be prohibited in chemical laboratories.

Within a nuclear medicine department the main areas of concern relate to the use of centrifuges and liquid scintillation solvents, the latter being both a toxic and a fire hazard. All chemicals must be clearly labelled.

40.6. Biological safety

As in any hospital department high standards of hygiene must be maintained. In nuclear medicine the biological risks are mainly connected with the collection and handling of blood samples. Whilst the use of disposable syringes and needles has largely overcome the danger of directly transmitting infection from patient to patient the risk to the operator through accidental inoculation remains. Extreme care is necessary when transferring blood from the syringe to the container and the needles must be disposed of safely. Any spillages should be treated with disinfectant.

Specimens from known or suspected cases of viral hepatitis must be handled with extreme care and be distinctly marked. Care is also needed in the disposal of used needles and syringes. Preferably these should be burnt.

40.7. Fire

In all cases of fire, the fire alarm should be raised by the designated procedure for your department. Speed is essential at this stage. Any patients should be removed from the vicinity of the fire, doors and windows closed, electrical equipment (including ventilation) switched off and preferably unplugged, and suitable fire extinguishers applied.

Circumstances will dictate the order in which these actions shall be carried out.

The most likely cause of fire is faulty electrical equipment. Should it occur, immediately switch off all equipment and use either a CO_2 or a bromochlorodifluoromethane (BCF) extinguisher—water must not be used.

Prevention is better than cure. Overloading of electrical circuits can be highly dangerous; only working stocks of flammable solvents should be kept within the department, and these should be kept in non-flammable containers away from strong acids or alkalis and electrical equipment.

40.8. First aid and medical emergencies

Clearly labelled first aid boxes must be provided in readily accessible positions; they must be regularly checked and any deficiencies made good. Any laboratory where chemical or radioactive procedures are carried out should also be equipped with emergency eye wash equipment and instructions for dealing with hazardous chemicals.

Medical emergency equipment should be available, as in any other area where patients are treated.

Appendices

Appendix 1

Revision of basic mathematics

The mathematics required to understand the basic science of nuclear medicine is neither extensive nor difficult. However the topics presented in this Appendix are important and should be clearly understood. Anybody who has not encountered these topics before should consult a suitable introductory text.

A1.1. Exponents or indices

The use of exponents is a convenient way of writing down a number multiplied by itself several times. For example, $2 \times 2 \times 2 \times 2 = 2^4$, where 4 is called the exponent or index of 2. The expression '2 raised to the fourth power' can be used to describe 2^4.

In general
$$a \times a \times a \ldots n \text{ times} = a^n$$

This notation is also valuable in writing large numbers, for example, the velocity of light is 300 000 000 metres per second; it is more convenient to write this as 3×10^8. More important, it leads to simpler calculations and is the basis of logarithms. There are four rules governing indices:

Rule 1. $a^m \times a^n = a^{m+n}$ (e.g. $3^2 \times 3^3 = 3^5$)
Rule 2. $a^m \div a^n = a^{m-n}$ (e.g. $2^4 \div 2^3 = 2$)
Rule 3. $a^0 = 1$ (put $m = n$ in Rule 2)
Rule 4. $a^{-n} = a^{1/n}$

The nth root of a number, a, $\sqrt[n]{a}$, is $a^{1/n}$. For the example the cube root of 9, $\sqrt[3]{9}$, can be written $9^{1/3}$.

A1.2. Logarithms

This is a simple extension of the use of exponents and is a method of multiplication by addition, and division by subtraction.

For example:

$\left.\begin{array}{l} 16 = 2^4 \\ 8 = 2^3 \end{array}\right\}$ $\therefore$ To multiply 16 by 8
$16 \times 8 = 2^4 \times 2^3 = 2^7 = 128$

399

When a number N is written in the form a^x then the index x is called the logarithm to the base of a of N.

$$N = a^x$$
$$x = \log_a N$$

The two basic rules of logarithms are:

Rule 1. $\log_a(XY) = \log_a X + \log_a Y$
Rule 2. $\log_a(X/Y) = \log_a X - \log_a Y$

These are the same as Rules 1 and 2 in A1.1 above, except they are written using logarithmic notation. In addition to these two rules there is one covering the situation where X is raised to the power p:

Rule 3. $\log_a X^p = p\log_a X$

Common logarithms
With our decimal system, it is natural to standardise and use 10 as the base, written '$\log_{10}$' or 'log', where the subscript is implied.

Number	Log
$1000 = 10^3$	3
$1000 = 10^2$	2
$10 = 10^1$	1
$1 = 10^0$	0
$0.1 = 10^{-1}$	-1
$0.01 = 10^{-2}$	-2

The logarithm of an intermediate number will be a fraction and can be looked up in tables of logarithms. In order to convert a logarithm to the corresponding number we use a table of antilogarithms (or antilogs).

Worked example. Calculate 3.452×26.2

Taking logs:

$\log_{10} 3.452 = 0.5381$ (from tables)
$\log_{10} 26.2 \ \ = 1.4183$
add: $\quad\quad\quad 1.9564$

Taking the antilog of 1.9564 we obtain the value of 90.45

$(\log_{10} 90.45 = 1.9564)$

Thus the answer is 90.45.

The number before the decimal point is called the characteristic and that after is called the mantissa. When taking the logarithm of a number the characteristic is determined by inspection and the mantissa from tables. When looking up antilogs only the mantissa is used and the characteristic determines the position of the decimal point. For example:

$$\log_{10} 26 \cdot 2 = 1 \cdot 4183$$

characteristic   mantissa

Numbers less than 1. The system used can best be explained with an example:

Number	Log	
$481 = 4 \cdot 81 \times 10^2$	$0 \cdot 6821 + 2 = 2 \cdot 6821$	mantissa
$4 \cdot 81 = 4 \cdot 81 \times 10^0$	$0 \cdot 6821 + 0 = 0 \cdot 6821$	is the same
$0 \cdot 481 = 4 \cdot 81 \times 10^{-1}$	$0 \cdot 6821 - 1 = -0 \cdot 3179$	

This last number involves a change of mantissa and would require a separate set of tables for each power of ten. It is therefore written as $\bar{1} \cdot 6821$ and similarly

$$0 \cdot 0481 = 4 \cdot 81 \times 10^{-2} \qquad 0 \cdot 6821 - 2 = \bar{2} \cdot 6821$$

$$- 2 + 0 \cdot 6821$$

The characteristic is given by the number of zeros after the decimal point plus one.

Worked example.   Divide $0 \cdot 240$ by $0 \cdot 00044$

$$\log_{10} 0 \cdot 240 \qquad = \bar{1} \cdot 3802$$
$$\log_{10} 0 \cdot 000444 = \bar{4} \cdot 6434$$
$$545 \cdot 5 \leftarrow 2 \cdot 7368 \quad \text{(subtracting)}$$

Care is required as the numbers after the decimal point are positive, whilst those before the characteristic are negative. The subtraction in full is:

$$(-1 + 0 \cdot 3802) - (-4 + 0 \cdot 6434)$$

Natural or naperian logarithms

Instead of using a base of 10 a base e, where $e = 2 \cdot 718$, can be used. The logarithm is written either $\log_e$ or $\ln$. The value of e is given by:

$$e = 1 + \frac{1}{1} + \frac{1}{1 \times 2} + \frac{1}{1 \times 2 \times 3} + \frac{1}{1 \times 2 \times 3 \times 4} + \cdots$$

$$= 1 + 1 + 0 \cdot 5 + 0 \cdot 1666 + 0 \cdot 0416$$

$$= 2 \cdot 718 \ldots$$

The constant e is of importance in calculus as the integral of $\dfrac{1}{N}$ is $\log_e N$.

$$\int \frac{dN}{N} = \log_e N$$

It occurs in several equations used in nuclear medicine, such as radioactive decay, $A = A_0 e^{-\lambda t}$.

Conversion from naperian to common logarithms.

Let $N = e^x$

Take $\log_{10}$

$$\log_{10} N = \log_{10} e^x = x \log_{10} e \qquad \text{(using Rule 3)}.$$

Now $x = \log_e N$

and from $\log_{10}$ tables, $\log_{10} e = 0.4343$.

$$\therefore \quad \log_{10} N = 0.4343 \log_e N$$

or $\log_e N = 2.303 \log_{10} N$

A1.3.   Graphs and equations

If two quantities, x and y, are directly proportional to each other, then if x is plotted against y a straight line is obtained (Fig. A1.1).

The equation of the line is

$$y = mx + c$$

$$m \text{ gives the slope} = \frac{y_1 - c}{x_1}$$

and c is the value of the intercept on the y axis.

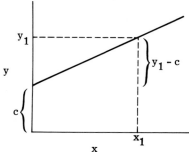

Fig. A1.1 Graph of the equation $y = mx + c$.

A linear relationship between x and y is the simplest relationship but in many cases the relationship is an exponential one. This means that y is proportional to e raised to the xth power.

$$y = ae^x \qquad a = \text{constant}$$

Two similar equations are

$$y = ae^{-x}$$

$$\text{and } y = a(1 - e^{-x})$$

Calculating $y(a = 1)$

x	e^x	e^{-x}	$(1 - e^{-x})$
0	1·00	1·00	0·0
0·5	1·65	0·61	0·39
1	2·72	0·37	0·63
2	7·39	0·13	0·865
3	20·1	0·050	0·95
4	54·6	0·018	0·98
5	148	0·007	0·993

Figure A1.2 shows these three equations plotted out using normal linear graph paper. It will be noted that $y = e^{-x}$ never actually reaches zero but is said to tend to zero. Similarly $y = a(1 - e^{-x})$ tends to a. The slope of the lines is steadily changing, either increasing ($y = ae^x$) or decreasing ($y = ae^{-x}$ and $y = a(1 - e^{-x})$).

These equations are encountered in

1. Absorption of X and γ radiation (Ch. 7)

$$I = I_0 e^{-\mu x}$$

2. Radioactive decay (Ch. 4)

$$A = A_0 e^{-\lambda t}$$

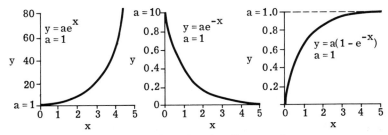

Fig. A1.2 Three exponential equations plotted on linear graph paper.

3. Build up of activity in targets irradiated with neutrons (Ch. 8).
4. Biological situations, e.g. clearance of activity from blood (Ch. 12).

It is valuable to plot exponential changes as a straight line graph.

Consider $y = ae^x$

Take $\log_{10}$

$$\log_{10}y = \log_{10}(ae^x) = \log_{10}a + \log_{10}e^x$$

$$= \log_{10}a + x\log_{10}e$$

$$= \log_{10}a + 0{\cdot}4343x$$

This is the same form as

$$y = mx + c$$

where $c \equiv \log_{10}a$

$y \equiv \log_{10}y$

and $m \equiv 0{\cdot}4343$

Therefore if $\log_{10}y$ is plotted against x a straight line is obtained (Fig. A1.3).

All the graphs plotted so far in this Appendix have been on linear-linear paper, that is the x and y scales have regular intervals. To simplify the plotting of exponential equations and to save using log tables, log-linear graph paper is available. With this type of paper the x-axis has a regular scale as before but the y-axis is logarithmic (Fig. A1.4). This enables y to be plotted directly onto the paper without having to look up tables of logarithms. The range of the y-axis, in terms of powers of ten, is called the number of cycles.

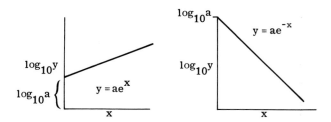

Fig. A1.3 The equations $y = ae^x$ and $y = ae^{-x}$ plotted as straight lines by plotting $\log_{10}y$ against x on linear graph paper.

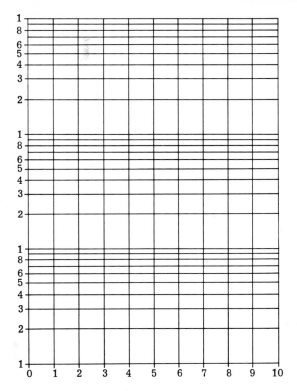

Fig. A1.4 An example of 3 cycle log-linear graph paper.

Appendix 2

Mathematical derivations

A2.1. The exponential law of radioactivity decay (Ch. 4)

Consider N atoms of a radioactive substance at time t. Let λ be the transformation constant, the chance which each radioactive atom has of decaying per unit of time.

In a very short interval of time, Δt (immediately after time t), a certain number of atoms, ΔN, will decay.

$$\Delta N = -N\lambda\Delta t \qquad \text{(equation 4.1)}$$

The negative sign indicates that there is a decrease in the number of radioactive atoms. Replacing the increments ΔN and Δt by their differentials:

$$dN = -N\lambda dt$$

Rearrange
$$\frac{dN}{N} = -\lambda dt$$

Integrate
$$\int \frac{dN}{N} = -\lambda \int dt \ .$$

Now remembering that

$$\int \frac{dx}{x} = \log_e x + c$$

$$\log_e N = -\lambda t + c \qquad \text{(A2.1)}$$

where c is a constant.

Let N_0 be the number of radioactive atoms at time $t = 0$.
Put $t = 0$ in the above equation (A2.1)

$$\log_e N_0 = c$$

Substituting back into equation (A2.1) for c gives

$$\log_e N = -\lambda t + \log_e N_0$$

Rearrange

$$\log_e N - \log_e N_0 = -\lambda t$$

$$\log_e \left(\frac{N}{N_0} \right) = -\lambda t \qquad \text{(equation 4.3)}$$

Hence

$$\frac{N}{N_0} = e^{-\lambda t} \qquad \text{(see Appendix A1)}$$

and

$$N = N_0 e^{-\lambda t}$$

A2.2. The exponential law of attenuation of electromagnetic radiation (Ch. 7)

The mathematics involved are identical to that used to derive the exponential law of radioactive decay.

Let I be the intensity of a narrow beam of electromagnetic radiation after passing through material of thickness x and let μ be the linear attenuation coefficient. If the beam passes through a further very thin thickness, Δx, its intensity will decrease by ΔI.

$$\Delta I = -I \mu \Delta x$$

Replace ΔI and Δx by their corresponding differentials and rearranging:

$$\frac{dI}{I} = -\mu dx$$

Integrate

$$\int \frac{dI}{I} = -\int \mu dx$$

$$\log_e I = -\mu x + c \qquad \text{(A2.2)}$$

If the intensity of the beam before passing through the material ($x = 0$) is I_0 then substituting into equation (A2.2)

$$\log_e I_0 = c$$

Substitute for c in (A2.2) and rearrange

$$\log_e \left(\frac{I}{I_0} \right) = -\mu x$$

Therefore

$$I = I_0 e^{-\mu x}$$

A2.3.   Build up of activity in target bombarded by neutrons (Ch. 8)

Let B atoms of the radionuclide of interest (transformation constant λ) be formed per unit time and let the number of radioactive atoms present in the target at time t be N and the corresponding activity be A.

Rate of change of number of radioactive atoms in target $= \dfrac{dN}{dt}$

$$\frac{dN}{dt} = \text{Rate of formation} - \text{Rate of decay.}$$

$$\frac{dN}{dt} = B - \lambda N$$

Multiply by $e^{\lambda t}$

$$e^{\lambda t}\frac{dN}{dt} = Be^{\lambda t} - \lambda N e^{\lambda t}$$

$$e^{\lambda t}\frac{dN}{dt} + \lambda N e^{\lambda t} = Be^{\lambda t}$$

or

$$\frac{d}{dt}(Ne^{\lambda t}) = Be^{\lambda t} \qquad \left[\text{N.B.}\,\frac{d}{dt}(XY) = Y\frac{dX}{dt} + X\frac{dY}{dt}\right]$$

Integrate

$$Ne^{\lambda t} = \frac{B}{\lambda}e^{\lambda t} + c$$

where $c = $ constant of integration.
Multiply by $e^{-\lambda t}$:

$$N = \frac{B}{\lambda} + ce^{-\lambda t}$$

At $t = 0$ there will be no radioactivity in the target and therefore $N = 0$

$$c = -\frac{B}{\lambda}$$

Therefore

$$N = \frac{B}{\lambda} - \frac{B}{\lambda}e^{-\lambda t}$$

$$N = \frac{B}{\lambda}(1 - e^{-\lambda t})$$

At $t = \infty$ the rate of formation will equal the rate of decay and the number of radioactive atoms will be constant, N_s, and the corresponding activity A_s.

$$N_s = \frac{B}{\lambda}$$

Substitute for $\dfrac{B}{\lambda}$

$$N = N_s(1 - e^{-\lambda t})$$

Now

$$A = \lambda N$$

Therefore

$$A = A_s(1 - e^{-\lambda t})$$

A2.4.   Parent-daughter relationships (Ch. 37)

This is a similar but more complex example of the problem dealt with in A2.3.

Consider N_1 atoms of a parent radionuclide, at time t, which is decaying into a radioactive daughter. Let there be N_2 atoms of the daughter at time t. λ_1 and λ_2 are the transformation constants and A_1 and A_2 their activities (Fig. A2.1). If N_1^0 is the initial number (at $t = 0$) of the parent atoms then the basic decay equation for the parent is

$$N_1 = N_1^0 e^{-\lambda_1 t} \tag{A2.3}$$

Rate of change of parent. The rate of change of the number of atoms of the parent, $\dfrac{dN_1}{dt}$, is equal to the rate of decay of the parent, $-\lambda_1 N_1$

$$\frac{dN_1}{dt} = -\lambda_1 N_1 \tag{A2.4}$$

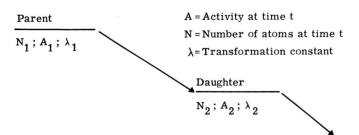

Parent

$N_1 ; A_1 ; \lambda_1$

A = Activity at time t

N = Number of atoms at time t

λ = Transformation constant

Daughter

$N_2 ; A_2 ; \lambda_2$

Fig. A2.1 Decay of parent radionuclide into radioactive daughter nuclide.

Rate of change of daughter. The rate of change of the number of atoms of the daughter, $\dfrac{dN_2}{dt}$, equals the rate of formation minus the rate of decay:

$$\frac{dN_2}{dt} = \lambda_1 N_1 - \lambda_2 N_2 \qquad (A2.5)$$

Substitute for N_1 in A2.5 using A2.3

$$\frac{dN_2}{dt} = \lambda_1 N_1^0 e^{-\lambda_1 t} - \lambda_2 N_2$$

Multiply by $e^{\lambda_2 t}$ and rearrange:

$$e^{\lambda_2 t}\frac{dN_2}{dt} + \lambda_2 N_2 e^{\lambda_2 t} = \lambda_1 N_1^0 e^{(\lambda_2 - \lambda_1)t}$$

or

$$\frac{d}{dt}(N_2 e^{\lambda_2 t}) = \lambda_1 N_1^0 e^{(\lambda_2 - \lambda_1)t}\left[\; \text{N.B.} \; \frac{d}{dt}(XY) = \frac{YdX}{dt} + \frac{XdY}{dt}\right]$$

Integrate

$$N_2 e^{\lambda_2 t} = \frac{\lambda_1}{\lambda_2 - \lambda_1} N_1^0 e^{(\lambda_2 - \lambda_1)t} + c$$

where c is the constant of integration.
Multiply by $e^{-\lambda_2 t}$:

$$N_2 = \frac{\lambda_1}{\lambda_2 - \lambda_1} N_1^0 e^{-\lambda_1 t} + c e^{-\lambda_2 t} \qquad (A2.6)$$

If at $t = 0$ there are zero atoms of the daughter, for example immediately after elution, then by substituting $t = 0$ into equation A2.6

$$c = \frac{-\lambda_1}{\lambda_2 - \lambda_1} N_1^0$$

Substituting into A2.6 and rearranging:

$$N_2 = \frac{\lambda_1}{\lambda_2 - \lambda_1} N_1^0 (e^{-\lambda_1 t} - e^{-\lambda_2 t}) \qquad (A2.7)$$

The number of atoms N_1 and N_2 are related to their corresponding activities A_1 and A_2 by

$$A_1 = \lambda_1 N_2 \quad \text{and} \quad A_2 = \lambda_2 N_2$$

Substituting for N_1^0 and N_2 in A2.7

$$A_2 = \frac{\lambda_2}{\lambda_2 - \lambda_1} A_1^0 (e^{-\lambda_1 t} - e^{-\lambda_2 t}) \tag{A2.8}$$

Maximum activity of daughter. Differentiate A2.8 with respect to time.

$$\frac{dA_2}{dt} = \frac{\lambda_2}{\lambda_2 - \lambda_1} A_1^0 (-\lambda_1 e^{-\lambda_1 t} + \lambda_2 e^{-\lambda_2 t})$$

The maximum activity of the daughter will occur when

$$\frac{dA_2}{dt} = 0$$

Hence,

$$\lambda_1 e^{-\lambda_1 t} = \lambda_2 e^{-\lambda_2 t}$$

$$e^{(\lambda_2 - \lambda_1)t} = \frac{\lambda_2}{\lambda_1}$$

Take the ln

$$t(\lambda_2 - \lambda_1) = \ln\frac{\lambda_2}{\lambda_1}$$

$$\therefore \quad t = \frac{1}{(\lambda_2 - \lambda_1)} \ln\frac{\lambda_2}{\lambda_1}$$

A2.5.   Fourier analysis (Ch. 28)

A temporal function $f(t)$ can be expressed in terms of the sum of a series of cosine waves.

$$f(t) = a_0 + a_1 (\cos \omega t - \Phi_1)$$
$$+ a_2 (\cos 2\omega t - \Phi_2)$$
$$+ a_3 (\cos 3\omega t - \Phi_3)$$
$$+ \cdots\cdots\cdots ,$$
$$= a_0 + \sum_{n=1}^{\infty} a_n (\cos n\omega t - \Phi_n)$$

where ω is the frequency of the function $\left(= \dfrac{2\pi}{T}, \text{where } T \text{ is the period}\right.$

of the function $f(t)\Big)$.

a_n are the amplitudes

and

Φ_n are the phases.

The process of determining the amplitudes and phases is called Fourier transformation:

$$F(\omega) = \mathrm{F}(f(t))$$

where F denotes the Fourier transform operation and $F(\omega)$ is the Fourier transform. The reverse process (from frequency domain to time domain) is called inverse Fourier transformation.

Appendix 3

S.I. units

The International System of Units (SI) has been adopted by most countries and is being steadily introduced. The system is based on seven basic physical quantities, the metre, kilogram, second, ampere (for electric current), candela (for luminous intensity) kelvin (for thermodynamic temperature) and mole (for amount of substance) as listed in Table A3.1. Decimal fractions and multiples of these basic units may be constructed by using the prefixes listed in Table A3.2.

Only one unit for any one physical quantity is permitted as an SI unit and all other physical quantities are regarded as being derived

Table A3.1 Names and symbols for basic SI units

Physical quantity	Name of SI unit	Symbol for SI unit
length	metre	m
mass	kilogram	kg
time	second	s
electric current	ampere	A
thermodynamic temperature	kelvin	K
luminous intensity	candela	cd
amount of substance	mole	mol

Table A3.2 Prefixes for SI units

The following prefixes may be used to indicate decimal fractions or multiples of the basic (Table A3.1) or derived (Table A3.3) SI units

Fraction	Prefix	Symbol	Multiple	Prefix	Symbol
10^{-1}	deci	d	10	deka	da
10^{-2}	centi	c	10^2	hecto	h
10^{-3}	milli	m	10^3	kilo	k
10^{-6}	micro	μ	10^6	mega	M
19^{-9}	nano	n	10^9	giga	G
10^{-12}	pico	p	10^{12}	tera	T
10^{-15}	femto	f	10^{15}	peta	P
10^{-18}	atto	a	10^{18}	exa	E

from the seven basic units by multiplication or division without numerical factors being involved. Many of these derived units have special names and those relevant to this book are listed in Table A3.3. Those with no special names are tabulated in Table A3.4.

Table A3.5 lists decimal fractions or multiples of SI units having special names; many of these are widely used but, with the exception of the litre, are not officially recognised and will be progressively abandoned. Table A3.6 gives conversion factors from non-SI units into the correct SI unit.

Table A3.3 Special names and symbols for derived SI units

Physical quantity	Name of SI unit	Symbol for SI unit	Definition of SI unit
energy, work, quantity of heat	joule	J	$\mathrm{kg\,m^2\,s^{-2}}$
force	newton	N	$\mathrm{kg\,m\,s^{-2}} = \mathrm{J\,m^{-1}}$
power	watt	W	$\mathrm{kg\,m^2\,s^{-3}} = \mathrm{J\,s^{-1}}$
pressure	pascal	Pa	$\mathrm{kg\,m^{-1}\,s^{-2}} = \mathrm{N\,m^{-2}}$
frequency	hertz	Hz	$\mathrm{s^{-1}}$
Electricity			
electric charge	coulomb	C	$\mathrm{A\,s}$
electric potential difference	volt	V	$\mathrm{kg\,m^2\,s^{-3}\,A^{-1}} = \mathrm{J\,A^{-1}\,s^{-1}}$
electric resistance	ohm	Ω	$\mathrm{kg\,m^2\,s^{-3}\,A^{-2}} = \mathrm{V\,A^{-1}}$
electric capacitance	farad	F	$\mathrm{A^2\,s^4\,kg^{-1}\,m^{-2}} = \mathrm{A\,s\,V^{-1}}$
inductance	henry	H	$\mathrm{kg\,m^2\,s^{-2}\,A^{-2}} = \mathrm{V\,A^{-1}\,s}$
Radiation			
activity	becquerel	Bq	$\mathrm{s^{-1}}$
absorbed dose	gray	Gy	$\mathrm{J\,kg^{-1}}$
dose equivalent	sievert	Sv	$\mathrm{J\,kg^{-1}}$

Table A3.4 Some examples of derived SI units and unit symbols for other quantities

Physical quantity	SI unit	Symbol or definition of SI unit
area	square metre	$\mathrm{m^2}$
volume	cubic metre	$\mathrm{m^3}$
density	kilogram per cubic metre	$\mathrm{kg\,m^{-3}}$
velocity	metre per second	$\mathrm{m\,s^{-1}}$
acceleration	metre per square second	$\mathrm{m\,s^{-2}}$
electric field strength	volt per metre	$\mathrm{V\,m^{-1}}$
magnetic field strength	ampere per metre	$\mathrm{A\,m^{-1}}$
wave number	1 per metre	$\mathrm{m^{-1}}$
molality	mole per kilogram	$\mathrm{mol\,kg^{-1}}$
concentration	mole per cubic decimetre	$\mathrm{mol\,dm^{-3}}$
exposure	coulomb per kilogram	$\mathrm{C\,kg^{-1}}$

Table A3.5 Decimal fractions and multiples of SI units having special names

Physical quantity	Name of unit	Symbol for unit	Definition of unit
length	micron	μm	10^{-6} m
area	barn	b	10^{-28} m^2
volume	litre	l	10^{-3} m^3 = dm^3
force	dyne	dyn	10^{-5} N
pressure	bar	bar	10^5 Pa
energy	erg	erg	10^{-7} J

Table A3.6 Other units defined in terms of SI units

Physical quantity	Name of unit	Symbol for unit	Definition of unit
length	inch	in	$2\cdot54 \times 10^{-2}$ m
mass	pound	lb	$0\cdot454*$ kg
pressure	atmosphere	atm	$101*$kPa
energy	electron volt	eV	$1\cdot6 \times 10^{-19}*$J
Radiation:			
absorbed dose	rad	rad	10^{-2} Gy = 10^{-2} J kg^{-1}
activity	curie	Ci	$3\cdot7 \times 10^{10}$ Bq
exposure	roentgen	R	$2\cdot58 \times 10^{-4}$ C kg^{-1} air

* Approximate

A3.1.   Guidance on use of SI units

1. *SI unit of time.* The SI unit is the second (s) but the minute (min), hour (h) and day (d) have been approved for use although they are not coherent with SI.

2. *Prefixes.* Only one prefix may be used at a time with each unit. However more than one prefix may be used in expressions containing several units, for example a radionuclide concentration may be expressed in megabecquerels per millilitre, MBq ml^{-1}.

3. *Units.* Names of units are written in full with lower case letters (except when a unit begins a sentence) even if they are taken from a personal name, e.g. becquerel.

4. *Symbols.* Symbols for units do not take a plural form and should not be followed by a full stop. Symbols taken from personal names are written with the first letter in upper case, e.g. Bq, others are written with the first letter in lower case.

5. *Working units.* These should provide for convenient numerical values in relation to common usage:

Nuclear medicine. The megabecquerel has been generally adopted as $0\cdot01$ to 1000 MBq covers most situations in practice, although the prefix, giga, is widely used when dealing with higher activity sources, such as ^{99}Mo/^{99}Tc^m generators.

Radiation protection. In practice the millisievert (mSv) is a convenient unit.

Appendix 4

Symbols used in nuclear medicine

A4.1. Some Greek letters used as symbols

Letter	Name	Used for
α	Alpha	Name of nuclear particle
β	Beta	Name of nuclear particle
γ	Gamma	Name of nuclear electromagnetic radiation
		Slope of photographic density dose curve
Δ	Delta	Mean energy of radiation per nuclear transformation (dosimetry—previously called equilibrium dose constant)
		A small increment
θ	Theta	Symbol for an angle
λ	Lambda	Wavelength of electromagnetic radiation
		Decay constant
μ	Mu	Coefficient of attenuation
ν	Nu	Frequency of electromagnetic radiation
		Neutrino
π	Pi	Ratio of circumference to diameter of circle
ρ	Rho	Density of matter
σ	Sigma	Standard deviation
Σ	Sigma	The sum of, e.g. $\sum_i a_1 = a_1 + a_2 + a_3 \dots$
τ	Tau	Symbol for an angle
ϕ	Phi	Absorbed fraction (dosimetry)
Φ	Phi	Specific absorbed fraction (dosimetry)

Appendix 5

Physical data for dosimetric calculations (see Ch. 9)

Table A5.1 Summarised and simplified nuclear data for some common nuclides. All the gamma rays above 100 keV have been grouped together. $\Delta_s = \sum \Delta_i$.— This is used for non-penetrating radiation and where several X or γ-Rays have been summed. For complete data refer to MIRD pamphlet 10 and ICRU report 32 (see Appendix 8).

Element	Nuclide	Half-life	Type of decay	Type of radiation	Mean number per transformation (n_i)	Mean* Energy (MeV) $(\bar{E}_i)$	Δ_i or Δ_s $\text{fJ Bq}^{-1}\,\text{s}^{-1}$	Δ_i or Δ_s $\text{g rad}\,\mu\text{Ci}^{-1}\,\text{h}^{-1}$
Hydrogen	^{3}H	12.3y	β^-	Non-penetrating	1·00	0·006	0.9	0·012
Carbon	^{14}C	5730y	β^-	Non-penetrating	1·00	0·049	7.9	0·105
Phosphorus	^{32}P	14·3d	β^-	Non-penetrating	1·00	0·695	111·1	1·480
Chromium	^{51}Cr	27·8d	EC	Non-penetrating			0.7	0·010
				Penetrating	0·10	0·320	5.2	0·069
Iron	^{59}Fe	45d	β^-	Non-penetrating			18·8	0·251
				Non-penetrating	0·04†	0·14–0·38	1·3	0·017
				Penetrating	1·00†	1·10–1·48	188·8	2·516
Gallium	^{67}Ga	78h	EC	Non-penetrating			6·5	0·086
				Non-penetrating	0·41†	0·093‡	6·2	0·082
				Penetrating	0·47†	0·18–0·89	18·7	0·249
Selenium	^{75}Se	120d	EC	Non-penetrating			3·2	0·042
				Non-penetrating	0·01	0·066	0·1	0·001
				Penetrating	0·03	0·097	0·5	0·006
				Penetrating	1·65†	0·12–0·57‡	58·1	0·774
Yttrium	^{90}Y	64h	β^-	Non-penetrating	1·00	0·931	148·9	1·984
Technetium	^{99}Tc^{m}	6h	IT	Non-penetrating			2·8	0·037
				Non-penetrating	0·08	0·019‡	0·2	0·003
				Penetrating	0·88	0·140	19·7	0·263
Indium	^{113}In^{m}	99m	IT	Non-penetrating			22·8	0·304
				Non-penetrating	0·25†	0·025‡	0·9	0·012
				Penetrating	0·62	0·392	38·9	0·518

Table A5.1 (continued)

Element	Nuclide	Half-life	Type of Decay	Type of radiation	Mean number per transformation (n_i)	Mean* Energy (MeV) ($\bar{E}_i$)	Δ_i or Δ_s fJ Bq⁻¹ s⁻¹	Δ_i or Δ_s g rad μCi⁻¹ h⁻¹
Iodine	^{123}I	13h	EC	Non-penetrating	0·87†	0·028‡	4·6	0·061
				Penetrating	0·86†	0·16–0·78	3·9	0·052
							23·1	0·308
Iodine	^{125}I	60d	EC	Non-penetrating	1·40†	0·028‡	3·2	0·043
				Penetrating	0·07	0·035	6·2	0·083
							0·4	0·005
Iodine	^{131}I	8d	β^-	Non-penetrating	0·05†	0·030‡	30·6	0·408
					0·03	0·080	0·2	0·003
				Penetrating	0·97†	0·17–0·73	0·3	0·004
Gold	^{198}Au	2·7d	β^-	Non-penetrating	0·03†	0·072‡	59·8	0·797
							52·5	0·699
				Penetrating	0·97	0·41–1·09	0·3	0·004
							64·4	0·858

* The range of energies given where γ-Rays have been grouped together.
† Sum of several X or γ-Ray
‡ Weighted mean of several X or γ-Rays

Table A5.2 Absorbed fractions, ϕ, for uniform sources in various organs. From MIRD pamphlet 5. Adapted with permission of the publisher.

Photon energies, E (MeV)

Target Organ	0·020	0·030	0·050	0·100	0·500	1·00
			Source Organ—Bladder			
Bladder	0·745	0·464	0·201	0·117	0·116	0·107
Marrow	0·138E-03	0·577E-02	0·202E-01	0·181E-01	0·895E-02	0·760E-02
Ovaries*	0·259E-04	0·229E-04	0·344E-03	0·252E-03	0·200E-03	0·174E-03
Testes*	0·813E-04	0·799E-03	0·126E-02	0·941E-03	0·754E-03	0·648E-03
Kidneys			0·102E-03	0·360E-03	0·390E-03	0·473E-03
			Source Organ—Kidneys			
Kidneys	0·582	0·298	0·112	0·661E-01	0·730E-01	0·670E-01
Liver	0·808E-02	0·264E-01	0·359E-01	0·282E-01	0·229E-01	0·218E-01
Lung	0·284E-04	0·101E-02	0·317E-02	0·332E-02	0·339E-02	0·357E-02
Marrow	0·966E-02	0·376E-01	0·515E-01	0·308E-01	0·154E-01	0·145E-01
Ovaries*		0·260E-05	0·247E-04	0·289E-04	0·357E-04	0·305E-04
Spleen	0·592E-02	0·113E-01	0·871E-02	0·612E-02	0·531E-02	0·457E-02
Testes*				0·512E-05	0·198E-04	0·269E-04
			Source Organ—Liver			
Kidneys	0·106E-02	0·437E-02	0·556E-02	0·437E-02	0·386E-02	0·335E-02
Liver	0·784	0·543	0·278	0·165	0·157	0·144
Lung	0·859E-02	0·165E-01	0·147E-01	0·101E-01	0·838E-02	0·825E-02
Marrow	0·819E-02	0·228E-01	0·325E-01	0·206E-01	0·107E-01	0·935E-02
Ovaries*		0·169E-05	0·112E-04	0·157E-04	0·186E-04	0·196E-04
Spleen		0·617E-04	0·533E-03	0·606E-03	0·619E-03	0·633E-03
Testes*			0·100E-05	0·346E-05	0·100E-04	0·115E-04

Table A5.2 (continued)

Target Organ	0·020	0·030	0·050	0·100	0·500	1·00
			Source Organ—Lung			
Kidneys		0·326E-03	0·923E-03	0·901E-03	0·116E-02	0·814E-03
Liver	0·142E-01	0·258E-01	0·239E-01	0·173E-01	0·154E-01	0·138E-01
Lung	0·475	0·231	0·829E-01	0·493E-01	0·514E-01	0·452E-01
Marrow	0·133E-01	0·386E-01	0·466E-01	0·254E-01	0·133E-01	0·125E-01
Ovaries*			0·482E-06	0·202E-05	0·418E-05	0·465E-05
Spleen	0·891E-03	0·182E-02	0·205E-02	0·146E-02	0·119E-02	0·113E-02
Testes*					0·270E-05	0·479E-05
			Source Organ—Skeleton			
Marrow	0·324	0·266	0·159	0·629E-01	0·466E-01	0·430E-01
Skeleton	0·830	0·681	0·400	0·173	0·118	0·110
Total body	0·917	0·847	0·608	0·374	0·335	0·315
			Source Organ—Spleen			
Liver		0·866E-03	0·545E-02	0·718E-02	0·566E-02	0·651E-02
Ovaries*			0·580E-05	0·152E-04	0·192E-04	0·166E-04
Marrow	0·652E-02	0·652E-01	0·336E-01	0·212E-01	0·110E-01	0·105E-01
Testes*					0·130E-04	
Spleen	0·625	0·331	0·128	0·709E-01	0·769E-01	0·699E-01
			Source Organ—Thyroid			
Lung		0·137E-02	0·374E-02	0·364E-02	0·406E-02	0·383E-02
Marrow	0·592E-03	0·668E-02	0·165E-01	0·126E-01	0·738E-02	0·717E-02
Thyroid	0·366	0·149	0·480E-01	0·278E-01	0·319E-01	0·295E-01
Total body	0·944	0·756	0·481	0·327	0·313	0·296
			Source Organ—Total Body			
Marrow	0·655E-01	0·740E-01	0·613E-01	0·329E-01	0·194E-01	0·182E-01
Total Body	0·892	0·774	0·548	0·370	0·340	0·321

Notes 1: Absorbed fractions are written in exponential notation, e.g. $0·502E-02 = 0·502 \times 10^{-2}$

2: Blank spaces indicate that there is more than a fifty per cent uncertainty in the figure and it has therefore been omitted.

Appendix 6

Physical data on radionuclides used in nuclear medicine

Table A6.1 The data listed below are largely based on the MIRD pamphlet No. 10. Note that nuclides decaying by EC or where IC occurs will emit X-Rays characteristic of the daughter element. The figures in brackets represent the number of particles or unconverted photons emitted per 100 nuclear transformations.

Isotope	Half-life	Type of decay	Maximum energies of principal particles (MeV)	Principal γ-ray energies (MeV)	Typical production process
^{3}H	12.3y	β^-	0·019 (100)	No γ's	^{6}Li(n, α)^{3}H
^{14}C	5730y	β^-	0·16 (100)	No γ's	^{14}N(n, p)^{14}C
^{18}F	110m	β^+, EC	0·633 (97); EC (3)	0·51 from β^+ (194)	^{16}O (α, np)^{18}F
^{24}Na	15h	β^-	1·39 (100)	1·37 (100); 2·75 (100)	^{23}Na(n, γ)^{24}Na
^{32}P	14·3d	β^-	1·71 (100)	No γ's	^{31}P (n, γ)^{32}P
^{35}S	87d	β^-	0·167 (100)	No γ's	^{35}Cl (n, p)^{35}S
^{42}K	12·4d	β^-	2·00 (18); 3·52 (82)	1·52 (18)	^{41}K (n, γ)^{42}K
^{51}Cr	27·8d	EC	EC (100)	0·32 (10)	^{50}Cr (n, γ)^{51}Cr
^{52}Fe	8.3h	EC, β^+	EC (42); 0·80 (58)	0·51 from β^+ (115); 0·169 (99)	^{50}Cr (α, 2n)^{52}Fe
^{59}Fe	45d	β^-	0·27 (46); 0·47 (52)	1·10 (55); 1·29 (44)	^{58}Fe (n, γ)^{59}Fe
^{57}Co	270d	EC	EC (100)	0·122 (86); 0·136 (10)	^{60}Ni (p, α)^{57}Co
^{58}Co	71d	β^+, EC	0·47 (15); EC (85)	0·51 from β^+ (31); 0·81 (99)	^{58}Ni (n, p)^{58}Co
^{67}Ga	78h	EC	EC (100)	0·093 (38); 0·185 (24); 0·30 (16); 0·39 (4)	^{65}Cu (α, 2n)^{67}Ga
^{68}Ga	68m	EC, β^+	EC (11); 1·90 (88)	0·51 from β^+ (178); 1·07 (3)	^{66}Zn (α, 2n)^{68}Ge $\rightarrow$ ^{68}Ga
^{75}Se	120d	EC	EC (100)	0·121 (16); 0·136 (54); 0·265 (57); 0·280 (24); 0·401 (12)	^{74}Se(n, γ)^{75}Se
^{81}Rb	4.58h	EC, β^+	1·05 (29); EC (68)	0·51 from β^+ (62); 0·191 (66)	^{79}Br (α, 2n)^{81}Rb
Daughter: ^{81}Kr^{rm}	13s	IT	IT (100)		

Table A6.1 (*continued*)

Isotope	Half-life	Type of decay	Maximum energies of principal particles (MeV)	Principal γ-ray energies (MeV)	Typical production process
^{99}Mo	66.7h	β^-	0.46 (18.5); 1.23 (80)	0.18 (7); 0.74 (14), 0.78 (5)	^{98}Mo (n, γ)^{99}Mo
Daughter: ^{99}Tc^m	6.0h	IT	IT (100)	0.140 (88)	
^{113}Sn	118d	EC	EC (100)	0.26 (2)	^{112}Sn (n, γ)^{113}Sn
Daughter: ^{113}In^m	100m	IT	IT (100)	0.391 (62)	
^{123}I	13h	EC	EC (100)	0.159 (84)	^{121}Sb (α, 2n)^{231}I
^{125}I	60d	EC	EC (100)	0.035 (7); 0.027 (X-rays, 136 %)	^{124}Xe (n, γ)^{124} Xe $\rightarrow$ ^{125}I
^{131}I	8.06d	β^-	0.33 (7); 0.61 (90)	0.364 (82); 0.637 (7)	^{130}Te (n, γ)^{131}Te $\rightarrow$ ^{131}I
^{133}Xe	5.31d	β^-	0.346 (98)	0.081 (36)	fission
^{137}Cs	30.0y	β^-	0.51 (95); 1.18 (5)	No γ's	fission
Daughter: ^{137}Ba^m	2.55m	IT	IT (100)	0.662 (90)	
^{198}Au	2.70d	β^-	0.96 (99)	0.412 (96)	^{197}Au (n, γ)^{198}Au
^{201}Tl	73.5h	EC	EC (100)	0.135(3); 0.167(10) 0.068–0.080 (X-Rays 95 %)	^{203}Tl (p, 3n)^{201}Pb $\rightarrow$ ^{201}Tl

425

Appendix 7

Problems and answers

A7.1. Problems

Chapter 4. Radioactivity
Required half-lives given in Appendix 6.
1. The activity of a radionuclide is measured as function of time and the following results obtained:

Activity	Time
8·51 MBq	
7·84	20 min
7·21	40 min
6·66	1 hour
5·18	2 hours
3·14	4 hours
1·92	6 hours

Plot the activity as a function of time using linear-linear graph paper and using log-linear graph paper. What is the half-life and transformation constant of this radionuclide?
2. A sample of Fluorine-18 has an activity of 480 MBq at 0900 hours. What will the activity be at 14.30 hours?
3. A patient is to be given 200 MBq of Technetium-99m at 14.00 hours. What activity should be dispensed at 10.00 hours?
4. A bottle contains 15 MBq of Selenium-75. How many days must elapse before the activity is only 6 MBq?
5. A bottle contained 400 MBq of ^{51}Cr in 1 ml on January 1st. 150 MBq were removed from the bottle on January 15th and the remaining activity diluted to 10 ml. On January 22nd it is required to give a patient 10 MBq. What volume should be used?

Chapter 7. Interaction of X and γ radiation with matter
1. The mass attenuation coefficient of lead for 350 keV photons is $0.245 \, \text{cm}^2 \, \text{g}^{-1}$. What is the linear attenuation coefficient at this energy? (Density of lead, ρ, = $11.3 \, \text{g cm}^{-3}$).

2. The mass attenuation coefficient in water for 300 keV photons is $0.11\,cm^2\,g^{-1}$. What is the half-value thickness?

3. Calculate the reduction in intensity of radiation from a $^{99}Tc^m$ source by (a) 2 mm, and (b) 1 cm thickness of lead. What would be the values if ^{131}I were used?

Assume: Mass attenuation coefficient of lead for $^{99}Tc^m$ is $2.0\,cm^2\,g^{-1}$ and for ^{131}I is $0.25\,cm^2\,g^{-1}$. The density of lead, ρ, is $11.3\,g\,cm^{-3}$.

4. What thickness crystals of sodium iodide are required to absorb ninety per cent of photons of (a) 25. (b) 150 and (c) 500 keV photons. The respective linear attenuation coefficients are 30, 2 and $0.35\,cm^{-1}$.

Chapter 9. Dosimetry
The assumptions are not valid in all cases and the data have been modified in order to simplify the calculation. Any further assumptions required should be stated.

1. The skeleton uniformly absorbs 15 J of energy. What is the absorbed dose in grays?

2. Calculate the absorbed fraction of 100 keV gamma rays by the lung from activity in the kidneys given the absorbed fraction in the kidneys from activity in the lung is 0.901×10^{-3}.

3. The clearance of activity of a radiopharmaceutical from the blood is found to have a biological half-life of 20 hours. If the physical half-life is 10 hours what is the effective half-life?

4. Four MBq of ^{51}Cr labelled red cells, which have been damaged, are injected into a patient. If it is assumed that all the cells are taken up immediately by the spleen and the effective half-life is equal to the physical half-life what is the absorbed dose to the spleen?

5. Calculate the absorbed dose, per MBq injected, to the liver from $^{99}Tc^m$ sulphur colloid. Assume 90 per cent of the radionuclide is taken up by the liver and 10 per cent by the spleen. Also assume the effective half-life is equal to the physical half-life.

6. Calculate the absorbed dose, per MBq injected, to the lung and liver from $^{99}Tc^m$ macro-aggregates. Assume instantaneous uptake by the lung of 90 per cent of the macro-aggregates, the remainder being deposited in the liver. The biological half-life of the aggregates in the lungs is 10 hours and infinite for those in the liver. Ignore the contribution to the absorbed dose from the $^{99}Tc^m$ after leaving the lung and also the dose to the lung from activity in the liver.

7. Half a megabecquerel of ^{131}I labelled human serum albumin is administered to measure plasma volume. What is the absorbed dose to the blood? Assume the labelled albumin stays entirely within the vascular compartment until it has physically decayed.

8. Estimate the absorbed dose to the thyroid from a therapeutic administration of 200 MBq of ^{131}I as sodium iodide. The following information is provided:

Wt. of patient: 70 kg

Time	Percentage uptake* in the thyroid
5h	20
12h	40
24h	65
2d	50
5d	6

Chapter 37. Generators

1. A 4 GBq ^{99}Mo–^{99}Tc^m generator column is eluted. Calculate the approximate mass of ^{99}Tc (^{99}Tc + ^{99}Tc^m) on the column 24 hours after the elution. If the column is re-eluted at the end of this period with 20 ml of saline, what is the molarity of the NaTcO$_4$ solution? Assume 100 per cent elution efficiency and refer to Chapter 24 for Avogadro's number.

2. A ^{99}Mo–^{99}Tc^m generator has an activity of 10 GBq at 1200 h on Monday. The generator (not previously eluted) is eluted Tuesday morning at 0900 h. What would the activity of the eluate be if the elution efficiency was eighty per cent? If the volume of the eluate is 15 ml what volume must be dispersed to give a patient a dose of 400 MBq at 1300 h on the same day?

3. After elution of a ^{113}Sn–^{113}In^m generator what period of time must be allowed for the activity of the daughter to build-up to eighty per cent of that of the parent?

(Use Table 37.1 for required data).

4. Calculate the activity of the eluate from a ^{132}Te–^{132}I generator (80 MBqi^{132}Te at 1200 h on Monday) when eluted on Wednesday at 0900 h. If the column is re-eluted 4 hours later what activity would be expected? Assume 80 per elution efficiency.

There is 100 per cent conversion from parent to daughter. Other data from Table 37.1.

5. What activity ^{99}Mo–^{99}Tc^m generator is required (calibrated 1200 h Monday) to prepare the following doses on Friday to be administered to patients?

1 × 800 MBq at 0930 h
6 × 200 MBq at 1030 h
3 × 400 MBq at 1200 h
3 × 400 MBq at 1500 h

---

* Corrected for physical decay.

It requires a minimum of 30 minutes to prepare the dose after elution. Assume eighty per cent elution efficiency. Calculate your answer for both a single elution on Friday and also assuming two elutions, the second one at 1430 h.

A7.2. Answers
Chapter 4
(1) 2 h 50 m; $0.24 \, h^{-1}$
(2) 60 MBq
(3) 317 MBq
(4) 160 d
(5) 0.92 ml

Chapter 7
(1) $2.77 \, cm^{-1}$
(2) 6.3 cm
(3) $^{99}Tc^m$ (a) 0.01
              (b) $<2 \times 10^{-10}$
       ^{131}I (a) 0.57
              (b) 0.06
(4) (a) 0.077 cm
     (b) 1.2 cm
     (c) 6.6 cm

Chapter 9
(1) 1.5 Gy
(2) 3.11×10^{-3}
(3) 6.66 h
(4) 0.897 mGy
(5) 0.095 mGy per MBq injected
(6) Lung: 0.068 mGy per MBq injected
     Liver: 0.014 mGy per MBq injected
(7) 3.22 mGy
(8) 7.35 Gy

Chapter 32
(1) 8×10^{-8} g
     2×10^{-8} molar
(2) 640 MBq
     1.5 ml
(3) 3.9 h
(4) 44.4 MBq
     30.4 MBq
(5) 20.8 GBq
     13.0 GBq

Appendix 8

Further reading

The following bibliography is by no means exhaustive, but is intended as a guide for those students desirous of a more detailed knowledge of the subjects dealt with in this book.

A8.1. General

1. Belcher, E. M. & Vetter, H. (Eds) (1971) *Radioisotope Techniques in Medical Diagnosis*, London: Butterworth.
2. Freeman, L. M. & Johnson, P. M. (eds) (1975) *Clinical Scintillation Imaging*, 2nd edn. New York: Grune & Stratton.
3. Wagner, H. (Ed.) (1968) *Principles of Nuclear Medicine*, Philadelphia: Saunders.
4. *Seminars in Nuclear Medicine*, (1971), quarterly, New York: Grune & Stratton.
5. McAlister, J. M. (1979) *Radionuclide Techniques in Medicine*, Techniques of measurement in medicine 3, Cambridge University Press.
6. Maisey, M. (1980) *Nuclear Medicine—A Clinical Introduction*, London: Update Books.
7. *Diagnostic Imaging* British Medical Bulletin. Volume 36, Number 3, 1980.
8. Moores, B. M., Parker, R. P. & Pullan, B. R. (Eds) (1981). *Physical Aspects of Medical Imaging*, New York: Wiley.
9. Maisey, M. N., Britton, K. E. and Gildoy, D. L. (Eds.) (1983) *Clinical Nuclear Medicine*, London: Chapman and Hall.

A8.2. Radiation and radioisotope physics

1. Evans, R. D. (1955) *The Atomic Nucleus*, New York: McGraw-Hill.
2. Johns, H. E. & Cunningham, J. R. (1974) *The Physics of Radiology* 3rd edn. Springfield, Illinois: Thomas.
3. Meredith, W. & Massey, J. (1972) *Fundamental Physics of Radiology*, 2nd edn. Bristol: Wright.

A8.3. Decay schemes and dosimetry

1. Attix, F. H. & Roesch, W. C. (Eds) (1966, 1968, 1969) 2nd edn. *Radiation Dosimetry*, 3 Vols. New York: Academic Press.
2. Lederer, C. M., and Shirley, V. S. I. (1978) *Table of Isotopes*, 7th edn. New York: Wiley.
3. Reports of the Society of Nuclear Medicine Incorporated (New York) Medical Internal Radiation Dose Committee (MIRD): Pamphlet No. 1 (revised). *A Revised Scheme for calculating the Absorbed Dose from Biologically Distributed Radionuclides;* Pamphlet No. 5 *Absorbed Fractions for Photon Dosimetry;* Pamphlet No. 5 (revised) *Estimates of Specific Absorbed Fractions for Photon Sources Uniformly Distributed in Various Organs of a Heterogenous Phantom;* Pamphlet No. 10 *Radionuclide Decay Schemes and Nuclear Parameters for Use in Radiation-Dose Estimation;* Pamphlet No. 11. *'S' Absorbed Dose per Unit*

Cumulated Activity for Selected Radionuclides and Organs. Also Pamphlets 2, 3, 7 and 8.
4. Kenenakes, J. G. *et al.* (1972) *Radiopharmaceutical Dosimetry in Paediatrics,* Seminars in Nuclear Medicine **2**, 316. New York: Grune & Stratton.
5. International Commission on Radiation Units and Measurements (ICRU) Report 32 (1979) *Method of Assessment of Absorbed Dose in Clinical Use of Radionuclides* Washington: ICRU.

A8.4.   Instrumentation

1. Dyer, A. (1974) *An introduction to Liquid Scintillation Counting.* London: Heyden.
2. Hine, G. J. (Ed) (1967, 1974) *Instrumentation in Nuclear Medicine,* Vol. 1, Vol. 2, New York: Academic Press.
3. Hospital Physicists' Association (1977) *The Theory, Specification and Testing of Anger-type Gamma Cameras.* London: Hospital Physicists' Association.

A8.5.   Chemistry

1. Adam, N. K. (1956) *Physical Chemistry.* Oxford: Clarendon Press.
2. Bandtock, J. & Hanson, P. (1974) *Success in Cemistry.* London: John Murray.
3. Kneen, W. R., Rogers, M. J. W. & Simpson, P. (1972) *Chemistry.* London: Addison Wesley.
4. Lehninger, A. L. (1970) *Biochemistry—The Molecular Basis of Cell Structure and Function.* New York: Worth Publishers Inc.
5. Mahan, B. H. (1966) *College Chemistry.* London: Addison Wesley.
6. Sheka, I. A. & Mityuseva, T. T. (1966) *The Chemistry of Gallium.* Amsterdam: Elsevier.

A8.6.   Radioisotope and radiopharmaceutical production

1. *Guidelines for the Preparation of Radiopharmaceuticals in Hospitals* (revised 1979). Special Report No. 11. London: British Institute of Radiology.
2. Croll, M. N., Brady, L. W., Honda, T. & Wallner, R. J. (1974) *New Techniques in Tumour Localisation and Radioimmunoassay.* New York: Wiley.
3. Horton, P. W. (1975) *Preparation of radiopharmaceuticals.* In *Recent Advances in Clinical Nuclear Medicine,* (Eds) Greig, W. R. & Gillespie, F. C. Edinburgh: Churchill Livingstone.
4. Lovett, D. E. (1974) *Radiopharmaceuticals.* In *Advances in Pharmaceutical Sciences* ed. Bean, H. S., Beckett, A. H. & Carlos, J. E. **4**, p. 263. New York: Academic Press.
5. Sönksen, P. H. (Ed) (1974) Radioimmunoassay and saturation analysis. *British Medical Bulletin,* **30**, 11.
6. Subramanian, G., Rhodes, B. A., Cooper, J. F. & Sodd, V. J. (Ed) (1975) *Radiopharmaceuticals.* New York: Society of Nuclear Medicine.
7. Kristensen, K. (1979) *Preparation and Control of Radiopharmaceuticals in Hospitals.* Vienna: International Atomic Energy Agency.
8. Tubis, M. & Wolf, W. (1976) *Radiopharmacy.* New York: Wiley.
9. Welch, M. J. (Ed) (1977) *Radiopharmaceuticals and other Compounds Labelled with Short-lived Radionuclides.* Oxford: Pergamon Press.
10. Faires, R. A. & Boswell, G. G. J. (4th Edition 1981) *Radioisotope Laboratory Techniques.* London: Butterworths.

A8.7.   Safety

1. International Commission on Radiological Protection Publications (Oxford: Pergamon Press) particularly: No. 17. *Protection of the Patient in Radionuclide Investigations* (1971); No. 25. *The Handling, Storage, Use and Disposal of Unsealed Radionuclides in Hospitals and Medical Research Establishments* (1977); No. 26. *Recommendations of ICRP* (1977).

2. Department of Health and Social Security (1972) *Code of Practice for the Protection of Persons against Ionizing Radiations arising from Medical and Dental Use.* 3rd edn. London: Her Majesty's Stationery Office.
3. Department of Health and Social Security. (1978) *Code of Practice for the Prevention of Infection in Clinical Laboratories and Post Mortem Rooms.* HMSO.
4. Everett, K. & Hughes, D. (1975) *A Guide to Laboratory Design.* London: Butterworth.
5. Martin, A. & Harbison, S. A. (1980) *An Introduction to Radiation Protection.* London: Chapman and Hall.

Index

433

Baby Bliss

Your One-Stop Guide for the
First Three Months and Beyond

DR HARVEY KARP

PENGUIN BOOKS

PENGUIN BOOKS

Published by the Penguin Group
Penguin Books Ltd, 80 Strand, London WC2R 0RL, England
Penguin Group (USA) Inc., 375 Hudson Street, New York, New York 10014, USA
Penguin Books Australia Ltd, 250 Camberwell Road, Camberwell, Victoria 3124, Australia
Penguin Books Canada Ltd, 10 Alcorn Avenue, Toronto, Ontario, Canada M4V 3B2
Penguin Books India (P) Ltd, 11 Community Centre, Panchsheel Park, New Delhi – 110 017, India
Penguin Group (NZ), cnr Airborne and Rosedale Roads, Albany, Auckland 1310, New Zealand
Penguin Books (South Africa) (Pty) Ltd, 24 Sturdee Avenue, Rosebank 2196, South Africa

Penguin Books Ltd, Registered Offices: 80 Strand, London WC2R 0RL, England

www.penguin.com

Published in the United States of America by Bantam as *The Happiest Baby on the Block* 2002
Published in Great Britain by Michael Joseph as *The Happiest Baby* 2002
Published in Penguin Books as *Baby Bliss* 2004

1

Printed in England by Clays Ltd, St Ives plc

To the generous hearts
of new parents everywhere
and to our sweet babies
who come into the world
with such trust

Contents

PART TWO

Learning the Ancient Art of Soothing a Baby

Conclusion

The Rainbow at the End of the Tunnel 233

Appendices

Index
261

This book contains advice and information relating to the care of infants. It is not intended to substitute for medical advice and should be used to supplement rather than replace the regular advice and care of your child's pediatrician. Since every child is different, you should consult your child's pediatrician on questions specific to your child.

Acknowledgments

The real voyage of discovery consists, not in seeking out new lands, but in having a new vision.

Marcel Proust

I am a pediatrician—and I love it. I am privileged to practice a field of medicine where I get to be part-biologist, part-psychologist, part-anthropologist, part–animal impersonator, and most especially part-grandmother.

In this book, I also wear all those hats. I hope not only to show what the best parents in history have done to soothe their babies but also to explain why it works and how to have some fun, too! In doing this, my greatest goal is to teach parents, grandparents, and everyone who cares about babies how to translate their messages of love into the language all babies understand.

This book took a number of years to prepare and may never have been completed had it not been for the support and encouragement of a small group of people, to whom I owe my profound gratitude and appreciation:

- To all the kind mothers and fathers in my practice who allowed me to touch their wonderful children, to be a part of their families, and to learn along with them.

- To my beloved mother Sophie, who taught me to marvel at the beauty and order in the world, and to my father Joe, whose patience is my model and whose selfless generosity sheltered me and gave me the gift of education.

- To my extraordinary wife Nina, my soulmate, who opened my heart and eyes and is my greatest friend, teacher, and compass. To my mother-in-law Desa, who is a unique and courageous woman. And to my daughter Lexi, who graciously tolerated my long hours of work.

- To my teachers Arthur H. Parmelee, Jr., and T. Berry Brazelton. Their brilliant talent for making the complex seem simple helped me learn how to observe and understand children. To the curious minds of Ronald Barr, Julius Richmond, Tiffany Field, Barry Lester, and many other honest explorers of science whose road signs guided me on this wonderful path into the inner world of babies.

- To my colleagues who reviewed this book and so generously gave of their time and knowledge: Marty Stein, Jim McKenna, Neal Kaufman, Sandra Steffes, Constance Keeffer, and Stan Inkelis.

- To my friends who counseled and helped me during the long process of bookmaking: Toby Berlin and Michael Grecco, Laurie David, Eric Weissler, Peter Gardner, Bart Walker, Richard Grant, Sylvie Rabineau, Katy Arnoldi, Laurel and Tom Barrack, and Jonathan Feldman.

- To the capable help of deputy publisher Nita Taublib, the sharp intellect and pencil of my editor Robin Michaelson, the witty imagination of Jennifer Kalis, and the savvy advice of my agent Suzanne Gluck.

Thank you all!

Introduction

How I Rediscovered the Ancient Secrets
for Calming Crying Babies

I certainly didn't realize how easy it was to calm crying babies when I began my pediatric studies in the early 1970s. During my medical-school training at Albert Einstein College of Medicine, my professors taught me that babies scream due to gas pains, so there were two valid approaches for soothing colic. First, try Grandmother's advice of holding, rocking, and pacifiers. If that failed, try medicine: *sedatives* (to push a baby into sleep), *anti-spasm medicines* (to treat stomach cramps), or *anti-gas drops* (to help get out burps).

By the late 1970s, however, these three medical approaches were called into question. Sedating babies was considered inappropriate. Doctors stopped using anti-spasm medicines after several babies treated with them lapsed into comas and died. And anti-gas drops lost their appeal when research proved them to be no more effective than water.

Although my medical education was excellent, I felt helpless when it came to caring for colicky newborns. As a resident, I worked for three years at Childrens Hospital of Los Angeles, one of the world's busiest pediatric hospitals. I was fully trained as a "baby doctor," yet I still couldn't help distraught parents soothe their babies' screams. In 1980, as a Fellow in Child Development at the UCLA School of Medicine, my frustration turned into shock and alarm. As a member of the UCLA Child Abuse Team, I treated several severely injured babies whose parents had committed horrible acts of abuse after being unable to calm their infants' persistent screaming.

I became outraged that our sophisticated medical system didn't have a single effective solution for babies with this common yet terribly disturbing problem. During the two years of my fellowship, I read everything I could about colic. I was determined to unearth every clue to explain why so many children were plagued by this mysterious condition.

I soon uncovered two facts that turned my alarm into hope.

First, I learned about the profound differences between the brain of a three-month-old baby and that of a newborn. A brilliant paper published in 1977 by one of America's preeminent pediatricians, Dr. Arthur H. Parmelee, Jr., described how sophisticated and complex the brains of babies become over the first months of life. He illustrated this point by showing pictures of two babies: a fussing newborn and a smiling three-month-old (shown below). Dr. Parmelee observed that most parents-to-be dreamed of giving birth to a smiling baby like the one on the left, while in reality they ended up with a fussy "fetus-like" newborn like the one seen on the right, at least for the first few months.

These pictures powerfully demonstrated the massive developmental leap babies make during the first

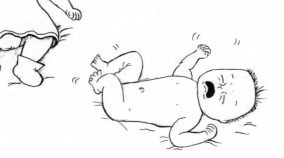

three months of life as well as the huge gap between how parents in our society expect new babies to look and act and their true behavior and nature.

My second pivotal discovery came when I read about child-rearing in other societies. As I explored the musty shelves of old books and journals stored at the UCLA Medical Library, I was shocked to learn that the colicky screaming that afflicted so many of my patients was *absent* in the babies of several cultures around the world!

The more I investigated this issue, the more it dawned on me that our culture, advanced in so many ways, was quite backward when it came to understanding the needs of babies. Somehow, somewhere, we had taken a wrong turn. Once I realized our ideas about babies' crying had been built upon centuries of myth and misconception, the solution to the prehistoric puzzle of why babies cry and how to soothe them suddenly became crystal clear. Our babies are born three months too soon.

I invite you to learn how your baby experiences the world, as well as my program of extremely effective techniques used to calm thousands of my patients over the last twenty years. These techniques may seem a little odd at first, but once you get the hang of them you'll see how wonderfully simple they are. Parents around the world have successfully used these methods to soothe their babies for thousands of years . . . and soon, you will, too!

—*Harvey Karp*

PART ONE

Look Who's Squawking:
Why Babies Cry—
And Why Some Cry
So Much

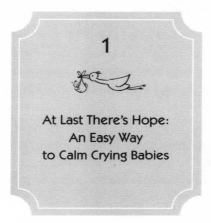

1

At Last There's Hope: An Easy Way to Calm Crying Babies

Main Points:

- All babies cry, but most new parents have little experience soothing them
- The Basic Problem: In many ways, babies are born three months too soon
- The Calming Reflex: Nature's *Off* switch for a baby's crying
- The 5 "S's": How to turn on your baby's calming reflex
- The Cuddle Cure: Combining the 5 "S's" to help any fussy baby

Suzanne was worried and exhausted. Her two-month-old baby, Sean, was a nonstop screamer. He could cry for hours. One afternoon her sister came to watch the baby, and Suzanne bolted to the bathroom for a hot shower and a quick "escape." Forty-five minutes later she awoke, curled up in a ball on the blue tile floor, being sprayed with ice-cold water!

Meanwhile, half a world away in the rugged Kalahari plains of northern Botswana, Nisa gave birth to a tiny girl named Chuko. Chuko was thin and delicate but despite her dainty size, she, too, was a challenging baby who cried frequently.

Nisa carried Chuko in a leather sling everywhere she went. Unlike Suzanne, she never worried when Chuko cried, because like all mothers of the !Kung San tribe, she knew exactly how to calm her baby's crying—in seconds.

Why did Suzanne have such trouble soothing Sean's screams?

What ancient secrets did Nisa know that helped her calm her baby so easily?

As you are about to learn, the answers to these two questions will change the way you think about babies forever! They will show you the world through your baby's eyes and, most important, they will teach you how to calm your baby's cries in minutes and help prolong her sleep.

Your Baby Is Born

When perfectly dry, his flesh sweet and pure, he is the most kissable object in nature.
Marion Harland, *Common Sense in the Nursery*, 1886

Congratulations! You've done a great job already! You've nurtured your baby from the moment of conception to your baby's "birth"day. Having a baby is a wonderful—and wonder-full—experience that makes you laugh, cry, and stare in amazement . . . all at the same time.

Your top job as a new parent is to love your baby like crazy. After showering her with affection, your next two important jobs are to feed her and to calm her when she cries.

I can tell you from my twenty-five years as a pediatrician, parents who succeed at these two tasks feel proud, confident, on top of the world! They have the happiest babies and they feel like the best parents on the block. However, mothers and fathers who struggle with these tasks often end up feeling distraught.

Fortunately, feeding a baby is *usually* pretty straightforward. Most newborns take to sucking like they have a Ph.D. in chowing-down! Soothing a crying baby, on the other hand, can be unexpectedly challenging.

No couple expects their sweet newborn to be "difficult." Who really lis-

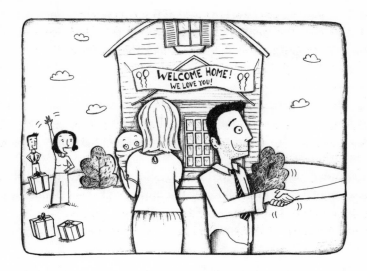

tens to horror stories friends and family share? We assume *our* child will be an "easy" baby. That's why so many new parents are shocked to discover how tough calming their baby's cries can be.

Please don't misunderstand me. I'm not saying crying is bad. In fact, it's brilliant! Leave it to nature to find such an effective way for helpless babies to get our attention. And once your baby has your attention, you probably zip down a checklist of questions and solutions:

- Is she hungry? Feed her.
- Is she wet? Change her diaper.
- Is she lonely? Pick her up.
- Is she gassy? Burp her.
- Is she cold? Bundle her up.

The trouble comes when *nothing* works.

Estimates are that one out of every five babies has repeated bouts of terrible fussiness—*for no apparent reason.* That adds up to almost one million sweet new babies born in the U.S. each year who suffer from hours of red-faced, eyes-clenched screaming.

This is why parents of unhappy babies are such heroes! A baby's scream is an incredibly heart-wrenching sound. Bone-tired and bewildered moms and dads lovingly cuddle their frantic babies for hours, trying to calm them, yet the continued crying can corrode their confidence: "Is my baby in pain?" "Am I spoiling her?" "Does she feel abandoned?" "Am I a terrible mother?"

Confronted by this barrage, sometimes the most loving parent may find herself pushed into frustration and depression. A baby's unrelenting shrieks can even drive desperate caregivers over the edge—into the tragedy of child abuse.

Exhausted parents are often told they must wait for their babies to "grow out of it." Yet most of us feel that can't be right. There must be some way to help our babies.

I'm going to show you how.

Help Wanted: Who Do New Parents Turn to When Their Baby Cries a Lot?

Although a network of clinics and specialists exists to help mothers solve their infant's feeding problems, there is little support for the parents of screaming babies. That's unfortunate because while the urge to quiet a baby is instinctual, the ability to do it is a skill that must be learned.

Today's parents have less experience caring for babies than any previous generation. (Amazingly, our culture requires more training to get a driver's license than to have a baby.)

That's not to say that inexperienced moms and dads are abandoned. On the contrary, they're bombarded with suggestions. In my experience, America's favorite pastime is not baseball but giving unasked-for advice to new parents. "It's boredom." "It's the heat." "Put a hat on him." Or "It's gas."

It can be so confusing! Who should you believe?

In frustration and concern, parents often turn to their doctor for help. Studies show that one in six couples visit a doctor because of their baby's persistent crying. When these babies are examined and found to be healthy, most doctors have little to offer but sympathy. "I know it's hard, but be patient; it won't last forever." Advice like this often sends worried parents to look for help in baby books.

Parents of colicky babies spend hours scanning books for "the answer" to their infant's distress. Yet, often the advice can be equally confusing: "Hold your baby—but be careful not to spoil him." "Love your baby—but let him cry himself to sleep."

Even these experts confess that for *really* fussy babies, they have nothing to offer:

> *Very often, you may not even be able to quiet the screaming.*
> What to Expect the First Year, Eisenberg, Murkoff, and Hathaway

> *The whole episode goes on at least an hour and perhaps for three or four hours.*
> Your Baby and Child, Penelope Leach

> *It's completely all right to set the baby in the bassinet while trying to drown out the noise with the running water of a hot shower.*
> The Girlfriend's Guide to Surviving the First Year of Motherhood, Vicki Iovine

But a hot shower is cold comfort for the parents of a screaming baby.

Many exhausted parents I meet have been persuaded, against their better judgment, that they can only stand by and endure their baby's screaming. But I tell them otherwise. Unhappy babies *can* be calmed—in minutes!

The Four Principles of Soothing Babies

In many ways, the people living in primitive cultures are backward compared to Western societies. However, in some areas their wisdom is great . . . and we are the "primitive" ones. This is particularly true when it comes to soothing crying newborns.

I teased out shreds of wisdom from the past and wove them with cutting-edge modern research and some unique observations made during my years of caring for more than five thousand infants. From this, I distilled four principles that are crucial for anyone who wants to understand babies better and be skillful at comforting them and improving their sleep:

- The Missing Fourth Trimester
- The Calming Reflex
- The 5 "S's"
- The Cuddle Cure

The Missing Fourth Trimester—Many Babies Cry Because They're Born Three Months Too Soon!

Did you ever see a baby horse or a baby cow? These newborn animals can walk, even run, on their very first day of life. In fact, they must be able to run—their survival depends upon it.

By comparison, our newborns are quite immature. They can't run, walk, or even roll over. One British mum told me her new daughter seemed so unready for the world she and her husband affectionately nicknamed her "The Little Creature." They're not alone in seeing babies that way; the Spanish use the word *criatura,* meaning *creature,* to describe babies.

In many ways your new baby is more a fetus than an infant, spending most of her time sleeping and being fed. Had you delayed your delivery just three more months, your baby would have been born with the ability to smile, coo, and flirt. (Who wouldn't want *that* on their baby's first day of life!) However, I've never been able to talk a woman into keeping her infant inside for a fourth trimester . . . and for good reason. It's already a tight squeeze getting a baby's head out after nine months of pregnancy; by twelve months it would be impossible.

Why are our babies so immature at birth? The reason is simple. Unlike baby horses whose survival depends on their big strong bodies, a human baby's survival depends on big smart brains. In fact, our babies' brains are so huge we have to "evict" fetuses from the womb well before they're fully ready for the world to keep their heads from getting stuck in the birth canal.

Newborns have some abilities that demonstrate their readiness to be in the world, but these notwithstanding, for the first three months, our babies are so immature they would really benefit if they could hop back inside whenever they get overwhelmed. However, since we're not kangaroos, the least we can do as loving, compassionate parents is to make our little

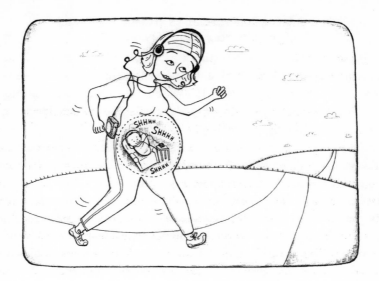

criaturas feel at home by surrounding them with the comforting sensations they enjoyed twenty-four hours a day in the womb. However, in order to give babies a fourth trimester, parents need to answer one important question: What exactly was it like in there?

In your womb, your baby was packed tight into the fetal position enveloped by the warm wall of the uterus and rocked and jiggled for much of the day. She was also surrounded by a constant shushing sound a little louder than a vacuum cleaner!

For thousands of years, parents have known that mimicking conditions in the uterus comforts newborns. That's why almost every traditional baby-calming technique around the world imitates the sensations of the womb. From swaddling to swings to shushing, these methods return babies to a cuddly, rhythmic, womblike world until they are ready to coo, smile, and join the family. As helpful as this fourth-trimester experience is for calm babies, it is *essential* for fussy ones.

Most parents assume that this imitation soothes their baby simply by making her feel "back home." Actually, these experiences trigger a profound neurological response never before recognized or reported—until today. This ancient and very powerful baby reflex is *the calming reflex.*

The Calming Reflex: Nature's Brilliant "*Off* Switch" for Your Baby's Crying

This automatic reset switch stills a baby's crying and is truly a baby's (and parent's) best friend. Why did nature choose imitating the uterus as the trigger for this blessed reflex? The reason may surprise you: As important as it was for our ancestors to be able to quiet their babies, it was triply important for them to be able to quiet their *fetuses!*

Just imagine what it would feel like if your fetus threw a temper tantrum inside you. Not only could pounding fists and kicking feet make you sore, they could damage the fragile placenta or rip the umbilical cord, causing a fatal hemorrhage. Perhaps even more deadly than the risk of accidental injury was the chance that a squirming baby might get stuck sideways in the uterus and be unable to slide out, thus killing herself and her mother.

I'm convinced that the survival of our fetuses, and perhaps even the survival of our species, depended on this ancient calming reflex. Over millions of years, fetuses who became entranced by the sensations inside the uterus didn't thrash about and thus were most likely to stay alive. Our babies today are direct descendants of those "Zen" fetuses who were so easily pacified by the womb.

The 5 "S's": Five Steps to Turn On Your Baby's Calming Reflex

How is a vacuum cleaner like a lullaby? How is a Volvo like a flannel blanket? They all help switch on your baby's calming reflex by imitating some quality of your womb.

Although our ancient ancestors intuitively understood how to turn off their baby's crying and turn on their baby's calming, recognition of the calming reflex itself remained completely overlooked until I identified it during the mid-1990s while studying the characteristics of hundreds of crying babies in my practice.

I was struck by the fact that many traditional baby-calming methods failed to work unless they were done *exactly right*. I realized that, similar to a doctor setting off a knee reflex with a precise whack of a little hammer, the calming reflex could only be triggered by certain very specific actions. When presented correctly, however, the sounds and feelings of the womb had such a powerful effect that they could carry an infant from tears to tranquillity, sometimes even in mid-cry.

Parents and grandparents traditionally have used five different characteristics of the womb to soothe their babies. I refer to these time-honored "ingredients" of calm as the 5 "S's":

1. *S*waddling—tight wrapping
2. *S*ide/Stomach—laying a baby on her side or stomach
3. *S*hushing—loud white noise
4. *S*winging—rhythmic, jiggly motion
5. *S*ucking—sucking on anything from your nipple or finger to a pacifier

These five methods are extremely effective but only when performed *exactly* right. When done without the right technique and vigor, they do nothing. (Detailed descriptions of how to perform each "S" are in Chapters 8 through 12.)

The Cuddle Cure: Combining the 5 "S's" into a Perfect Recipe for Your Baby's Bliss

You don't have to be a rocket scientist to be a terrific parent, but there are some little tricks that can help you do your job better. Most infant-care books list these calming tips, but that's as unhelpful as listing the ingredients of a recipe without giving the instructions for how to combine and cook them.

Each individual "S" may be effective for soothing a mildly fussy baby. Your "easy" baby may only need to suck or to be danced around the room in order to be calmed. However, doing all five together can switch on the calming reflex so irresistibly that they soothe even the most frantic newborns. This layering of one "S" on top of another is so successful at making unhappy babies feel cozy and calm that one of my patients dubbed it "the Cuddle Cure."

If the Cuddle Cure were indeed a cake recipe made from the 5 "S's," I think it would be for a layer cake.

Swaddling is the first step of calming and the first layer in this comfort cake. Next is the Side/Stomach position. These initial "S's" prepare your baby to be calmed. Swaddling sets the stage for success by keeping her from flailing and accidentally overstimulating herself; the side or stomach position also stops the flailing, by taking away your baby's feeling that she's falling and by activating the calming reflex.

The next layer is Shhhh, followed immediately by Swinging. Both activate the calming reflex so your baby pays attention to you and the wonderful cuddling you're giving her. These get her more and more relaxed.

Last, but not least, Sucking is the icing on the cake! It works best after the other layers have calmed your baby down. It, too, triggers the calming reflex and keeps it turned on to make your baby feel deeply and profoundly at peace. (Of course, from your baby's point of view, you aren't making a cake, but she will feel like you have popped her back inside the "oven" for a little fourth-trimester time!)

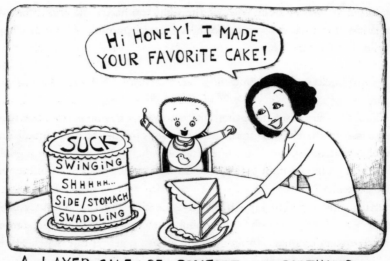

A LAYER-CAKE OF COMFORT AND SOOTHING

The Cuddle Cure to the Rescue: The Story of Sean

These five principles form the most effective program for soothing agitated infants that has ever been discovered. It works on even the most challenging of babies, like Sean. . . .

Remember Sean? He's the boy whose crying so exhausted his mother that she fell asleep in the shower.

Don and Suzanne had expected that having a new baby might sometimes feel like motoring down a bumpy road, but they never imagined it would feel like driving off a cliff! Sean was a typical colicky baby, and his parents were the typical loving, bewildered, exhausted parents of a colicky child.

Here's how Suzanne described the early days with Sean:

"When I was growing up, my mother often told me what a colicky baby I had been. Shortly after Sean was born, I knew it was payback time. My handsome, dark-haired boy was born a week early but, like a racehorse, he was 'out of the gate' at a gallop!

"From almost the second week of his life, Sean had fits of uncontrollable screaming for hours every day. I felt like a terrible mother as I watched him writhe in pain. Nothing worked to settle him, and usually I ended up crying right along with him.

"Equally distressing was my secret fear that Sean's cries were the result of some injury he suffered at birth. His delivery was very difficult. After one and a half hours of hard pushing, the obstetrician yanked him out with a vacuum suction. My first memory is of Sean's poor head looking like a black and blue banana.

"For the first month, our pediatrician advised us that Sean's wailing was just his need to 'blow off some steam.' He warned that always responding to our baby could spoil him and accidentally teach him to cry even more! We thought his advice sounded logical, but leaving Sean to shriek made our baby even crazier—plus it was agonizing for us.

"Don and I read every baby book we could find. Day after day, we tried new approaches: swaddling—a failure; pacifier—useless; a change in my diet—futile; a swing—like waving to a jet thirty thousand feet overhead. We even tried a device that imitated a car's noise and vibration. This, too, was a bust.

"Exhausted and demoralized, we returned to our doctor. He was sympathetic but reiterated that we had no option other than to endure Sean's shrieking until he outgrew this phase. That afternoon, when Don and I got home, we agreed that it would be unbearable to wait, both for our suffering baby and for us.

"The next morning was terrible too. At our wit's end, we took our six-week-old baby to meet a new pediatrician. Dr. Karp asked us many questions, and once he was convinced that Sean's crying wasn't the sign of a serious medical condition, he taught us a technique he called the 'Cuddle Cure.'

"The Cuddle was a very specific mix of tight wrapping, vigorous rocking, and loud shushing. Dr. Karp explained that these sensations mimicked the baby's life in the womb. He said most babies cry because 'They're just not ready to be born. In a way they still need to be in the protected world of the uterus for another three months!'

"To be honest, my skeptical self thought, *This is too simple to be true.* After all, I had attempted wrapping, rocking, and white noise and ended up as squashed as a bug under a fly swatter. But after watching Dr. Karp's technique I realized I was doing them only halfway.

"Don and I decided to try the Cuddle. As incredible as it sounds, that afternoon was the last time Sean cried uncontrollably! The Cuddle cured Sean's crying. Whenever he began going berserk, we would do all the steps of the Cuddle, and within minutes his little body would relax and melt into our arms. We finally found the comfort Sean had been begging us for for so many weeks." 🍼

The Cuddle worked quickly for Suzanne and Don; however, like most techniques, it may take you some practice to get the hang of it. But don't worry: If you follow the advice in this book, step by step, you should master it within five to ten tries.

Some parents I speak with are hesitant to use the 5 "S's." They've been warned not to spoil their newborns and they fear that using the 5 "S's" will accidentally give their babies bad habits. Is that possible? Can young babies inadvertently be turned into brats who demand constant holding and attention?

Thankfully, the answer to that question is . . . *No!* During the first three months of life (the fourth trimester), it's impossible to spoil your baby by letting her suck or stay in your arms for hours. Does that surprise you? It really shouldn't when you remember that you were lavishing her with these sensations twenty-four hours a day—up until the moment of birth. Even if you hold your baby twelve hours a day now, it's a giant reduction from *her* point of view. What you will see is that by three to four months your baby will be increasingly able to calm herself with cooing, moving around, and sucking her hands. Since she will no longer need so much of your help, you will be able to rapidly wean her off the five "S's" at that time.

Parenting Crying Babies in the 21st Century

I hope you are beginning to get excited that there *are* fast and effective ways of soothing your baby when she gets fussy! My goal is to teach you the tricks that the best parents around the world have used for centuries.

The first part of the book will answer the questions:

- Why do babies cry?
- What is colic and how can you tell if your baby has it?
- Why are gas pains, anxiety, immaturity, and temperament rarely the causes of colic?
- What is the missing fourth trimester and why is it the *true* cause of colic?

The second part of the book will discuss:

- The calming reflex and how to trigger it by imitating the uterus
- The 5 "S's" and why they must be done vigorously to be effective
- Exact instructions to help you become an expert at swaddling, side/stomach position, shushing, swinging, and sucking
- The Cuddle Cure and how you can work wonders by doing all 5 "S's" together
- Other techniques that can help you soothe your fussy baby
- Tricks and tips to get your baby to sleep more at night
- Medical problems that can mimic colic

Once you understand your baby's need for a fourth trimester, the 5 "S's," and the Cuddle, you will be able to prevent countless hours of screaming. It is my sincere hope that once this knowledge is shared, *colic* will be found only in dictionaries.

You have been blessed with one of the most amazing experiences a person can ever have—the birth of a baby. It's an exciting ride, so strap yourself in . . . and enjoy. Please don't worry when your baby cries. Consider it an opportunity to perfect your new parenting skills as you learn how to turn your fussy infant into *the happiest baby on the block!*

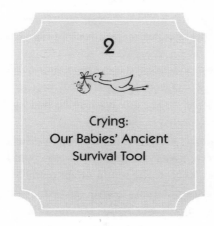

2

Crying:
Our Babies' Ancient
Survival Tool

Main Points:

- The Crying Reflex: Your baby's brilliant attention-getting tool
- How a baby's crying can make you feel
- Do different baby cries have different meanings? Some babies scream even for little problems

At delivery, your baby's powerful wails are a welcome sign that you've given birth to a healthy child. However, if after the first week or two your infant continues to scream, his crying may become the last thing you want to hear! But we should be grateful for our babies' crying—it's one of their most wonderful abilities.

During the first few months of life, your baby will have no problem getting by without the foggiest idea of how to smile or talk, but he would be in terrible danger if he couldn't call out to you. Getting your attention is so important that your newborn can cry from the moment his head pops out of you. This great ability is called the "crying reflex."

The Crying Reflex: Nature's Brilliant Solution for Getting a Cavewoman's Attention!

A baby's cry . . . cries to be turned off.
Peter Ostwald, *Soundmaking: The Acoustic Communication of Emotion*

My guess is that millions of years ago, a Stone Age baby accidentally was born with a perfect way for getting his mother to come to him—screaming. Even if he yelped just because he had hiccups or had scared himself, his mom appeared in seconds.

Other baby animals also need to get their mother's attention quickly, but they would never *scream* for it. Loud crying could be fatal for a young rabbit or a monkey, because the sound might reveal his location to a hungry lion. For this reason, kittens meekly meow for help, squirrel monkeys make soft beeping sounds when they fall out of trees, and baby gorillas barely even whimper when they need their moms.

Baby humans, on the other hand, gave up such caution a long time ago. Whenever they needed their cavemom's attention, they wailed! Perhaps such brash, demanding babies were safe because their parents were able to fight off dangerous animals. Or perhaps a powerful cry was the only sound that could carry far enough for a baby's mom to hear him while working or chatting with friends outside the cave. Some scientists even believe that

---

Why are babies born with a cry reflex . . . but not a laugh reflex?

Wouldn't it be fun if babies were born laughing? Of course it would, but there are two very good reasons why newborns can cry up a storm yet can't giggle.

First, crying is easier than laughing. It takes less coordination, because it's one continuous sound made with each breath. Laughter, on the other hand, is a series of rapid, short sounds strung together like pearls on a single breath.

And while laughter is helpful for social play when your baby is older, crying is crucial for a baby's minute-to-minute survival, from his first day of life.

---

successive generations of babies began to shriek louder and louder because such noisy infants received more food and attention to keep them quiet, and thus were more likely to survive.

We may never know exactly when or how ancient human babies began to cry, yet it's clear that the cave babies who survived and passed their genes on to us were those who could "raise a ruckus."

Your baby's shrill cry is powerful enough to yank you out of bed or hoist you off the toilet with your pants down. (Not bad for a ten-pound weakling!) However, it is a mistake to think your baby is crying because he's *trying* to call you for help. During the first few months, trying to get your attention is the furthest thing from your crying baby's mind. In fact, your baby has absolutely no idea he's even sending you a message.

When you hear your two-week-old scream, you're not getting a communication from him; rather you're *accidentally eavesdropping* on his conversation . . . with himself. His cries are like agitated complaints he's muttering to himself, "Gosh, I'm hungry," or "Boy, I'm cold." Since you're right next to him, you hear his grumbles and want to lovingly respond, "What's the matter, sweetheart? You sound upset."

In a few months, your baby will begin to figure out that crying makes you come. By four to six months your baby will develop a vocabulary of

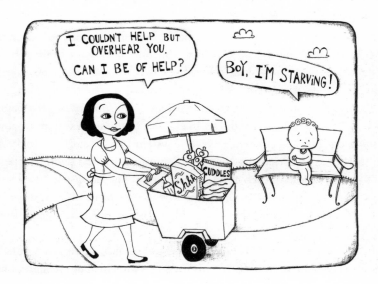

coos, bleats, and yells to communicate specific needs. This is when you may get the sense that your baby is beginning to make "phony" little shrieks to get you to come. But for now, don't worry that responding to his cries will teach him bad habits. Training your baby not to be manipulative will become an important lesson during the second six months of his life. For the moment you *want* him to learn that you'll come whenever he cries. This message of predictable, consistent love and support is *exactly* what will nurture his trust in you.

How a Baby's Cry Makes Us Feel

And, still Caroline cried, and Martha's nerves vibrated in extraordinary response, as if the child were connected to her flesh by innumerable invisible fibers.

Doris Lessing, A Proper Marriage

Just as your baby is born with certain automatic, built-in reflexes (like crying) you too are equipped with many automatic and irresistible feelings about your baby. Researchers proved years ago that adults are naturally attracted to an infant's face. Your baby's heart-shaped face, upturned nose, big eyes, and full forehead give you the urge to kiss and cuddle him for hours!

You also have special instincts to help you tell whether your infant is babbling or if he needs you urgently. Not only does your brain get the message but your body does too. That's why your baby's screams can really "get under your skin." You feel your nervous system snap into "red alert" as your heart begins to race, your blood pressure soars, your palms sweat, and your stomach tightens like a fist. Studies show that a baby's piercing cry can jolt a parent's nervous system like an electric shock. As you might expect, scientists have also demonstrated that parents experiencing other stresses—such as fatigue, isolation, marital discord, financial stress, hormonal imbalance, problems with family or neighbors, or other serious strains—are especially susceptible to feeling overwhelmed by their baby's cries.

It's not just the *sound* of your baby's cry that makes you want to help him, it's how he looks too. Seeing his little fists punching at the air and his face twist in apparent pain can penetrate your heart like an arrow. Every loving fiber in your body will compel you to comfort your crying baby. This powerful biological impulse is *exactly* why it feels so wrong to wait outside the nursery door and let your baby cry it out.

Not only parents tune in to a baby's cries. Single adults and children, too, find the sound of a baby crying upsetting. But new parents, especially ones without prior infant-care experience, find their baby's crying exceptionally disturbing.

Your baby's cry may even rekindle forgotten emotional trauma from your past. You may suddenly recall memories of prior failures or humiliations, like someone who was unfair to you, or remember people who criticized and attacked you. The crying may make you feel that you are being punished for some past misdeed. For some parents, this sense of helplessness is so intolerable that it makes them turn away from their babies' screams and ignore their needs. (See Appendix B for more practical advice about how to survive these difficult days.)

Of course, your baby isn't intentionally trying to make you feel guilty or inadequate. During the first few months of life, his cries are *never, never, never* manipulative, mean, rude, or critical. Nevertheless, those feelings may bubble up inside you when your baby screams on and on.

"Tell Mommy What's the Matter": Your Baby's Three-Word Vocabulary

Our tiny baby's first word to us wasn't Mama <u>or</u> Dada. It sounded more like . . . well, a smoke alarm! She just <u>blasted</u>! It was scary because we had no idea exactly what she was trying to tell us.
Marty and Debbie, parents of two-week-old Sarah Rose

When you first bring your baby home from the hospital, every fuss can sound like a problem and every cry an urgent alarm. All parents dedicate themselves to meeting their newborn's needs, but when your baby cries, can you tell exactly what he needs? Should you be able to figure out why your baby is upset from the sound of his cry? Is the "I'm sleepy" cry of a one-month-old different from his "I'm starving" yell?

Some baby books tell parents that with careful observation they can decipher their baby's message from the way he cries; however, forty years of studies by the world's leading colic researchers have taught us that's not really true.

In a 1990 University of Connecticut study, mothers listened to the audiotaped yells of two different babies, a hungry one-month-old and a newborn who was just circumcised. They were asked if the babies were hungry, sleepy, in pain, angry, startled, or wet. Only twenty-five percent correctly identified the cry of the unfed baby as sounding like hunger (forty percent thought it was an overtired cry). Only forty percent of moms identified the cries of the recently circumcised baby as a pain cry (thirty percent thought he was either startled or angry).

You might wonder if these mothers would better understand their babies' cries if they were more experienced. However, the evidence shows that is not the case either. Researchers in Finland asked eighty experienced baby nurses to listen to the recorded sounds of babies at the moment of birth, when hungry, when in pain, and when gurgling in pleasure. Surprisingly, even these seasoned pros only correctly identified why the baby was crying about fifty percent of the time—barely better than by chance alone.

By three months your baby will learn to make many different noises, making it easier to decipher some messages from the sound of his cry alone. However, at birth, your infant's compact brain simply doesn't have enough room for a repertoire of grunts and whines. That's why during the first few months, most babies only make three simple but distinct sounds: whimpering, crying, and shrieking.

> **Whimpering:** This mild fussing sounds more requesting than complaining, like a call from a neighbor asking to borrow some sugar.
> **Crying:** This good strong yelp demands your attention, like when your kitchen timer goes off.
> **Shrieking:** This last "word" is a piercing, glass-shattering wail, as shrill and unbearable as a burglar alarm.

If asked what each sound signified, you'd probably guess that whimpering means a slight unhappiness like hunger pangs or getting sleepy;

crying indicates some greater distress like being very hungry, thirsty, or cold; and shrieking signals pain, fear, anger, or irritation (if earlier cries got no response).

If your baby is an easy, relatively calm child, your guesses are probably correct. As a rule, the more intense and shrill your baby's cry is—and the quicker it escalates to a shriek—the more likely he's in pain or needs your help right away.

And by adding a few more visual clues to the sound he's making, you'll increase your accuracy. For example:

- Is your baby opening his mouth and rooting? (This could indicate hunger.)
- Is he yawning, rubbing his eyes, moving his head from side to side, or staring out with droopy eyelids? (This could indicate fatigue.)
- Does he seem to be intentionally looking away from you or starting to hiccup? (This could indicate overstimulation.)
- Is he making facial grimaces and trying to bear down? (This could indicate intestinal discomfort.)

In short, when an *easy* baby is a little upset he whimpers, like a puppy whining outside the door. Usually his protests only get louder if his cries are ignored or if he is in great distress.

The needs of *fussy* babies, on the other hand, are often impossible to decipher from the sound of their cries alone. These little ones lack the self-control to proceed patiently through their three-"word" vocabulary, especially when tired or overstimulated. They blow by whimpering and crying, and shift immediately into loud, piercing shrieks that make it impossible to tell whether or not they have an urgent problem. These babies often get so upset by their own screaming that it snowballs and they are crying because they're crying! The gas or loud noise that started the wailin' and flailin' is almost forgotten.

Even when scientists use sophisticated acoustic analyzers to study the cries of fussy babies, they cannot find any differences between their shrieks of hunger, pain, overstimulation, boredom, startling, and even impatience. These intense babies blast out the same one-size-fits-all scream *regardless of what's bothering them.*

> Pam, the mother of two high-powered little boys, Matthew
> and Austin, told me when her boys were babies she joked
> with her husband that their screams were like the blasts of
> a smoke alarm. She said, "When you hear a smoke alarm go off,
> it's <u>impossible</u> to tell from the sound whether it's signaling a
> minor problem—burnt toast—or a calamity—your house is
> burning down. Likewise, with my boys, it was impossible for
> us to tell from the intensity of their cries if they were very ill
> or merely announcing a burp."

Most of the time, even a baby's most terrible shrieks are merely his way of telling you he's hungry, wet, soiled, or lonely, and he will quiet once you give him what he needs. But what if your baby's yelping persists even though his diaper is dry and you're holding him? What happens if you try *everything* and he still doesn't stop screaming?

That's when parents start to wonder if their baby has COLIC.

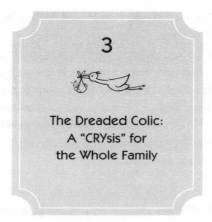

3

The Dreaded Colic:
A "CRYsis" for
the Whole Family

Main Points:

- What is colic?
- The top ten ancient theories about colic
- The Colic Clues: Ten universal facts about colic
- Today's top five colic theories

> *The sound of a crying baby is just about the most disturbing,*
> *demanding, shattering noise we can hear. In the baby's crying*
> *there is no future or past, only now. There is no appeasement, no*
> *negotiations possible, no reasonableness.*
>
> Sheila Kitzinger, *The Crying Baby*

Waaaa . . . waaaa . . . waaaaaa . . . WAAAAAAAAAAAAAAAAAAA!!!!!!!!
The word *infant* derives from Latin and means "without a voice." However, many colicky babies wail so powerfully that their parents think a better name for them would be *mega*-fants or *rant*-fants!

There's no doubt that colicky infants can cry louder and longer than any adult. We would drop from exhaustion after five minutes of full-out screaming, but these little cuties can go and go, with the tenacity of the Energizer bunny.

The word *colic* derives from the Greek word *kolikos,* meaning "large intestine or colon." In ancient Greece, parents believed that intestinal pain caused their babies' crying. (While a gas twinge may start a baby's screaming fit, at other times these very same babies have gas and noisy stomachs yet they don't even make a peep. More on this in Chapter 4.)

All babies have short periods of crying that usually last for a few minutes, totaling about a half hour a day. These babies settle quickly once fed, picked up, or carried. However, once colicky babies start their frantic screaming, they can yell, on and off, for hours.

How Can You Tell If Your Baby Has Colic?

In 1982, Dr. T. Berry Brazelton asked eighty-two new mothers to record how much their normal, healthy infants cried each day during their first three months of life.

The results of this study are shown in the figure below. When Dr. Brazelton did the math, he discovered that at two weeks of age, twenty-

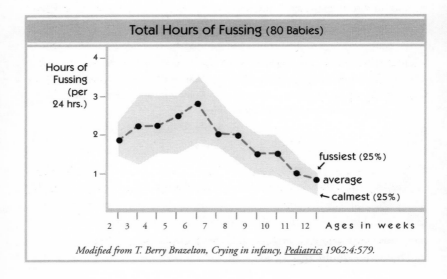

Modified from T. Berry Brazelton, Crying in infancy, Pediatrics 1962:4:579.

five percent of the babies cried for more than two hours each day. By six weeks, twenty-five percent cried for more than three hours each day. Reassuringly, he found that by three months almost all had recovered from their fussy period and few cried more than one hour a day. (Persistent crying tends to vanish after three months which is why some doctors refer to it as "three-month" colic.)

When a baby is brought to me because of crying fits, I first ask about the parents' family history and the baby's birth, feeding habits, and general behavior. Next I examine the baby to make sure she's healthy and thriving. Once I'm sure that the baby is well, I consider if her crying pattern fits the "Rule of Threes," the formal medical definition of colic first formulated by Dr. Morris Wessel, a private pediatrician from Connecticut.

The "Rule of Threes" states that a baby has colic if she cries at least: three hours a day . . . three days a week . . . three weeks in a row.

Some doctors call babies colicky even if they don't fit the "Rule of Threes" but still frequently scream uncontrollably for no obvious reason.

Some parents in my practice also think that the "Rule of Threes" should be revised. They say the true definition of colic is when a baby cries so much her poor mom needs three nannies, three margaritas, and . . . six hands! (Okay, there's an exception to every rule.)

Parents often ask me if there's a way to predict which babies will have colic. While many doctors have tried to find a pattern to this problem, no consistent association has been found between colic and a baby's gender, prematurity, birth order, or their parents' age, income, or education. Colic can happen to anybody's baby. It is truly an equal-opportunity parental nightmare!

What Really Causes Colic?

Nine times out of ten, parents of colicky babies believe that their infants are suffering from some kind of pain. This would seem to be a reasonable guess, since colicky babies:

- are not relieved by the comforts of feeding and holding
- often writhe and grunt

- may start and stop their screaming very abruptly
- have a shrill cry that resembles the sound they make when they're in pain (like after getting a shot)

Pain was what was on Sherry's mind when she brought her baby in to see me for a consultation about his incessant crying.

Charlie, a robust two-month-old, had a normal examination. This surprised his mother who was convinced that his daily frenzies must be the result of pain. When I asked her how she could be so sure, Sherry sheepishly admitted that she'd accidentally hit Charlie's head with the telephone receiver. She said, "When that happened, I realized that his cry after getting whacked sounded <u>exactly</u> the same as his normal afternoon screamfest. I thought, <u>That proves it, he's been in pain this whole time.</u>"

Was Sherry right? Was Charlie's crying caused by pain? Or had she somehow misread the situation? As you can imagine, since time immemorial, parents of crying babies have been analyzing their child's shrieks, trying to come up with an explanation for why their contented little infant at times suddenly "morphs" into one of the unhappiest babies on the block.

The "Evil Eye" (and Other Theories): How Our Ancestors Explained Colic

Before I got married I had six theories about bringing up children; now I have six children and no theories.

John Wilmot

It wasn't so long ago that people believed leeches could cure diseases and babies were born blind. Likewise, our ancestors made many guesses about why some infants cried so much. Deciphering a Stone Age baby's cry may well have been one of the first multiple-choice questions in history:

Your cave baby is crying because:

a. She's hungry.

b. She's cold.

c. She needs a fresh loincloth.

d. A witch cast a spell on her.

Over the centuries, wild theories have abounded about the cause of prolonged crying. Here are a few:

The Top Ten Ancient Theories of the Cause of Colicky Crying

1. Someone who dislikes the mother gave the baby the "evil eye."
2. The baby caught a draft.
3. The baby's spirit is unhappy because her father denied the baby was his.
4. The baby is possessed by the devil.
5. The baby is communicating with the spirits of unborn babies.
6. The daytime is for adults to make noise, and at night it's the baby's turn.
7. The baby's crying is a punishment for Adam and Eve's original sin.
8. The mother's milk is too thin.
9. The mother's milk is too rich.
10. A trauma during pregnancy made the baby fearful.

Even Shakespeare tossed in his two cents about why babies cry. In *King Lear* he guessed: *When we are born, we cry that we are come to this great stage of fools.* Babies are amazing, but I'm afraid Shakespeare was giving them more credit than they deserve.

The Myth of "Blowing Off Steam"

Crying is good for the lungs the way bleeding is good for the veins!

Lee Salk

Parents have long noticed that fussy infants eventually cry themselves to sleep. Some experts have guessed that these babies *need* to scream to exercise their lungs or unwind from the day's thrills before they surrender to sleep.

I strongly disagree. The idea that screaming is good for babies is illogical from both a biological and evolutionary point of view. First, the lungs of calm babies are as healthy and strong as the lungs of colicky babies. Second, colicky prehistoric infants might well have put themselves in danger. Their screaming could have attracted enemies to their family's hiding place. And it might have enraged their Neanderthal parents, leading to abandonment, abuse, and even infanticide.

Now, I freely admit . . .

Yes . . . babies can get wound up by a full day's excitement.

Yes . . . some babies ignore their parents' best attempts to calm them.

Yes . . . screaming babies eventually conk out from sheer exhaustion.

But your baby is not a little pressure cooker that needs to "blow off steam" before cooling down. Letting your baby cry it out makes as little sense as closing your ears to your screeching car alarm while you wait for the battery to die.

At this point, you may be thinking, "But *I* often feel better after I have a good cry." Of course that's true; however, while adults may sob for minutes, colicky babies can wail for hours!

I believe that most parents who let their babies shriek until they collapse do this only because they feel desperate and exhausted. It's a last resort that goes against every parental instinct. Can it stop the crying? Yes. However, the real question is whether or not this climate of inconsistency—sometimes you answer her cry and sometimes you don't—is what you want to teach your baby to expect from you. Most parents answer that question with a resounding no.

All baby experts agree that our children do best when we are *consistent* in our responses. You know how frustrating it can be when some days you can calm your baby yet other days nothing works. Well, that's how your baby feels when her cry in the morning brings a prompt reward of touching and warm milk yet in the afternoon it's ignored.

Is it *ever* okay to let your baby yell? I don't believe it's a tragedy if your little one cries for ten minutes while you are in the bathroom or preparing dinner. The loving and cuddling you've been giving her all day easily out-weighs that short-lived frustration. But fussy infants are not like toddlers. If your two-year-old screams because she wants to yank your earrings, you may have to let her cry so she can learn that when you say, "No!" you mean it. The time will come when lessons of discipline will become im-portant, even lifesaving. But you're jumping the gun if you think you need to teach discipline to your two-month-old!

For the first few months, you should soothe your baby whenever she yells. Infants rarely cry unless they're upset about something, and it's our challenge and duty to figure out what they need and how to give it to them.

The Colic Clues—
Ten Universal Facts About Colic

In order to understand what causes colic, we first must agree on what it is. Researchers analyzing babies from all around the world have discovered ten fundamental traits of colic and colicky babies:

1. *Colicky crying usually starts at two weeks, peaks at six weeks, and ends by three to four months of age.*

2. *Preemies are no more likely to have colic than full-term babies. (And their colic doesn't start until they are about two weeks past their due date.)*

3. *Colicky babies have twisted faces and piercing wails, like a person in pain. Often, their cries come in waves (like cramps) and stop abruptly.*

4. *Their screams frequently begin during or just after a feeding.*

5. *They often double up, grunt, strain, and seem relieved by passing gas or pooping.*

6. *Colic is often much worse in the evening (the "witching hour").*

7. *Colic is as likely to occur with a couple's fifth baby as with their first.*

8. *Colicky crying often improves with rocking, holding, shhhhing, and gentle abdominal pressure.*

9. *Babies are healthy and happy between crying bouts.*

10. *In many cultures around the world, babies never get colic.*

Once scientists determined the colic clues, they compared them to the popular colic theories to determine which, if any, explained them best. The researchers immediately excluded many of the crazy old ideas and what remained are today's top five colic theories:

1. *Tiny Tummy Troubles*—babies suffer from severe discomfort caused by simple digestive problems (such as gas, constipation, cramps).
2. *Big Tummy Troubles*—babies suffer severe pain from true intestinal illness (such as food intolerance or stomach acid reflux).
3. *Maternal Anxiety*—babies wail because of anxiety they pick up from their mothers.
4. *Brain Immaturity*—immaturity of a baby's nervous system causes her to get overwhelmed and scream.
5. *Challenging Temperament*—a baby's intense or sensitive temperament makes her shriek even in response to minor upsets.

Each of these theories has its group of followers, but is any one of them the true cause of colic? Can any one of these theories explain all ten of the universal characteristics of colic?

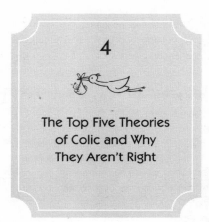

4

The Top Five Theories of Colic and Why They Aren't Right

Main Points:

- Gas, constipation and overactive intestines: Why these Tiny Tummy Troubles are not the cause of severe crying
- Food sensitivities and stomach acid reflux: Why these Big Tummy Troubles are rarely the cause of persistent crying
- Why maternal anxiety isn't the cause of colic
- The ways in which a baby's brain is immature, and why that can't be the entire explanation for uncontrollable crying
- What is meant by challenging temperament and why it fails to explain why babies get colic

Theory #1: Do Tiny Tummy Troubles Cause Colic?

For thousands of years, many parents have had a "gut feeling" that their infants were crying from bad stomach pain. The three tummy-twisting problems that became the prime suspects of causing colic were intestinal "gas"; pooping problems; and "overactive" intestines.

Burping with the Best of Them

Babies often gulp down air during their feedings. Here are tips to help your baby swallow less air and to burp up what does get in:

1. Don't lay your baby flat during a feeding. (Imagine how hard it would be for you to drink lying down, without swallowing a lot of air.)

2. If your baby is a noisy eater, stop and burp him frequently during the meal.

3. Before burping your baby, sit him in your right hand, with your left hand cupped under his chin. Then bounce him up and down a few times. This gets the bubbles to float to the top of the stomach for easy burping. (Don't worry, it won't make him spit up.)

4. The best burping position: Sit down with your baby on your lap, with his chin resting comfortably in your cupped hand. (I never burp babies over my shoulder, because their spit-up goes right down my back.) Next, lean him forward so he's doubled over a little. Give his back ten to twenty firm thumps. Babies' stomachs are like glasses of soda, with little "bubblettes" stuck to the sides. So thump your baby like a drum to jiggle these free.

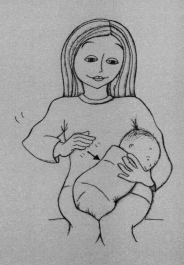

Let's examine each individually and then I will explain why none of these nuisances is the real cause of colic.

Do Babies Cry from Intestinal "Gas" . . . or Is That Just a Lot of Hot Air?

Most infants have gas—often. I'm sure you've witnessed virtuoso performances of burping, tooting, and grunting several times a day. Many parents are convinced this intestinal grumbling causes their baby's cries.

Parents who think colic is a gas problem have two powerful allies: grandmas and doctors. For generations, grandmothers have advised new moms to treat their baby's colic by avoiding gassy foods, burping them well, and feeding them sips of tummy-soothing teas. For decades, doctors have suggested that mothers alter their diet or their child's formula, or give burping drops (simethicone) to reduce a baby's intestinal gas.

However, with all due respect to grandmothers and doctors, fussy newborns have no more gas in their intestines than calm babies. In 1954, Dr. Ronald Illingworth, England's preeminent pediatrician, compared the stomach X rays of normal babies with colicky babies and found *no* difference in the amount of gas the calm and cranky babies had at their peaks of crying. In addition, repeated scientific experiments have shown that simethicone burping drops (Mylicon and Phazyme) are no more helpful for crying babies than plain water. It turns out that the gas in your baby's intestine comes mostly from digested food, not from swallowed air.

Pooping Problems: Can Constipation Trigger Colicky Crying?

Some parents worry that constipation is causing their baby's colic. Babies struggling to poop can look like they're in a wrestling match. However, constipation really means hard poop, and only a few, fussy, formula-fed babies suffer from that. Most infants who groan and twist usually pass soft or even runny stools.

If grunting babies aren't constipated, why are they straining so hard?

1. To poop, an infant has to simultaneously tighten his stomach and relax his anus. This can be hard for a young baby to do. Many accidentally clench both at the same time and try to force their poop through a closed anus.

Black Tar to Scrambled Eggs: What Are Normal Baby Poops Like?

Few new parents are prepared for how weird baby poops are. For starters, there's the almost extraterrestrial first poop—meconium. (Robin Williams described its tarry consistency as a cross between Velcro and toxic waste!) Within days, meconium's green-black color changes to light green and then to bright, mustard yellow with a seedy texture. (The seeds are miniature milk curds.)

In breast-fed babies, poops then turn into runny scrambled eggs that squirt out four to twelve times a day. Over the next month or two, the poop gradually becomes thicker, like oatmeal, and may only come out once a day or less. (The longest period I've ever seen a healthy, breast-fed baby go without a stool has been twenty-one days. However, if your baby is skipping more than three days without a stool, call your pediatrician to make sure he's okay.)

For bottle-fed babies, poop may be loose, claylike, or hard in the first weeks. The particular formula a baby drinks can affect this consistency. Some infants get constipated from cow's milk formula, while others get stopped up by soy. A few are even sensitive to whether the formula is made from powder or concentrate.

2. They're lying flat on their backs. Just think of the trouble you'd have trying to poop in that position!

Babies grunt and frown when they poop because they're working so hard to overcome these two challenges, *not* because they're in pain! (For more on infant constipation, see Chapter 14.)

"Overactive" Intestines—Crying, Cramps, and the Gastro-colic Reflex

Does your baby cry and double up shortly after you start a feeding? This twisting and grunting may look like indigestion, but it's usually just an overreaction to a *normal* intestinal reflex called the "gastro-colic reflex" (literally, the stomach-colon reflex).

This valuable reflex is the stomach's way of telling the colon: "Time to

How Your Baby's Tummy Works

A baby's digestive system is like a long conveyor belt. At one end, milk is loaded into the mouth five to eight times a day. It is quickly delivered to the stomach, and then is slowly carried through the intestines, where it is digested and absorbed. Whatever milk isn't absorbed gets turned into poop and is temporarily stored in the colon.

When the next meal begins, the stomach telegraphs a message to the lower intestines, commanding them to squeeze. The squeezing pushes the poop out, making room for the next load of food. This message from the stomach to the colon is to constrict the gastro-colic reflex.

get rid of the poop and make room for the new food that was just eaten!" If you've noticed that your baby poops during or after eating, this is why.

Most infants are unaware when this reflex is happening. Others feel a mild spasm after a big feeding or if they're frazzled at day's end. But for a few babies, this squeezing of the intestine feels like a punch in the belly! These infants writhe as if in terrible pain.

As you might imagine, the gastro-colic reflex can be even more uncomfortable if your baby is constipated and his colon must strain to push out firm poop. However, most babies who cry from this reflex have soft, pasty poops. They cry because they are overly sensitive to this weird sensation.

The Reasons Why Tiny Tummy Troubles Cannot Be the True Cause of Colic

It's not what we don't know that gets us into the most trouble, it's what we know . . . that just ain't so!

Josh Billings, *Everybody's Friend*, 1874

Despite the fact that many people think gas causes colic, it and the other Tiny Tummy Troubles (TTT's) don't explain this terrible crying because:

- Most colicky babies burp and pass wind many times a day without a whimper.

Anti-Spasm Medicines:
Soothing Crying Babies into a Stupor

From the 1950s to the 1980s, doctors armed parents with millions of prescriptions of anti-cramp medicine. Some doctors used Donnatal (a mix of anti-cramp medicine plus phenobarbitol) while others preferred Levisin (hyocyamine). Both are cramp-relieving and sedating, and both are still occasionally prescribed by doctors today.

However, of all the anti-spasm drugs recommended for colic, Bentyl was by far and away the most popular. In 1984, 74 million doses of it were sold in Britain alone. But Bentyl turned out to be the most dangerous of all the tummy drugs. In 1985, doctors were horrified to discover that a number of colicky babies being treated with it suffered convulsions, coma—even death.

In retrospect, it's likely that anti-cramp medicines work *not* because of any tummy effect, but because they induce sedation as an incidental side effect.

- Adults double up when they have stomachaches, but babies snap into this fetal position *whenever* they are upset, regardless of the cause.

- Many babies shriek even when they only are experiencing a minor discomfort.

The TTT's also fail to explain five of the ten universal characteristics of colic and colicky babies:

- *Colicky crying usually starts at two weeks, peaks at six weeks, and ends by three to four months of age.* Neither gas nor the gastro-colic reflex fit this clue because both are present from birth (before colic starts) and continue long past three months (when colic is over).

- *Colic in preemies doesn't start until two weeks after their due date.* Preemies have lots of gas and a vigorous gastro-colic reflex. If these sensations truly caused colic, crying in preemies would start immediately, not be delayed for months.

- *Colic is often much worse in the evening.* Babies poop and have stomach rumblings twenty-four hours a day, so if they caused colic, crying would be as common in the morning as it is at night.

- *Colicky crying often improves with rocking, wrapping, shhhhing, and tummy pressure.* It doesn't make any sense that rocking, wrapping, or shhhhing could stop bad stomach pain.

- *There are many cultures around the world where babies never get colic.* All babies around the world experience TTT's. So if they were the basis of colic, why would there be cultures where prolonged crying is virtually nonexistent?

Theory #2: Do Big Tummy Troubles Cause Colic?

Over the past thirty years, scientists have discovered several new problems that cause stomach pain in adults. I call these conditions "Big Tummy Troubles" because they are actual medical illnesses, not merely burps and hiccups.

As each new illness was reported, pediatricians carefully considered if it might occur in infants and explain the inconsolable crying that plagues so many of our babies. Two of these Big Tummy Troubles have been scrutinized as possible keys to the mystery of colic: food sensitivities and stomach acid reflux.

Food Sensitivity—Warning!
Some Foods May Be Hazardous to Your Baby's Smile

If you are breast-feeding, you may have been counseled to avoid foods that are too hot, too cold, too strong, too weak, as well as to steer clear of spices, dairy products, acidic fruit and "gassy" vegetables.

Likewise, mothers of colicky, bottle-fed babies are often advised to switch their child's formula to remove an ingredient that may cause fussiness.

Over the years, experts have considered three ways a baby's diet might trigger uncontrollable crying: indigestion, allergies, and caffeine-type stimulation.

Indigestion: Are Garlic and Onions Risky or the Spices of Life?

Passing up garlic, onions, and beans seems reasonable to most people. These foods can make *us* gassy. But if gassy foods are hard on a baby's tummy, why can breast-feeding moms in Mexico eat *frijoles* (beans) and those in Korea munch *kim chee* (garlic-pickled cabbage) without their babies ever letting out a peep?

Nevertheless, I do think it's reasonable for the mother of an irritable baby to avoid "problem" foods (citrus, strawberries, tomatoes, beans, cabbage, broccoli, cauliflower, brussels sprouts, peppers, onion, garlic) for a few days to see if her baby cries less. However, in my experience, only a handful of infants improve when these foods are eliminated. Studies even show that babies love tasting a smorgasbord of flavors. So don't be surprised if your little one sucks on your breast *more* heartily after you've had a plate of lasagna loaded with garlic!

Food Allergies: Why Couldn't Babies with Allergies Just Sneeze Instead of Scream?

Allergies are part of our immune system, protecting us from unfamiliar proteins (like inhaled pollen or cat dander) that try to enter our bodies.

As a rule, if you have an allergic reaction you'll sneeze, because the fight between your body and the allergens typically takes place in your nose. With infants, however, the battleground between their bodies' immune system and the foreign protein is usually in the intestines. Your baby's intestine is not yet fully developed. Her immature intestinal lining allows large, allergy-triggering molecules to enter her bloodstream like flies zooming through a torn screen door. Over the first year of life, your baby's intestinal lining gradually becomes a much better barrier to these protein intruders.

For many years, doctors believed babies could be allergic to their own mother's milk. In 1983, Swedish scientists proved this impossible. They demonstrated that babies whose colic improved when they were taken off their mother's milk were sensitive *not* to their mom's milk itself but to traces of cow's milk that had floated across the lining of the mother's intestines and snuck into her milk.

Please don't be overly concerned about your diet troubling your child. As a rule, babies rarely develop allergies to the foods their moms eat. The two biggest exceptions to that rule, however, are cow's milk, the proverbial eight-hundred-pound gorilla of baby allergies, and soy, coming in a not-too-distant second place (about ten percent of babies who are milk allergic are soy allergic as well).

I tell my patients it should come as no surprise that some babies develop an allergic reaction to cow's milk. After all, this food is lovingly made by cows for their own babies, and it was never intended to feed our hungry tots.

Cow's milk protein starts passing into your breast milk within minutes of drinking a glass. It reaches its peak level about eight to twelve hours later and it's out of your milk in twenty-four to thirty-six hours. Fortunately, most babies have no problem tolerating this tiny bit of milk protein. However, sensitive babies begin reacting to it within two to thirty-six hours of consuming it.

Milk-allergic babies may suffer from a number of bothersome symptoms besides severe crying. I have cared for infants whose milk allergy gave them skin rashes, nose congestion, wheezing, vomiting, and watery stools. The intestines of some of my patients have gotten so irritated by allergies that they produced strings of bloody mucous that could be seen mixed in with their stools. Although blood in your baby's diaper will raise your heart rate, it is usually no more ominous than finding blood in your mucous when you blow your nose. Be sure to contact your baby's doctor, however, to discuss the problem.

Stimulant Food: Is Your Baby on a Caffeine Jag?

Some babies are supersensitive. They jump when the phone rings and cry when they smell strong perfume. It should come as no surprise that some babies also get hyper from caffeine (coffee, tea, cola, or chocolate) or from stimulant medicines (diet pills, decongestants, and certain Chinese herbs) in their mom's milk.

While many babies are unfazed when their mothers drink one or two cups of coffee, even that small amount of caffeine can rev a sensitive baby up into the "red zone." The caffeine collects in a woman's breast milk over four to six hours and can make a baby irritable within an hour of being eaten.

Stomach Acid Reflux:
Do Colicky Babies Cry from "Heartburn"?

Pediatricians have also examined stomach acid reflux (also known as Gastro-Esophageal Reflux, or GER) as a possible colic cause. This condition—where acidic stomach juice squirts up toward the mouth, irritating everything it touches—is a proven cause of heartburn in adults.

Now, for most babies, a little reflux is nothing new. We just call it by a different name: "spit-up." Since the muscle that keeps the stomach contents from moving "upstream" is weak in most babies, a bit of your baby's last meal can easily sneak back out when she burps or grunts, especially if she was overfed or swallowed air.

Most newborns don't spit up much, but some babies "urp" up prodigious amounts of their milk. Fortunately, most of these babies don't suffer any ill effects from all this regurgitation. The greatest problem caused by their vomiting is often milk stains on your sofa and clothes.

On the other hand, infants with severe GER are plagued with copious amounts of vomiting, poor weight gain, and occasional burning pain. (In some babies, stomach acid travels just partially up the esophagus, causing heartburn *without* vomiting.)

When should you suspect reflux as the cause of your baby's unhappiness? Look for these telltale signs:

- She vomits more than five times a day and more than an ounce each time.
- Her crying occurs with most meals, during the day *and* night.
- She often wails right after a burp or a spit-up.
- The bouts of crying are no better by the time she's three months old.
- She may have episodes of back arching, hoarseness, wheezing, choking, and/or excessive and even painful hiccuping.

Big Tummy Troubles Strike Out as the Major Cause of Colic

Food sensitivity and acid reflux can make some babies scream, but do the Big Tummy Troubles (BTT's) explain most cases of colic or just a small number of ultrafussy babies?

In my experience, five to ten percent of very fussy infants cry due to food sensitivity from cow's milk or soy, and one to three percent of them cry from the pain of acid reflux. That notwithstanding, Big Tummy Troubles (BTT's) are *not* the cause of colic for the majority of fussy infants:

- If food allergies caused colic, a mother would only have to change her baby's formula or her diet and, *poof,* the crying would stop. But this rarely helps.

- If allergies caused colic, formula-fed babies should be especially fussy because they eat hundreds of times more cow's milk protein than do breast-fed babies. Yet colic is equally common in both groups.

- Doctors in Melbourne, Australia, examined twenty-four babies under three months of age who were so irritable they had to be hospitalized. All were checked for acid reflux; only one baby had it.

- Most babies with severe reflux have *no* pain. A review of 219 young babies sent to a hospital clinic because of severe reflux found that thirty-three percent had severe vomiting, thirty percent were not gaining weight, but very few had excessive crying.

The BTT's also fail to explain five of the ten universal characteristics of colic and colicky babies:

- *Colicky crying usually starts at two weeks, peaks at six weeks, and ends by three to four months of age.* Newborns are continually exposed to spit-up and allergens in their diet. If the BTT's caused colic, crying would start right away and continue well past three months. (Babies with cow's milk allergy have problems that last for at least six to twelve months, and serious reflux usually causes heartburn complaints for nine months or more.)

- *Colic in preemies doesn't start until two weeks after their due date.* A preemie born two months early rarely shows colic before she's two and a half months old, despite her daily exposure to spit-up and allergenic proteins.

- *Colic is often much worse in the evening.* If the BTT's caused colic, crying would occur at any time of the day, because babies eat the same food—and spit it up—from morning to night.

- *Colicky crying often improves with rocking, holding, shhhhing, and tummy pressure.* Why would these actions soothe inflamed intestines or heartburn? Indeed, rocking and pressure might even squirt *more* acid up from the stomach, worsening reflux pain.

- *There are many cultures around the world where babies never get colic.* All babies, regardless of where they live, occasionally spit up and drink breast milk containing tiny samplings from their mommy's last meal. Yet, despite this, infants in some cultures around the world *never* suffer from colic.

Theory #3: Does Maternal Anxiety Cause Colic?

Any mother who has felt fear and anxiety surrounding the birth of her new baby might wonder if these disquieting feelings could affect her newborn. This was Trina's concern. . . .

With her ruby lips and lush, black hair, Tatiana was exquisite. But her delicacy in form was balanced by a strong and feisty temperament. She reflected her parents' passionate personalities, and Trina and Mirko could not have been more thrilled. However, as the weeks went by, they became more and more frustrated as Tatiana's feistiness turned into prolonged periods of screaming.

Trina called one afternoon after her four-week-old daughter had been particularly cranky. She confided, "I'm a very sensitive and intuitive person. Is it possible that Tatiana is too? Is it possible she's upset because of all the stress I'm under?"

It seems that the joy Trina and Mirko had felt after Tatiana's birth was tempered by Trina's painful recovery from a cesarean section and then the destruction of their possessions from a flood in the apartment above theirs, days after they brought Tatiana home.

"The nest we created for our baby collapsed like a house of cards and we had to move into our friend's living room. When Tatiana developed colic at three weeks of age, I couldn't help but think her screams stemmed from all the anxiety she felt from me during this terribly upsetting time."

The birth of an infant brings with it such a wonderful but weighty responsibility that it's a rare parent who doesn't feel some anxiety and self-doubt. Many new mothers confide in me that they feel overwhelmed because:

- *Caring for their baby is unexpectedly stressful.*
  No matter how much you thought that you were prepared for your new baby, it still may hit you like a ton of bricks.

- *They have little baby experience.*
  Most of us have had very few opportunities to care for small babies. That's why our generation may well be the least experienced . . . in history!

- *They feel like everybody is criticizing them.*
  New parents are very vulnerable to everyone's advice and criticisms. "Pick her up!" "Don't pick her up!" "Feed on demand!" "Feed on a schedule!" Getting peppered by all these comments can whittle down your confidence and magnify your self-doubts.

■ *The responsibility falls predominantly upon their shoulders.*
Mothers feel a pressure to know what they're doing because
they are the ones who are expected to be able to soothe their
baby when no one else can.

A New Mom's Feelings of Inadequacy

Aye, aye, aaaaaye! Am I really ready for this?

Mothering a baby is a magnificent experience, but it's neither automatic
nor instinctive. Unless you've spent lots of time baby-sitting or helping
with younger siblings, don't be surprised if your new baby makes you feel
you need six arms—like a Hindu deity. For most women, mothering their
newborn is the toughest job they've ever had!

After talking to thousands of new mothers, I've made an "Aye, Aye,
Aye" list of the top ten stresses that can undermine a new mom's self-
confidence—and make even a goddess start to crumble:

1. *I*ntense fatigue
2. *I*nexperience
3. *I*solation from loving family and friends
4. *I*nsufficient isolation from intrusive family and friends
5. *I*nconsolable crying (the baby's, that is)
6. *I*rritating arguments with your spouse
7. *I*nstant loss of job income and gratification
8. *I*nsecurity about your body
9. *I*nstability of your hormones
10. *I*ndelible barf stains on every piece of clothing you own

Of course, these problems pale when compared to the vivid joy and feeling of purpose your baby brings into your life. However, new mothers enter
a vulnerable psychological space after giving birth, and fatigue and fear can
even further distort your perceptions. You're in the midst of one of life's
most intense experiences and, particularly if you have a colicky baby, waves
of anxiety and depression may repeatedly wash over you during these initial
months. (For more on postpartum depression, see Appendix B.)

Fortunately, the pressures you feel today will soon melt into a warm love that will probably be more powerful and profound than any other you have ever felt. In the meantime, please be tolerant of yourself, your husband, and, especially, your baby.

A Mom's Anxiety "Ain't" the Answer for Colic

Colicky infants are born, not made.
Dr. Martin Stein, *Encounters with Children*

It's common for mothers of irritable babies to feel jealous and self-critical when they see other moms with easy-to-calm infants. Those feelings can cast a shadow over a woman's confidence and make her wonder if her anxiety causes her baby's crying.

Fortunately, during the first few months of life babies aren't able to tell when their mothers are distressed and worried. Remember, *babies are just babies!* They are not born with the ability to read their mother's feelings as if they were messages written on her forehead in lipstick. These little prehistoric creatures even have trouble . . . burping. So don't worry about your baby being affected by your anxiety.

Also, new parents sometimes mistakenly assume their newborns are nervous because their hands tremble, their chins quiver, and they startle at sudden sounds or movements. However, those reactions are normal signs of a newborn's undeveloped nervous system and automatically disappear after about three months.

In my experience, however, there are a few ways a mother's anxiety about her fussy infant could unintentionally nudge her baby into more crying:

- Anxiety might lessen the mother's breast-milk supply or interfere with her milk letdown, thus frustrating a hungry baby. (See Chapter 14 to remedy these feeding problems.)

- A mother may be so distracted and depressed that she's emotionally unavailable to comfort her crying infant.

- An anxious mother may be afraid to handle her baby as vigorously as is necessary to calm the screaming. (See the discussion about "Vigor" in Chapter 7.)

- Nervous moms tend to jump impatiently from one calming method to another. They can get so lost in their anxiety they don't notice they're upsetting their babies even more.

However, when you carefully study the issue of maternal anxiety, it's clear that it can't be making a million of our babies cry for hours every day. The nervous-mommy theory fails to explain three colic characteristics:

- *Colic in preemies starts about two weeks past their due date.* If a mother's anxiety caused her baby's colic, crying would occur earlier and more often in preemies. After all, these fragile babies can turn even calm parents into nervous wrecks.

- *Colicky babies seem to be in pain.* Even if your baby could sense your anxiety, why would she cry as if she had pain?

- *Colic is as likely to occur with a couple's fifth baby as with their first.* This is the most powerful argument against a connection between anxiety and colic. Since experienced parents are more confident, their fifth baby should be less prone to colic than their first, but that just isn't the case.

Trina didn't need to worry that her stress had invaded Tatiana's tender psyche. In reality, the opposite is usually the case. Your baby's wail can trigger red alert in *your* nervous system, making *you* feel tense and anxious!

Theory #4: Is a Baby's Immature Brain the Cause of Colic?

During medical school, I was taught colic was an intestinal problem. Soon thereafter, that theory was pushed aside by the concept of brain immaturity. As we discovered more about our babies' nervous systems, we came to believe colic resulted from their immature brains getting overstimulated by all the new experiences babies encountered after birth. It's no wonder this theory became popular because, let's face it, babies are so . . . immature!

Babies have the coordination of drunken sailors and the quick wits of, well, newborns. But what *exactly* is immature in your baby's brain, and how might that predispose him to uncontrollable crying?

Mental Abilities Your Baby Was Born With

Imagine you're taking a very long trip but can only bring one suitcase with you. Now imagine that your suitcase is tiny. In a funny way, that's the situation your baby was in as he was preparing for birth. He could only fit into his small brain the most basic abilities he would need to live outside the protection of your womb.

If you could have helped him pack, what abilities would you have considered important for him to be born with? Walking? Smiling? Saying "I love you, Mommy"?

Over millions of years, Mother Nature picked four indispensable survival tools to fit into our babies' apple-size brains:

1. *Life-support controls*—the ability to maintain blood pressure, breathing, etc.
2. *Reflexes*—dozens of important automatic behaviors that help newborns sneeze, suck, swallow, cry, and more.
3. *Limited control of muscles and senses*—once babies can breathe and eat, these very limited abilities allow them to touch, taste, look around, and interact with the world.
4. *State control*—after babies start interacting with their families and their exciting new world, state control helps them turn their attention on (to watch and learn) and off (to recover and sleep).

Of all of these abilities, state control is the most important in determining whether or not he gets colic.

State Control: Your Baby's Ability to Tune the World In . . . or Shut It Out

When doctors talk about your baby's state, we're not discussing whether you live in Ohio or Florida. State describes your baby's level of wakefulness or sleep—in other words, his state of alertness. States range from deep sleep to light sleep to fussiness to full-out screaming. Right in the middle

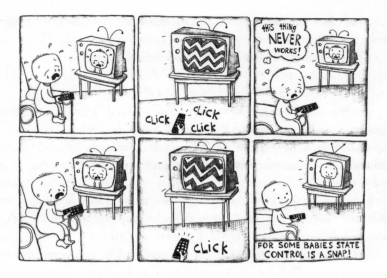

is perhaps the most magical state of all: quiet alertness. It's easy to tell when your baby is quietly alert: his eyes will be open and bright and his face peacefully relaxed as he surveys the sights around him.

Maintaining a state is one of the earliest jobs your baby's brain must accomplish. His ability to stop his crying, keep awake, or stay asleep is called his "state control." I like to think of state control as your baby's TV remote, which allows him to "keep a channel on" when something is interesting, to "change channels" when he gets bored, and to shut the "TV" off if it starts upsetting him or it's time to go to bed.

Many young infants have excellent state control. These "I can do it myself" babies focus intensely on something for a while then pull away whenever they want; they easily shift between sleeping, alertness, and crying. These self-calming babies are especially good at protecting themselves from getting overstimulated. When the world gets too chaotic, some stare into space, some rhythmically suck their lower lip, and others turn their heads as if to say, "You excite me sooo much, I just have to look away to catch my breath!"

You may also notice your baby settling himself by using an attention off-switch called "habituation." It is one of your baby's best tools for shielding himself from getting too much stimulation. Like a circuit breaker that cuts the electrical flow when the wires overload, habituation allows your baby to shut off his attention when his brain gets overloaded.

Habituation explains the extraordinary "sleep anywhere-anytime-despite-the-noise" ability that infants have. (It's also the tool baby boys use to help them sleep despite the pain of circumcision.)

You'll notice that your newborn follows a simple plan during his first few weeks of life: eating and sleeping! Then, as he acclimates to being out of your womb, he'll spend increasing time in quiet alertness. Unfortunately, many young babies can't handle the additional excitement that comes with this alertness. These babies are *poor* self-calmers with immature state control. They have trouble shutting off their alertness, so their circuits often overload. After a few weeks, as they begin to wake up to the world, their state control starts to get overwhelmed and fail.

These babies look exhausted but their eyes keep staring out, unable to close, as if held open by toothpicks. It's as if their remote control malfunctioned, stranding them on a channel showing a loud, upsetting movie.

One exasperated mom told me her colicky three-month-old, Owen, cried for several hours every day. He clearly needed to sleep, but he wouldn't close his eyes. She said, "I keep trying to get him off *The Crying Channel* and help him find the *Sleep Station* again."

When your little baby is locked into screaming, please don't despair. Much better state control will be coming to rescue you both in a few months. In the meantime, the second part of this book will teach you exactly how to soothe him when he's having a meltdown.

"Help Me . . . The World Is Too Big!" How *Overstimulation* Causes Crying

Avoid overstimulation with toys, lights, and colors; this fatigues the baby's senses.
Richard Lovell, *Essays on Practical Education*, 1789

Considering how exciting the world is, it's a wonder that all babies don't get overstimulated! Fortunately, most are great at shutting out the world when they need to. However, if your baby has poor state control, even a low activity level may push him into frantic crying. He may begin to sob because of a tiny upset, like a burp or loud noise, but then get so wound up—by his own yelling—that he's soon raging out of control.

These babies cry because they get overstimulated and then stuck in "cry mode." If we could translate their shrieks into English, we'd hear something like "Please . . . help me . . . the world is too big!"

"Help Me . . . I'm Stuck in a Closet!"
How *Understimulation* Causes Crying

Your baby is not crying to make you pick him up, but because you put him down in the first place.

Penelope Leach, *Your Baby and Child*

Our culture believes in the strange myth that a baby wants to be left in a quiet, dark room. But what is this stillness like for your new baby? Imagine you've been working in a noisy, hectic office for nine months. One morning you come to work and find yourself alone—no chatter, no ringing phones, no commotion. Soon, the stillness gets on your nerves. You begin pacing and muttering, until you lose it and scream, "Get me out of here!"

This scene is similar to the way babies experience the world when they come home from the hospital. Although *our* image of the perfect nursery is one where our little angel sleeps in serene quiet, to a newborn that feels a bit like being stuck in a closet.

As strange as it sounds, your baby doesn't want—or need—peace and quiet. What he yearns for are the pulsating rhythms that constantly surrounded him in his womb world. In fact, the understimulation and stillness of our homes can drive a sensitive newborn every bit as nuts as chaotic overstimulation can.

Does understimulation mean babies cry because they're bored? No. Unlike older children and adults, babies don't find monotonous repetition boring. (That's why your baby is happy drinking milk day after day.) Rather, they find the *absence* of monotonous repetition hard to tolerate. Their cries ask for a return to the constant, hypnotizing stimulation of the womb. Fussy babies often take three months before they become mature enough to cope with the world without this rhythmic reassurance.

Either understimulation or overstimulation can be terribly unsettling to young infants; however, even worse is to experience both at the same time. When an immature baby is subjected to chaos in the absence of calming, rhythmic sensations, it can drive him past his point of tolerance!

Is Immaturity the Long-Sought Cause of Colic? Close, but No Cigar!

Brain immaturity is a large piece of the colic puzzle. But this theory can't be the whole truth because it fails to explain two crucial colic clues:

- *Preemies are no more likely to have colic than full-term babies.* If brain immaturity were the underlying cause of a baby's screaming, preemies, with their superimmature brains, would be the fussiest of all babies. Yet these tiny babies never cry without a clear reason, and they stop promptly once their need is met.

- *There are many cultures around the world where babies never get colic.* This fact proves that brain immaturity cannot be the sole basis of persistent crying. There is no biological reason why the brains of infants in some cultures would be so much more mature than those in others.

Theory #5: Does Challenging Temperament Cause Colic?

> A few years ago, I spoke at a Lamaze class. During the talk, a pregnant woman named Ronnie told the class about her plan to have an "easy" child. She said, "I have two friends with young children. Angela has twin two-year-olds who scream and fight like little savages, but Lateisha's child is an angel. I don't want to make the same mistakes Angela did; I want my baby to be like Lateisha's little princess!"

Anyone who has been lucky enough to spend time around infants knows that some babies are as gentle as a merry-go-round while others are as wild as a roller coaster! What makes some children so volatile and challenging? Was Ronnie right? Is an error committed by their parents, or are some babies just natural-born screamers?

Nature Versus Nurture: What Determines Your Baby's Personality?

There's an old story that as a boy handed his father a report card of all F's, he lowered his head and asked quietly, "Father, do you think my trouble is my heredity . . . or my upbringing?"

For generations, people have debated what predicts a child's temperament. Is it determined by his hereditary gifts (nature) or is personality gradually molded by one's upbringing (nurture)?

A thousand years ago, baby experts believed temperament was transferred to babies in the milk they were fed. That's why ancient experts warned parents never to give their baby milk from an animal or from a wet nurse with a weak mind, poor scruples, or a crazy family.

Today it is widely accepted that many personality traits are direct genetic hand-me-downs from our parents. For this reason, shy parents usually have shy children, and passionate parents tend to have babies who are little chili peppers.

> *Andrea was the spirited baby of Zoran, a former race-car driver, and Yelena, a mile-a-minute research psychiatrist. A real handful from the moment she was born, by two months of age Andrea shrieked her complaints almost twenty-four hours a day. As Zoran noted, "She's as tough as nails, but what else would you expect? Two Dobermans just don't give birth to a cocker spaniel!"*

Let's take a closer look at temperament and see why, even though it may contribute to colic, it's not the main cause.

Temperament: The Sea Your Child Sails On

> *People are wrong when they think that quiet babies are good and fussy babies are bad. The truth is that some gracious and softhearted babies fuss a lot because they can't handle the turbulence of the world around them.*
>
> Renée, mother of Marie-Claire, Esmé, and Didier

Your baby is like a boat and her temperament the sea she sails on. If her boat is stable (a good self-calming ability), and the sea is smooth (she has a calm temperament), she will sail through infancy. However, if the boat is

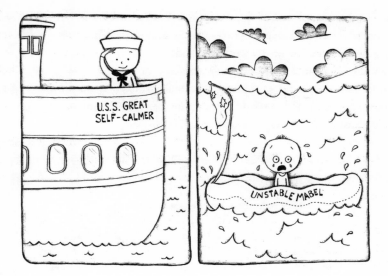

unstable (a poor self-calming ability), or the sea is rocky (she has a challenging temperament), she's in danger of getting tossed about. Once children get older and their self-calming ability becomes stable, the turbulence of their passions is no longer such an overpowering experience. But for young babies, a very intense temperament may be more than they can handle.

Luckily, most babies are mild-tempered and easy to calm, like sweet little lambs. But challenging babies are more like a mix of skittish cat and bucking bronco. These excessively sensitive and/or intense babies engage in a daily struggle to keep their balance during their first months of life.

Easy-Tempered Babies—"Mary Had a Little Lamb . . ."

Mild and mellow from the first moments of life, rather than scream at birth, an easy baby might shyly fuss, as if to say, "Please Mummy, it's a teensy bit too bright in here!"

Sabrina was one such undemanding baby:

> *Sabrina's dark lashes framed eyes the color of the sky. She was extremely alert, watching the world with the peaceful gaze of an old Zen master. Sabrina slept beautifully and hardly ever cried. Even when she was hungry, she rarely made a noise louder than a whimper to get her parents' attention.*

Easy-tempered babies have terrific state control and are great self-calmers. They are easygoing little "surfer dudes" who have no trouble taking all the craziness of the world in stride.

However, babies who are very sensitive or intense—or, Heaven help you, both—and who have poor self-calming skills may not be able to keep from screaming as the world's strange mixture of action and stillness toss them around like boats in a storm.

Infants with a Challenging Temperament—Little Babies with Big Personalities

> Lizzy and her twin sister Jennifer were like two peas in a pod, both super-sensitive to noise and sudden movements. When unhappy, their faces flushed and cries flew out of their mouths with deafening force.
>
> However, while Jenny was usually able to quiet her own crying, Lizzy's screams pulled her like a team of wild horses. Once she got rolling, she had no ability to rein herself in!
>
> Lizzy's mother, Cheryl, tried to regain control of her frenzied daughter with pacifiers, wrapping, and constant holding, but nothing helped. "For the first three months, I walked around every day not knowing when the 'train wreck' would occur."

Babies like Lizzy are tough. During the first few months of life, their personalities can be too big for them to handle. That's why parents often dub these babies with funny names to remind themselves not to take life too seriously. For example, Amanda's parents nicknamed her "Demanda," Natalie Rose's parents called her "Fussy Gassy Gussy," and Lachlan's parents referred to him as "General Fuss-ter."

Two types of temperament can be particularly challenging for new parents: sensitive and intense.

Sensitive Babies: Perceptive Infants Who Can Be as Fragile as Crystal

Of course, we all know that some people are much more sensitive than others. One person can sleep with the TV on while another is annoyed by any little sound. Some newborns also show signs of being extra sensitive, such as jumping when the telephone rings, grimacing at the taste of lanolin on your nipple, or turning her head to the smell of your breast.

Sensitive babies are wide-eyed and super-alert; their reactions to the world are as transparent and pure as crystal. But like crystal, sensitive infants are often fragile and require extra care. They are *so* open to everything around them they can easily become overloaded. That's why these babies have such a hard time settling themselves when they're left to cry it out. In other words, they can *go* bonkers from *being* bonkers!

If your newborn has a sensitive temperament, she may occasionally look away from you during her feeding or playtime. This is called "gaze aversion." Gaze aversion occurs when you get a little too close to your baby's eyes. Imagine a ten-foot face suddenly coming right in front of *your* nose. You, too, might need to look away or pull back a bit and check it out from a more comfortable distance! Don't mistake this for a sign that she doesn't like you or want to look at you. Just move back a foot or two and allow her to have slightly more space between her eyes and your face.

Intense Babies: A Cross Between Passionate . . . and Explosive

Throughout your baby's normal waking cycles, he's bound to experience tiny flashes of frustration, annoyance, and discomfort. Calm babies handle these with hardly a fuss, but intense babies handle these *intensely.* It's as if the "sparks" of everyday distress fall onto the "dynamite" of their volatile temperament, and "*Kapow!*" they explode. When babies lose control like that, they may get so carried away that they can't stop screaming even when they're given exactly what they want.

This intense crying was what Jackie experienced when she tried to feed her hungry—and passionate—baby. Two-month-old Jeffrey often began his feedings like this:

> "He would let out a shriek that sounded like, 'Feed me or I'm gonna die!' I would leap off the sofa, take out my breast, and insert it into his cavernous mouth. However, rather than gratefully taking it, he would often shake his head from side to side and wail around my dripping boob as if he were blind and didn't even know it was there. At times I worried that he thought my breast was a hand trying to silence him rather than my loving attempt to come to his rescue.
>
> "Fortunately, I had already figured out that Jeffrey couldn't stop himself from reacting that way. So, despite his protests, I

kept offering him my breast until he realized what I was trying
to do. Eventually, he would latch on and start suckling. And
then, lo and behold, he'd eat as if I hadn't fed him for months."

Jackie was smart. She realized Jeffrey wasn't intentionally ignoring her gift of food; he was just a little bitty baby trying to deal with his great big personality. Like a rookie cowboy on a rodeo bull, he was trying so hard to hold on that he didn't notice she was right there next to him, ready to help.

Does a Baby's Temperament Last a Lifetime?

As babies grow up, they don't get less intense or sensitive, but they do develop other skills to help themselves control their temperaments and better cope with the world. By three months they begin to smile, coo, roll, grab,

What's Your Baby's Temperament?

Even on the first days of your baby's life, you can get glimpses of his budding temperament. The answers to these questions may help you determine if your child's temperament is more placid or passionate:

1. Do bright lights, wet diapers, or cold air make your baby lightly whimper or full-out scream?
2. When you lay him down on his back, do his arms usually rest serenely at his sides or flail about?
3. Does he startle easily at loud noises and sudden movements?
4. When he's hungry, does he slowly get fussier and fussier or does he accelerate immediately into strong wailing?
5. When he's eating, is he like a little wine taster (calmly taking sips) or an all-you-can-eater (slurping the milk down with speedy precision)?
6. Once he works himself into a vigorous cry, how hard is it for you to get his attention? How long does it take to get him to settle back down?

These hints can't perfectly predict your child's lifelong temperament, but they *can* help you begin the exciting journey of getting to know and respect his uniqueness.

and chew. And shortly thereafter they add the extraordinarily effective self-calming techniques of laughter, mouthing objects, and moving about.

With time infants develop enough control over their immature bodies to allow them to direct the same zest that used to spill out into their shrieks into giggles and belly laughs. Passionate infants often turn into kids who are the biggest laughers and most talkative members of the family. ("Hey, Mom, look! *Look!* It's incredible!") And sensitive infants often grow into compassionate and perceptive children. ("No, Mom, it's not purple. It's *lavender.*")

So if you have a challenging baby, don't lose heart. These kids often become the sweetest and most enthusiastic children on the block!

Is Temperament the True Cause of Colic? Probably Not.

Is a baby's temperament the key factor that pushes him into inconsolable crying? No. This reasonable theory fails because it doesn't explain three of the universal colic clues:

■ *Colicky crying usually starts at two weeks, peaks at six weeks, and ends by three to four months of age.* Since temperament is present at birth and lasts a lifetime, colic caused by a challenging temperament should begin at birth and persist—or even worsen—after the fourth month of life. It doesn't.

Goodness of Fit—What happens when two cocker spaniels give birth to a Doberman?

Since temperament is largely an inherited trait, a baby's personality almost always reflects his parents'. However, just as brown-eyed parents may wind up with a blue-eyed child, mellow parents may unexpectedly give birth to a T. rex baby who makes them run for the hills!

Parents sometimes have difficulty handling a baby whose temperament differs dramatically from their own. They may hold their sensitive baby too roughly or their intense baby too gently. These parents need to learn their baby's unique temperament and nurture him exactly the way that suits him the best.

■ *Preemies are no more likely to have colic than full-term babies. (And it starts about two weeks past their due date.)* One would expect an immature preemie with a sensitive and/or intense personality to be *more* prone to colic than a mature full-term baby. Similarly, one would expect his colic to begin right away, not weeks to months later.

■ *There are many cultures around the world where babies never get colic.* Temperament can't be the cause of colic because in many cultures colic is nonexistent among their most intense and passionate infants.

So if one million U.S. babies aren't crying because of gas, acid reflux, maternal anxiety, brain immaturity, or inborn fussiness, what *is* the true cause of colic? As you will see in the next chapter, the only theory that fully explains the mystery of colic is . . . the missing fourth trimester.

5

The True Cause of Colic: The Missing Fourth Trimester

Main Points:

- The First Three Trimesters: Your baby's happy life in the womb
- The Great Eviction: Why babies are so immature at birth
- Why your baby wants (and needs) a fourth trimester
- A "Womb with a View": A parent's experience of the fourth trimester
- The Great American Myth: Young babies can be spoiled
- The connection between the fourth trimester and other colic theories
- Ten reasons why the missing fourth trimester is the true cause of colic

---

Once upon a time, in a faraway land, four blind wise men were asked to describe the true nature of an elephant. Each took a turn touching the beast. One by one, they spoke.

"This animal is long and curved like a spear," said the first blind man after grabbing a tusk. The next, clutching the giant's leg, raised his voice. "I disagree! This animal is thick and up-right—like a tree." As they began to argue, the next man

touched the ear and compared it to a giant leaf. Finally, the last man, wrapped up in the elephant's trunk, declared triumphantly that they were all wrong—the animal was like a big, fat snake.

What Is the Fourth Trimester and How Did It Become Missing?

In this story, each man described a *part* of the elephant. Yet, he was so sure his view was the whole truth, he didn't consider the possibility that there was another explanation that could account for all the different observations.

Similarly, wise men and women trying to solve the mystery of colic have focused on single bits of truth. Some heard grunting and thought gas was the culprit. Others saw a grimace and thought it was pain. Still others noticed that cuddling helped and assumed the infants were spoiled.

In recent years, colic has been blamed on pain, anxiety, immaturity, and temperament. Yet, while each is a piece of the puzzle, colic can only be understood by viewing all the pieces together. Only then does it become clear that the popular colic theories are linked by one previously overlooked concept: the missing fourth trimester.

Your baby's nine months—or three trimesters—inside you is a time of unbelievably complex development. Nevertheless, it takes most babies *an additional* three months to "wake up" and become active partners in the relationship. This time between birth and the end of your baby's third month is what I call your baby's fourth trimester.

Now let's see what a baby's life is like before they're born, why they must come into the world before they're fully mature, and the ways great parents soothe their babies by imitating the womb for the first three months of their baby's life.

The First Three Trimesters: Your Fetus's Happy Life in Your Womb

Did you think your baby was ready to be born after your nine months of pregnancy? God knows *you* were ready! But in many ways, your baby wasn't. Newborns can't smile, coo, or even suck their fingers. At birth, they're really still fetuses and for the next three months they want little more than to be carried, cuddled, and made to feel like they're still within the womb.

However, in order to mimic the sensations he enjoyed so much in your uterus, you need to know what it was like in there. Let's backtrack to the time when your fetus was still in the womb and see life through his eyes. Imagine you can look inside your pregnant uterus. What do you see? Just inside the muscular walls, silky membranes waft in a pool of tropical amniotic waters. Over there is your pulsating placenta; like a twenty-four-hour diner, it serves your fetus a constant feast of food and oxygen.

At the center, in the place of honor, is your precious baby. He's protected from hunger, germs, cold winds, mean animals, and rambunctious siblings by the velvet-soft walls of your womb. He looks part-astronaut–part-merman as he floats weightlessly in the golden fluid. Over these nine months, your fetus develops at lightning speed. His brain adds two hundred fifty thousand nerve cells a minute, and his body grows one billion times in weight and infinitely in complexity.

Let's zoom in on your baby's last month of life inside you. It's getting really tight in there. Like a little yoga expert, your fetus is nestled in, folded and secure. However, contrary to popular myth his cozy room is neither quiet nor still. It's jiggly (imagine your baby bouncing around when you hustle down the stairs) and loud (the blood whooshes through your arteries, creating a rhythmic din noisier than a vacuum cleaner).

Amazingly, all this commotion doesn't upset him. Rather, he finds it soothing. That's why unborn babies stay calm during the day but become restless in the still of the night. It's an ideal life in there—so why do babies pack up and pop out after just nine months, when they're still so immature?

The Great Eviction: Speculations on Why Our Babies Can't Stay in the Womb for a Fourth Trimester

Upon thee I was cast out from the womb.

Psalms 22:10

During the past century, archaeologists have pieced together a clearer picture of how humans evolved over the past five million years. They have studied such issues as why we switched from knuckle-walking to running upright and when we began using language and tools. However, what has not been fully appreciated until now is that over millions of years evolutionary changes gradually forced our ancestral mothers to deliver babies who were more and more immature. I believe that eventually, prehistoric human mothers had to *evict* their newborns three months early because their brains got so big!

In the very distant past, our ancestors likely had tiny-headed babies who didn't need to be evicted early from the womb. However, a few million years ago, our babies began going down a new branch of the evolutionary tree—the branch of supersmart people with big-brained babies. Pregnant mothers began stuffing new talents into their unborn babies' brains, filling them up like Christmas stockings. Eventually, their heads must have gotten so large that they began to get stuck during birth.

Perhaps that would have ended the evolution of our big brains, but four adaptations occurred that allowed our babies' brains to continue growing:

1. Our fetuses began to develop no-frills brains, containing only the most basic reflexes and skills needed to survive after birth (like sucking, pooping, and keeping the heart beating).

2. An ultrasleek head design slowly evolved to keep the big brain from getting wedged in the birth canal. On the outside it had slippery skin, squishable ears, and a tiny chin and nose. On the inside it had a compressible brain and a soft skull that could elongate and form itself into a narrower, easier to deliver cone shape.

3. Their big heads began to rotate as they exited the womb. (You've probably noticed it's easier to get a tight cork out of a bottle if you twist it as you pull it out.)

These three modifications helped tremendously. However, the crowning change that allowed the continued growth of our babies' brains was the fourth change—"eviction."

4. I believe that over hundreds of thousands of years, big-brained babies were less likely to get stuck in the birth canal—and more

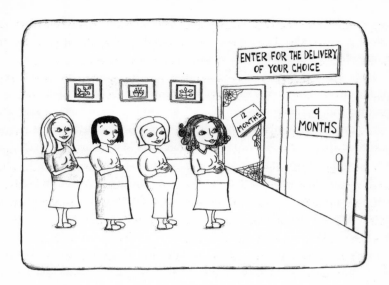

likely to survive—if they were born a little prematurely. In other words, if they were evicted.

Today, mothers give birth to their babies about three months before they're fully mature in order to guarantee a safe delivery.

However, as any mother can tell you, even with all these adaptations, giving birth is still a very tight squeeze. At eleven and a half centimeters across, our fetuses' heads have to compress quite a bit to get pushed through a ten centimeter, fully dilated cervix. No wonder midwives call the cervix at delivery the "ring of fire"!

Childbirth has always been a hazardous business occasionally putting both children and mothers in mortal peril. That's why, through the ages,

Imagine giving birth to a baby half the height or weight of an adult. Of course, a three-foot-long, eighty-pound newborn would be ridiculous. Now imagine giving birth to a baby with a head half the size of an adult's. That sounds even more absurd, but the fact is that such a head would be *small* for a new baby. At birth, our babies' noggins are almost two-thirds as big around as an adult head. (Ouch!)

many societies have honored childbirth as a heroic act. The Aztecs believed women who died giving birth entered the highest level of heaven, alongside courageous warriors who lost their lives in battle.

Early eviction lessened that risk and was made possible by the ability of prehistoric parents to protect their immature babies. Thanks to their upright posture and highly developed manual dexterity, early humans could walk while carrying their infants to keep them warm and cuddled. And our ancestors used their hands for more than holding. They created warm clothing and slinglike carriers that mimicked the security of the womb.

The hard work of imitating the uterus was the price our Stone Age relatives accepted in exchange for having safer early deliveries. However, in recent centuries, many parents have tried to wiggle out of this commitment to their babies.

They still wanted their babies to have big smart brains and be born early, but they didn't want to feed them so frequently or carry them around all day. Some misguided experts even insisted that newborns should be expected to sleep through the night and calm their own crying. Like kangaroos refusing their babies' entrance to the pouch, parents who subscribed to these theories denied what mothers and fathers for hundreds of thousands of years had promised to give their new infants.

Why Your Baby Wants (and Needs) a Fourth Trimester

The baby, assailed by eyes, ears, nose, skin, and intestines at once, feels it all as one great blooming, buzzing confusion.
William James, *The Principles of Psychology*, 1890

When you bring your soft, dimpled newborn home from the hospital, you may think your peaceful nursery is perfectly suited for his cherubic body and temperament, but that's not how your baby sees it. To him, it's a disorienting world—part Las Vegas casino, part dark closet!

His senses are bombarded by new experiences. From outside, he's assaulted by a jumble of lights, colors, and textures. From inside, he's flooded with waves of powerful new feelings like gas, hunger, and thirst. Yet, at the same time, the stillness of the room envelops him like a closet, devoid of the rhythms that were his constant comfort and companion for the past nine months. Imagine how strange the quiet of a hospital room must be to your baby after the loud, quadraphonic shhhh of the womb. No wonder babies look around as if they're thinking, *This just can't be real!*

Most infants can deal with these changes without a hitch. However, some babies can't. They need to be held, rocked, and suckled for large chunks of the day. These sensations duplicate the womb and form the basis of every infant-soothing method ever invented. This fourth-trimester experience calms babies *not* because they're spoiled and *not* because it tricks them into thinking they're back home, but because it triggers a powerful response inside our babies' brains that turns off their crying—the calming reflex.

The fourth trimester is the birthday present babies really hope their parents will give them.

A "Womb with a View": A Parent's Experience of the Fourth Trimester

> *When the baby comes out, the true umbilical cord is cut forever ... yet the baby is still, in that second, a fetus ... just a fetus one second older.*
>
> Peter Farb, *Humankind*

What an unforgettable moment the first time you see and touch your new baby. His sweet smell, open gaze, and downy soft skin capture your heart. But newborns can also be intimidating. Their floppy necks, irregular breathing, and tiny tremors make them seem so helpless.

This vulnerability is why I believe that a fourth-trimester period of imitating the womb is exactly what new babies need.

This need was probably obvious to you when your baby's sobs melted away the moment he was placed on your chest. Your ears and his cry will now become a virtual umbilical cord, an attachment, like an invisible bungee cord that stretches to allow you to walk around the house—until a sharp yelp yanks you back to his side.

> *"When Stuart came out of me, he didn't seem ready to be in the world," said Mary, a mother in my practice. "He required almost constant holding and rocking to keep him content. My husband, Phil, and I joked that he was like a squishy cupcake that needed to go back in the oven for a little more baking."*

In effect, what Mary and Phil realized was that Stuart needed a few more months of "womb service." But it's not so easy being a walking uterus! Bewildered new moms often observe that they're still in their pajamas at five P.M. Within days of delivery, you'll discover that it takes all day long to accomplish what your uncomplaining uterus did twenty-four hours a day for the past nine months.

From your baby's point of view, being in your arms for twelve hours a day is a disappointment, if not a rip-off. If he could talk, your infant would probably state with pouty disdain, "Hey, what's the big deal? You used to hold me twenty-four hours a day and feed me every single second!"

Unfortunately, many parents in our culture have been convinced that it's wrong to cuddle their babies so much. They have been misled into believing that their main job is to teach and educate their newborn. They treat their young child more like a brain to train than a spirit they are privileged to nurture. Other cultures consider an infant's needs differently. In Bali, babies are never allowed to sleep alone and they barely leave the arms of an adult for the first hundred and five days! The parents bury the placenta and nourish the burial spot with daily offerings of rice and vegetables. On the hundred and fifth day, a holy ceremony welcomes babies as new members of the human race; up until that point they still belong to the gods. In this ritual, babies receive their first sip of water, and an egg is rubbed on their arms and legs to give them vitality and strength. Only then are their feet finally allowed to touch Mother Earth.

It's no coincidence that in cultures like Bali, where colic is virtually nonexistent, parents give babies much more of a fourth-trimester experience than we do.

The Great American Myth:
Young Babies Can Be Spoiled

Hide not thine ear to my cry.
Lamentations 3:56

There are at least two things all parents know for sure:

1. There are a lot of spoiled kids out there.
2. You don't want your child to become one of them.

We all want to raise respectful children, and some experts warn us that being too attentive to our baby's cries will accidentally teach them to be manipulative. Can promptly answering your newborn's cries with holding, rocking, and sucking start a bad habit? Can cuddling your baby backfire on you?

Fortunately, the answers to these two questions are . . . no and no. It's impossible to spoil your baby during the first four months of life. Remember, he experienced a dramatic drop-off in holding time as soon as he was born. One mother told me, "I imagine new babies feel like someone who enters a detox program and has to go cold turkey from snuggling. No wonder they cry!"

Today's mothers and fathers aren't the only ones who have worried about turning their children into whining brats. In the early twentieth century, American parents were told not to mollycoddle their babies for fear of turning them into undisciplined little nuisances. The U.S. Children's Bureau issued a stern warning to a mother not to carry her infant too much, lest he become "a spoiled, fussy baby, and a household tyrant whose continual demands make a slave of a mother."

In 1972, however, Sylvia Bell and Mary Ainsworth of Johns Hopkins University shook those old ideas about spoiling to their very foundations. They found that babies whose mothers responded quickly to their cries during the first months of life *did not* become spoiled. On the contrary, infants whose needs were met rapidly and with tenderness fussed less and were more poised and patient when tested at one year of age! As Ainsworth and Bell proved—and most parents know in their hearts—the more you love and cuddle your little baby, the more confident and resilient he becomes.

Despite this evidence, many new parents still have nagging doubts about whether they're holding their babies too much. Although our natural parental instinct is to calm our baby as quickly as possible, the repeated warning, "Don't spoil your baby," has been drummed into our heads so much it makes us question ourselves.

Now, I admit it's easy to feel manipulated when your baby wakes up and screams every time you gently lower him into the crib. But letting him cry is no more likely to teach him to be independent than leaving him in a dirty diaper is likely to toughen his skin. (It's reassuring to know that traditionally many Native American parents held their babies all day and suckled them all night and still those babies grew up to be brave, respectful, and self-sufficient.)

Don't misunderstand me. I'm not arguing against establishing a flexible feeding/sleeping schedule for your baby. (See the discussion of scheduling in Chapter 15.) Some babies and families find scheduling very helpful. However, trying to mold passionate babies who have irregular sleeping and eating patterns into a fixed schedule usually leads to frustration for everyone.

As the Bible says, "To everything there is a season." I believe disciplining is a very important parental task—but not with young infants. The beginning of the fourth month is the earliest time concerns about accidentally spoiling your baby become an issue. However, before four months, you have a job that is *one hundred times* more important than preventing spoiling; your job is nurturing your baby's confidence in you and the world.

Building our child's faith is one of parenting's greatest privileges and responsibilities. I'm convinced that a rapid and sympathetic response to our baby's cries is the foundation of strong family values, not the undermining of them. When your loving arms cuddle your baby or warm milk satisfies him, you're telling him, "Don't worry. I'll always be there when you need me." This begins your baby's trust in you and becomes the bedrock of his faith in those closest to him.

Please treasure these amazing first months with your sweet, kissable baby. There will be plenty of time later on for training and disciplining, but now is the time for cuddling. Enjoy this time because, as any experienced parent will tell you, it will be over faster than you could imagine.

The Missing Fourth Trimester: The True Basis of Colic

There's no place like home.
Dorothy, *The Wizard of Oz*

After centuries of myths and confusion, I am convinced that the true basis of colic is simply that fussy babies need the sensations of the womb to help stay calm.

You might ask, "If all babies get evicted early and need a fourth trimester, why don't they all get colic?"

The reason is simple: Most babies can handle being born too soon because they have mild temperaments and good self-calming abilities. Thus, despite being exposed to waves of overstimulation and understimulation, they can soothe themselves.

Colicky babies, on the other hand, have big trouble with self-calming. They live through the same experiences as calm babies, but rather than taking them in stride, they overreact dramatically. These infants desperately need the sensations of the womb to help them turn on their calming reflex.

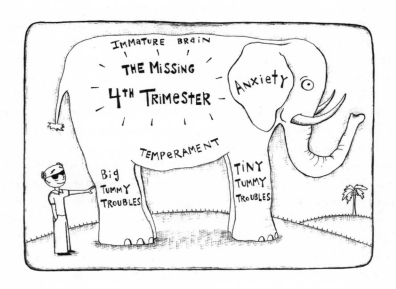

**The Colic Elephant: A Blend of the Fourth Trimester
and Other Colic Theories**

As we've discussed, experts have blamed colic on tummy troubles, anxiety, immaturity, and temperament. But, like the blind men and the elephant, these experts perceived only parts of the problem and overlooked the all-important common link—the missing fourth trimester.

The missing fourth trimester makes babies vulnerable to the unstable qualities of their individual natures (brain immaturity and challenging temperament) and to small daily upsets.

This is how I believe all the colic theories relate to one another:

1. Brain Immaturity—This inborn characteristic can greatly increase a baby's need for a fourth trimester. Fussy infants have such poor state control and self-calming ability that even small amounts of over- or understimulation can set off a chain reaction of escalating flailing and loud cries.

2. Temperament—A baby whose nature is extremely sensitive and/or intense often overreacts to small disturbances and needs a great deal of help turning on the calming reflex.

3. Big Tummy Troubles—Pain from food allergies or acid reflux can occasionally make a baby frantic. But these problems are much more distressing in babies whose self-calming ability is immature or who have challenging temperaments.

4. Tiny Tummy Troubles—Constipation and gas can spark discomfort that provokes crying in babies with brain immaturity and/or a challenging temperament.

5. Maternal Anxiety—Fussy babies sometimes cry more when their anxious mothers handle them too gently or jump chaotically from one ineffective soothing attempt to another.

Putting the Theory of Fourth Trimester to the Test

There's a reason behind everything in nature.
Aristotle

For a colic theory to be proven correct it must fit all ten colic clues. After long and exhaustive study, I have found the only theory that explains all ten and solves the centuries-old mystery of colic is the concept of the missing fourth trimester:

1. *Colicky crying usually starts at two weeks, peaks at six weeks, and ends by three to four months of age.*

For the first two weeks of life, newborns have little alert time. This helps keep them from getting over- or understimulated and thus delays the onset of colic.

After two weeks, babies start staying alert for longer periods. Mellow babies can easily handle the stimulation this increased alertness exposes them to. However, babies who are poor self-calmers or who have challenging temperaments may begin to get overwhelmed. Thus the crying starts.

By six weeks, these vulnerable babies are very alert and very overstimulated, yet they still have poor state control. They launch into bouts of screaming that can be soothed only by masterful imitations of the womb.

By three to four months, colic disappears. Now babies are skilled at cooing, laughing, sucking their fingers, and other self-calming tricks. They are mature enough to deal with the world without the constant holding, rocking, and shushing of the fourth trimester. At last, they are ready to be born!

2. *Preemies are no more likely to have colic than full-term babies. (And their colic doesn't start until they are about two weeks past their due date.)*

Preemies are good sleepers, even in noisy intensive-care units. Their immature brains have mastered the sleep state, but not the complex state of alertness. This near absence of alert time fools preemies into thinking they're still in the womb. They don't notice they're missing the fourth trimester until they're past their due date and become more awake and alert.

3. *Colicky babies have twisted faces and piercing wails. Often, their cries come in waves (like cramps) and stop abruptly.*

Your baby's colicky cries may sound identical to the wails he makes when he's in pain. However, many babies overreact to trivial experiences (loud noises, burps, etc.) with pain-like screams. They're like smoke alarms that go off even though only a little piece of toast burned.

The fact that these shrieks can be quieted by car rides or breast-feeding proves these babies aren't in agony. What they're really suffering from is the loss of their fourth trimester.

4. *Their screams frequently begin during or just after a feeding.*

Babies who cry during or right after meals are usually overre-acting to their gastro-colic reflex, the intestinal squeezing that oc-curs when the stomach fills with food. Most babies have no problem with this reflex, but for colicky babies, at the end of the day (and at the end of their patience), this sensation may be the last straw that launches them into hysterics.

That this distress vanishes after three months (while the gastro-colic reflex is still going strong) further supports the no-tion that this crampy feeling triggers screaming only in babies who need the calming sensations of the fourth trimester.

5. *They often double up, grunt, strain, and seem relieved by passing gas or pooping.*

All babies experience intestinal gas; however, this sensation triggers screaming only in infants with sensitive and/or intense temperaments. Even those babies usually stop crying when res-cued by the calming rhythms of the womb.

6. *Colic is often much worse in the evening (the "witching hour").*

Just as some harried moms crumble at the end of their tod-dlers' birthday parties, some young babies unravel after a full day's roller-coaster ride of activity. Without the fourth trimester to settle them down, these vulnerable infants bubble over each evening like pots of hot pudding.

7. *Colic is as likely to occur with a couple's fifth baby as with their first.*

Each new baby represents a reshuffling of their parents' per-sonal deck of genetic traits. That's why a couple's first four babies may be calm and easy to keep happy, while their fifth may inherit traits like sensitivity or poor state control that make him fall apart unless he's held and rocked all day.

These colicky babies require the sanctuary of the fourth trimester to help them cope until they're mature enough to soothe themselves.

8. *Colicky crying often improves with rocking, holding, shhhhing, and gentle abdominal pressure.*

This clue is compelling proof that the true cause of uncontrollable crying in babies is their need for a few more months in the uterus. That's because each of these calming tricks imitates the womb, and after three months they're no longer required.

9. *Babies are healthy and happy between crying bouts.*

If the only reason babies have colic is because they're born too soon, it's logical to expect immature infants to be healthy and happy until something pushes them over the edge.

10. *In many cultures around the world, babies never get colic.*

The babies of the villagers of Bali, the bushmen of Botswana, and the Manali tribesmen of the Himalayan foothills all share one trait: these babies never suffer from persistent crying. When anthropologists study "colic-free" cultures, they find that the mothers in those societies closely follow the fourth-trimester plan. Women hold their infants almost twenty-four hours a day, feed them frequently, and constantly rock and jiggle them. For several months, these moms give their babies an almost constant imitation of the womb.

Only the missing fourth trimester explains *all* the colic clues. However, if soothing a screaming baby is just a matter of imitating the womb with some wrapping and rocking, why do these approaches so often fail to calm colicky kids? The reason is quite simple: Parents in our culture are rarely taught how to do them correctly.

Thankfully, it's not too late to learn, and in the next part of this book, I will share with you detailed descriptions of the world's most effective methods for calming crying babies.

PART TWO

Learning the Ancient Art
of Soothing a Baby

6

The Woman Who Mistook Her Baby for a Horse: Modern Parents Who Forgot About the Fourth Trimester

Main Points:

- Unlike newborn horses, our babies are not up and running on the first day of life; they need a fourth trimester to finish getting ready for the world
- The striking differences between four-day-old and four-month-old babies
- Ancient lessons you can learn from some mothers whose children never get colic

That which was done is that which shall be done; and there is no new thing under the sun.

Ecclesiastes 1:9

Picture a crisp December day, gleaming like a jewel. Yesterday your life changed with the birth of a beautiful baby boy. Now, as the nurse wheels his bassinet into your room, your son lifts his fragile head, slowly turns to face you, and flashes a big grin! Then he vaults into your arms and, with a

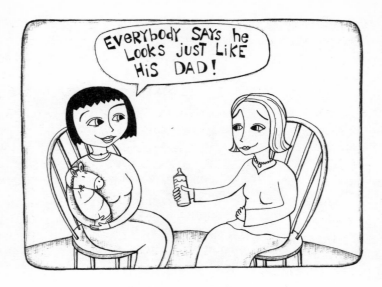

laugh that makes your heart melt, proclaims, "You're the best mom in the whole world!"

Of course, no one expects their baby to walk and talk right after birth. However, many modern parents are unprepared for how dependent and vulnerable newborns truly are. They expect their babies to be more mature, sort of like baby horses! Within minutes of birth, newborn horses can stand, walk, and even run. A baby horse's survival depends on these crucial abilities to keep away from hungry predators. By comparison, our new babies are still immature little fetuses.

The Surprising Truth: The Differences Between Four-Day-Old and Four-Month-Old Babies

After the first month, I wanted some recognition that my twin girls could distinguish me from the woman down the block. When Audrey was two months old, she peed on me, then suddenly smiled. I know it sounds crazy but I was ecstatic!

Debra, mother of Audrey and Sophia

When I teach prenatal classes I often ask the parents-to-be to describe the differences between four-day-old and four-month-old babies. Those without much baby experience usually answer that a four-month-old is like a newborn, except bigger and more alert.

In fact, there are *gigantic* differences between these two ages. As extraordinary as newborns are, their ability to interact with the world is extremely limited. While a four-day-old can't even coo or turn around to see who's speaking, a four-month-old's delicious smile and glowing eyes reach out like a personal invitation to join her on her amazing life journey.

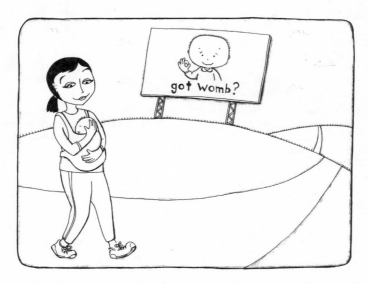

As noted earlier, baby horses depend on brawn for their survival, so their developed bodies are as big as they can possibly be when they pop out of their mothers' wombs. By contrast, our babies' survival depends on their brains. For that reason, at birth, their heads are as big as they could possibly be and not get stuck. Then amazingly, during the first three months, a baby's brain balloons an additional twenty percent in size. Accompanying that growth is an explosive advance in her brain's speed, organization, and complexity. No wonder parents notice their babies suddenly "wake up" as the fourth trimester draws to a close.

Our ancient relatives realized how immature their babies were at birth. Over the centuries, they discovered that the most effective way of caring for newborns during the early months of infancy was by imitating their previous home—the uterus!

Four-Day-Old Babies	Four-Month-Old Babies

Sensory Abilities

▥ Can focus only on objects eight to twelve inches away. ▥ Love looking at light/dark contrasts and designs.	▥ Easily focus on large objects across a room. ▥ Can turn their head to find where a sound comes from.

Social Abilities

▥ More attracted to the sound of the human voice than to music or noise. Can recognize their mother's voice from the muffled sounds they heard in the womb. ▥ Prefer looking at a person's face rather than an object. May be able to imitate facial expressions like a mom opening her mouth or sticking out her tongue.	▥ Patiently wait for you to stop talking before they take a turn in the conversation by releasing a symphony of coos, grunts, and giggles. ▥ Enamored with their parents' faces and brighten visibly when they enter the room. Smile and coo to make their parents smile and may become upset when ignored.

Motor Abilities

▥ Often get crossed eyes. Can follow only slowly moving objects and have very jerky eye movements. ▥ Hard for them to get their fingers to their mouths and *very* hard for them to keep them there for more than thirty seconds.	▥ No longer get crossed eyes. Can now follow objects swiftly and smoothly as they move around the room. ▥ Much more able to reach out and touch objects. Easily get their fingers to their mouths and keep them there for many minutes.

Physiological Characteristics

▥ Hands and feet are blue much of the time. ▥ Bodies occasionally get jolted by hiccups, jittery tremors, and irregular breathing. ▥ Have little ability to control body movements.	▥ No longer get blue hands and feet unless cold. ▥ Rarely hiccup, never tremor, and breathing is smooth and regular. ▥ Much better at controlling body movements. Can roll over, spin around, and lift head high off the mattress.

Out with the New, In with the Old: Rediscovering the Stone Age Wisdom of Imitating the Fourth Trimester

Do you remember how in *Star Wars* Luke Skywalker achieved victory by using the long forgotten powers of the Force? Well, over the last fifty years, our society has also advanced by returning to ancient wisdom such as getting more exercise, protecting the environment, and eating food grown with less pesticides. Technology is a blessing, but today we are relearning the value of living in harmony with nature; it's just common sense!

That's why there's logic in examining the past to understand ourselves better. Although our clothes and music are contemporary, our biology is clearly prehistoric, and that's especially true for babies.

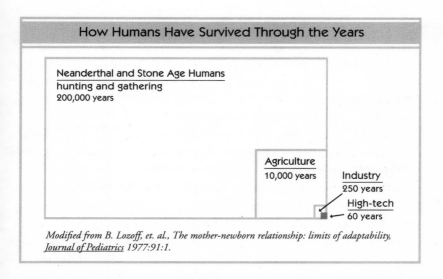

Modified from B. Lozoff, et. al., The mother-newborn relationship: limits of adaptability, *Journal of Pediatrics* 1977:91:1.

In the diagram above, we occupy the tiny bottom right corner, the technological age of man. Yet our babies are far from high-tech. In most respects, they haven't changed a hair in the past thirty thousand years! That's why, although most of us would never survive if suddenly sent back to the Stone Age, our infants would feel right at home. Babies expect to be born into a cave family, and they expect us to be as experienced at handling them as our Stone Age cousins were. Unfortunately, most of us are a little rusty—if not completely in the dark—when it comes to those prehistoric parenting tips. What valuable baby-care tricks could you learn if an experienced cave mother lived next door to you?

While we can't go back in time, we can get an idea of some calming techniques cave moms might have used by looking through a virtual "window" to the past, the study of primitive tribes living around the world today.

Please don't be fooled by the word *primitive*. Although it conjures up images of backward people, over the past eighty years research has shown that many so-called primitive peoples possess wisdom of the natural world about which we are ignorant. Some know the medicinal power of rare plants, some know how to find water in the desert—*and some even know how to prevent colic!*

Past Perfect: Lessons from the !Kung San

For hundreds if not thousands of years, the !Kung San (or African bushmen) have lived in isolation on the plains of the Kalahari Desert. Over the past forty years, however, the !Kung have graciously allowed scientists to observe their lives, including how they care for babies.

I've read reports of their newborn care with great interest because !Kung infants hardly ever cry. It's not that they never cry—it's that they never CRY! (And I know you understand that distinction.) While !Kung infants get upset as often as our babies do, their parents are so skilled at soothing them that the average fussy bout lasts only sixteen seconds, and more than ninety percent of their crying jags end in under a minute.

What's their secret? What ancient wisdom do the !Kung know that our culture has forgotten? I believe three facts account for much of this tribe's stunning success:

- !Kung mothers hold their babies almost twenty-four hours a day.
- !Kung mothers breast-feed their babies around the clock.
- !Kung parents usually respond to their babies' cries within ten seconds.

!Kung mothers carry their babies all day long in a leather sling and sleep next to them at night. This closeness makes it easy to soothe any fussiness the instant it starts.

In addition to holding and cuddling, the !Kung calm their babies by giving them quick little feedings on the breast—up to one hundred times a day! We in the West might think such snacking would spoil a baby, but that's not the case. Despite the lavish and immediate attention paid to their crying, !Kung children grow up to be happy, independent, and self-sufficient.

Now, don't worry. I'm not suggesting we adopt all the !Kung ways; they clearly don't fit our busy lives. However, I am suggesting that we study these highly successful parents to learn which of their solutions could be easily adopted by Western moms and dads.

I believe the biggest secret the !Kung know is that all their baby soothing methods share a common thread: They imitate the uterus and provide babies the comfort of the fourth trimester.

Compared to our infants, !Kung babies may be deprived of many material possessions, but compared to the !Kung, our babies are deprived of an important "maternal" possession—long hours of being in our arms. While !Kung mothers are with their infants almost nonstop, studies in the United States show that we leave our young babies alone for up to sixteen hours a day. I'm afraid that for many newborns, this abrupt transfer from cozy womb to empty room ends up making them terribly upset.

For the first few months of life, we need to treat our babies the way our ancient ancestors treated theirs thousands of years ago, with the reassuring rhythms of the fourth trimester. In other words, we should no longer mistake our newborns for little horses. Rather, we should treat them like little kangaroos! Kangaroos "know" their babies need a few more months of TLC before they're ready to get hoppin', so they welcome them into the pouch the moment they're born. Likewise, we need to offer our sweet newborns "pouches" of prolonged holding, rocking, shushing, and warmth. If you do this you'll be amazed. Once you master the skill of imitating the womb, you'll be able to do *exactly* what !Kung moms do: settle your baby's cries in minutes!

Imitating the womb to calm colic isn't the only ancient wisdom that has been ignored by our culture. Over the past fifty years, researchers have carefully proved the benefits of another prehistoric skill, breast-feeding, which was rescued from the brink.

Breast-Feeding Makes a Comeback

Within days of your baby's birth, your breast milk appears, as if by magic. It's exactly what the doctor, and your baby, ordered. This sweet, nutritious, easy-to-digest food gives your newborn an almost constant flow of nourishment, just like she had inside the womb.

Early in the 1900s, after millions of years of being developed to perfection, mother's milk was suddenly abandoned in many parts of the world. It was nudged aside by mass-produced artificial formula that was promoted as equally healthful and more hygienic than mother's milk. Many women were convinced that scientists knew better than nature. They fed their babies formula, mistakenly believing that the product of a chemist was better than the old-fashioned product of their own breasts.

Mothers asked their doctors for medicine to dry up their breast milk and to recommend their favorite commercial formula. By the 1950s, breast-feeding became so rare in America that the women who tried it were considered radical or eccentric.

Moms who still wanted to breast-feed often failed because they had no personal experience and little professional guidance. As unbelievable as it sounds, within two generations our culture almost lost this basic human ability that had sustained our species for millions of years! Fortunately, many committed women (and men) were appalled by this lack of support. Through their great efforts, groups like La Leche League were launched and specialists were trained to help new mothers rediscover this wonderful skill.

In recent years, public interest in breast-feeding has dramatically rebounded, spurred by an avalanche of research revealing the shortcomings of formula and the benefits of breast milk. Scientific studies show that breast milk helps build babies' brains, boosts their immunity, protects them against diabetes, and lowers a woman's risk of breast and ovarian cancer. Today, breast milk is so universally accepted as the preferred food for babies that even formula companies recommend women use their product only if they can't breast-feed.

I'm thankful we have excellent artificial formulas to feed babies who are unable to feed at their mother's breast. However, all medical groups agree, if you can do it, "breast is best" for feeding your baby.

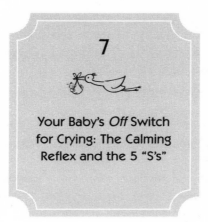

7

Your Baby's *Off* Switch for Crying: The Calming Reflex and the 5 "S's"

Main Points:

- What reflexes are, and the many built-in behaviors and skills all babies are born with
- The Calming Reflex: Your baby's *Off* switch for crying
- The 5 "S's": How to turn on your baby's calming reflex
- Vigor: The essential tip for calming your little cave baby
- Three reasons your baby may take time to respond to the 5 "S's"

Most people who have taken care of a fussy infant wonder at some point: "Wouldn't it be great if babies came with a secret button to turn off their crying?"

Now don't laugh, it's not such a wild idea. Since babies wail as loud as car alarms, shouldn't there also be a way to turn their "alarm" off?

Well, the good news is, there is! I call this *Off* switch the calming reflex, and, as you will soon learn, it works almost as quickly as the car-alarm reset button on your key chain. But first, let's review what reflexes are and how they work.

Reflexes: Incredible Things Your Baby Knows How to Do Automatically

Reflexes are your body's way of reacting automatically, such as blinking before something hits you in the eye or shooting out your arms when you're knocked off balance. Like a good buddy, reflexes reassure the brain: "Don't even think about it. I'll handle everything."

All reflexes have the following characteristics:

- *They are reliable.* Every time the doctor hits your knee to test your reflex, your foot jumps out. It can be done five hundred times in a row and always works.
- *They are automatic.* Reflexes work even when you're asleep.
- *They require a very specific triggering action.* The knee reflex is automatic and reliable *only* when it's done in exactly the right way. It won't work if your knee is hit too softly or an inch too high or low.

Could you imagine having to teach your baby how to suck or poop? Thankfully you don't have to, because these and more than seventy other automatic reflexes are packed away in your newborn's compact brain.

Most of these reflexes help your baby during the first months after birth. The rest are either fetal reflexes (useful only during his life inside you), leftover reflexes (valuable to our ancestors millions of years ago, but now just passed from generation to generation, like our intestinal appendix), or mystery reflexes (whose purposes are unknown).

Here's a list of some common reflexes you'll probably see your baby performing:

1. **Keeping-safe reflexes:** These protective reflexes help prevent accidental injury. (Most are so important they continue to work in adults.)

    Crying—Crying, the "mother" of all baby safety reflexes, can be triggered by any sudden distress and is extraordinarily effective at getting your attention.

    Sneezing—Your newborn's sneeze usually isn't a sign of a cold; rather, it's a response to irritating dust and mucous his body is trying to rid from the nose.

2. **Getting-a-meal reflexes:** Even though no food ever passed your fetus's lips, from the moment of birth he was ready to receive and enjoy your milk.

    Rooting—When you touch your baby's cheek or lips, his face will turn toward the touch and his mouth will open and then shut. This reflex helps your baby locate and grasp your nipple, even in the dark. But don't worry if you stroke your baby's cheek and he doesn't respond. This is a smart reflex: It's not there until he's hungry. That's why the rooting reflex is a great way for you to tell if your baby is crying because he wants to eat. If you touch his mouth and he doesn't root, he probably is not crying for food.

    Sucking—Your baby practiced this complex reflex even before birth. Many parents have ultrasound photos of their little cuties sucking their thumbs, weeks before delivery.

3. **Fetal and leftover reflexes:** These reflexes either help our fetuses before they are born or were useful only to our distant animal ancestors.

    Step—Holding your baby upright, let the sole of one foot press onto a flat surface. In a few seconds, that leg will straighten and the other will bend. This reflex helps babies move around a little during the last months of pregnancy, thus helping to prevent pressure sores and getting the fetus into position for delivery.

    Grasping—If you press your finger into the base of your baby's toes or fingers, he will grab on tightly, even when he's sleeping. This reflex is critically important for newborn apes! It helps them cling to their mother's fur while she's moving through the jungle. (Be careful. It works on dads with hairy chests too!)

    The Moro reflex—This extremely important leftover reflex protected our ancient relatives carrying their babies through the trees. It's the "I'm falling" reflex activated the second your baby gets startled (by a jolt, loud noise, or a dream).

The Moro reflex makes your baby's arms shoot out and around, as if he's trying to grab hold of you. This venerable response probably kept countless baby monkeys from falling out of their mother's arms. (Adults who fall asleep in a chair and whose heads suddenly drop back may also experience this reflex.)

As your baby matures his newborn reflexes will gradually get packed away and forgotten, like tattered old teddy bears. However, at the beginning of life, these invaluable responses are some of the best baby gifts a mother could ever hope for.

There is one more built-in, newborn response that parents in my practice think is the most wonderful reflex of all: the calming reflex.

The Calming Reflex: Nature's Automatic Shut-off Switch for a Baby's Crying

I believe once our ancestors began living in villages and cities, they forgot that, since the Stone Age, babies were almost constantly jiggled and wiggled as their moms walked up and down the mountains. Sadly, many babies deprived of these comforting movements began to startle and cry at every disturbance. I'm afraid that in order to explain that crying, modern parents began to mistakenly think that babies were so fragile they could only tolerate *quiet* sounds and *gentle* motion.

This new attitude undermined their confidence in triggering the calming reflex, because as you are about to learn it *can be activated only by vigorous actions*—especially in very fussy babies. Gradually, this ancient calming tool was forgotten.

As you will recall, reflexes require specific triggers. The triggers for your baby's calming reflex are the sensations he felt in the uterus. It is my belief that this precious reflex came about *not* as a way of soothing upset infants but rather as a way of soothing upset *fetuses!*

This vital response saved countless numbers of mothers and unborn babies by keeping fetuses entranced so that they wouldn't thrash around and kink their umbilical cords or get wedged into a position that made delivery impossible. How brilliant of Mother Nature to design this critical, lifesaving response to be automatically activated by the sensations fetuses are naturally surrounded by.

Not only are the rhythms of the uterus profoundly calming to babies, they're also comforting to adults. Think of how you're affected by hearing the ocean, rocking in a hammock, and cuddling in a warm bed. However, while we merely enjoy these sensations, our babies *need* them—and fussy babies need them desperately.

So if you've tried feeding, burping, and diaper changing and your baby is still yelling himself hoarse, it's time to try soothing him this "old" new way.

The Top Ten Ways You Can Imitate the Uterus
1. Holding
2. Dancing
3. Rocking
4. Wrapping
5. White noise or singing
6. Car rides
7. Walks outside
8. Feeding
9. Pacifiers
10. Swings

This list includes just a few of the dozens of ways clever parents have invented to calm their infants. But what you know now is something that no mom or dad throughout history realized, that these tricks relax newborns by switching on the ancient reflex that kept them in a protective, lifesaving trance when they were fetuses.

The most popular baby calming methods can be grouped into five basic categories: *S*waddling, *S*ide/*S*tomach position, *S*hhhhing sounds, *S*winging, and *S*ucking. I call these the 5 "S's"; they are the qualities of the uterus that help activate the calming reflex. However, like all reflexes, even these great techniques only switch on the calming reflex if they're done correctly.

The 5 "S's": Five Steps to Activate Your Baby's Calming Reflex

There should be a law requiring that the 5 S's be stamped onto every infant ID band in the hospital. For our frantic baby, they worked in seconds!

Nancy, mother of two-month-old Natalie

In the early 1900s, baby experts taught new parents to do the following when their infant cried: 1) feed them, 2) burp them, 3) change the diaper, and 4) check for an open safety pin. Authorities proclaimed that when these didn't work, babies had colic and there was nothing else a parent could do. Today, most doctors give similar recommendations.

But for parents of a frantic newborn, the nothing-you-can-do-but-wait advice is intolerable. *Few impulses are as powerful as a mother's desire to calm her crying baby. This instinct is as ancient as parenting itself.* Yet, the frustrating reality is while parents instinctively *want* to calm their babies, knowing *how* to do it is anything but instinctive. It's a skill. Luckily, it's a skill that is fairly easy to learn.

Peter, a high-powered attorney, is the father of Emily and Ted. When his kids were born, Pete and his wife, Judy, had very little baby experience. So, after the birth of each child, I sat down and reviewed the concepts of the fourth trimester and the 5 "S's." Several years later, Peter wrote:

It has been more than ten years since I was taught the 5 "S's" as a way to quiet my crying babies. Even today, I like to share them with clients who bring their infants into my office. It's great fun to see the amazed looks when a large, lumbering male like me happily collects their distraught baby and calms the delicate creature in seconds—with a vigorous swaddle, side, swing, shush, and suck. These simple techniques give any parent a true sense of accomplishment!

The 5 "S's" are the only tools you'll need to soothe your fussy infant.

1. *Swaddling: A Feeling of Pure "Wrap"ture*
   Tight swaddling is the cornerstone of calming, the essential first

step in soothing your fussy baby and keeping him soothed. That's why traditional cultures from Turkey to Tulsa (the Native Americans, that is) use swaddling to keep their babies happy.

Wrapping makes your baby feel magically returned to the womb and satisfies his longing for the continuous touching and tight fit of your uterus. This "S" doesn't actually trigger the calming reflex but it keeps your baby from flailing and helps him pay attention to the other "S's," which *do* activate the reflex.

Many irritable babies resist wrapping. However, it's a mistake to think this resistance means that your baby needs his hands free. Nothing could be further from the truth! Fussy young babies lack the coordination to control their arm flailing, so if their arms are unwrapped they may make themselves even more upset.

Here's how one grandmother learned the ancient tradition of swaddling and passed it along:

> *My youngest sister was born when I was nearly ten years old. I remember my mother teaching me how to swaddle her snugly in a warm blanket. That year, mothering and bundling began for me, and they have continued, without interruption, into my sixtieth year!*
>
> *When my grandchildren began to arrive, I faithfully taught my kids to wrap their babies very tightly in receiving blankets. My passion for swaddling often led to some good-humored discussion: "Watch out for Bubby and her bundling!" Yet somehow it always seemed to help.*
>
> *The babies in our family, although beautiful, talented, and brilliant, share a fussy, high-maintenance profile, if only for the first two or three months. But swaddling has always been a big help. I can't tell you how many times I've seen it change their faces from a scowl to serenity.*
>
> Barbara, "Bubby" of Olivia, Thomas,
> Michael, Molly, and Sawyer

2. Side/Stomach: Your Baby's Feel-Good Position

Swaddling stops your baby's uncontrolled arm and leg acrobatics that can lead into frenzied crying. In a similar fashion, the side/

stomach position stops an equally upsetting but invisible type of stimulation—the panicky feeling of falling!

Being dropped was such a serious threat to our ancient relatives that their babies developed a special alarm—the Moro reflex—that went off the moment they felt they were falling out of their mother's arms.

Most babies are content to be on their backs if they're in a good mood. However, when your baby is crying, putting him on his back may make him feel like he's in a free fall. That in turn can set off his Moro, which starts him thrashing and screaming.

The side or stomach positions soothe your screaming newborn by instantly shutting off the Moro. That's why these are the perfect feel-good positions for fussy babies. When it comes to putting your small one to sleep, however, the back is the safest position for all babies. Unless your doctor instructs you otherwise, *no baby should ever be put to sleep on his stomach.* (More on this in Chapter 9.)

3. Shhhhing: Your Baby's Favorite Soothing Sound

Believe it or not, a loud, harsh shushing sound is music to your baby's ears. Shhhhing comforts him by mimicking the whooshing noise of blood flowing through your arteries. This rough humming surrounded your baby every moment during his nine months inside you. That's why it is an essential part of the fourth trimester.

Many new parents mistakenly believe their babies prefer the gentle tinkling sounds of a brook or the distant hush of the wind. It seems counterintuitive that our tender infants would like such a loud noise; certainly we wouldn't. Yet babies love it! That's why many books recommend the use of roaring appliances to settle screaming infants.

I have never met a cranky baby who got overstimulated by the racket from these devices. On the contrary, the louder babies cry, the louder the shhhhing has to be in order to calm them.

 In a rush to get out of the house, Marjan put off feeding her hungry baby for a few minutes while she went into the bathroom and finished getting ready to leave. Two-week-old Bebe didn't care for this plan, and she wailed impatiently for food. However, after a few minutes Bebe suddenly quieted. Marjan panicked, was her tiny baby okay? When Marjan opened the

> *bathroom door, she was relieved to see that her daughter was*
> *fine. Then she realized that Bebe had stilled the very instant she*
> *turned on the hair dryer.*

Marjan shared this exciting discovery with her parents, but they were not supportive. They warned her it was dangerous to use the hair dryer to calm an infant: "It's so loud it will make her go crazy!"

Despite their concerns, Marjan used her new "trick" with 100% success whenever her baby was crying (but only when her family was not around).

4. Swinging: Rock-a-Bye Baby

Lying on a soft, motionless bed may appeal to you, but to your baby—fresh out of the womb—it's disorienting and unnatural. Newborns are like sailors who come to dry land after nine months at sea; the sudden stillness can drive them bananas. That's why rhythmic, monotonous, jiggly movement—what I call swinging—is one of the most common methods parents have always used to calm their babies. Swinging usually must be vigorous at first to get your baby to stop screaming, and then it can be reduced to a gentler motion to *keep* him calm.

In ancient times and in today's traditional cultures, babies are constantly jiggled and bounced. Many third-world parents use cradles or hammocks to keep their babies content, and they "wear" their infants in slings to give the soothing feeling of motion with every step and breath. Even in our culture, many tired parents use bouncy seats, car rides, and walks around the block to try to help their unhappy babies find some peace.

> *Mark, Emma, and their two kids were visiting Los Angeles from London. While I was examining four-year-old Rose, little Mary, their two-month-old baby, startled out of a deep sleep and immediately began to wail. Without missing a beat, Mark scooped her up so she sat securely in his arms. He began swinging her from side to side as if she were a circus performer and he the trapeze. Within twenty seconds, her eyes glazed over, her body melted into his chest, and we were able to finish our conversation as if Mary had never cried at all.*

5. Sucking: The Icing on the Cake

Once your cranky baby starts to settle down from the swaddle, side position, shushing, and swinging, he's ready for the fifth glorious "S": sucking. Sucking is the icing on the cake of calming. It takes a baby who is beginning to quiet and lulls him into a deep and profound state of tranquillity.

Obviously, it's hard for your baby to scream with a pacifier in his mouth, but that's not why sucking is so soothing. Sucking has its effect deep within your baby's nervous system. It triggers his calming reflex and releases natural chemicals within his brain, which leads in minutes to a rich and satisfying level of relaxation.

Some parents offer their infants bottles and pacifiers to suck on, but the all-time number-one sucking toy in the world is a mother's nipple. As was previously mentioned, mothers in some cultures help keep their babies calm by offering them the breast up to one hundred times a day.

Hannah thought her first son, Felix, was almost addicted to the pacifier. "He insisted on using it for years. So when my second child was born, I vowed to try not to use it. But once again it became an invaluable calming tool. Harmon was so miserable without it, and so content with it, that I couldn't bring myself to deny him that simple pleasure."

In summary, the first two "S's"—swaddling and side/stomach—start the calming process by muffling your baby's flailing movements, shutting off the Moro reflex and getting him to pay attention to what you're doing as you begin to activate the calming reflex. The third and fourth "S's"—shhhhing and swinging—break into the crying cycle by powerfully triggering the calming reflex and soothing your baby's nervous system. The fifth "S"—sucking—keeps the calming reflex turned on and allows your baby to guide himself to a profound level of relaxation.

The 5 "S's" are fantastic tools, but as with any tools, your skill in using them will increase with practice. Since the calming reflex works only when triggered in precisely the right way, you'll find that mastering these ancient techniques is one of the first important tasks of parenthood.

Interestingly, not only do parents get better with practice, so do babies. Many parents notice that after a few weeks of swaddling their babies straighten their arms and begin to calm the instant they're placed on the blanket. It's as if they're saying, "Hey, I remember this! I really like it!"

You might read about the 5 "S's" and think, "So what's new? Those soothing techniques have been known for centuries." And you would be partly right. The methods themselves are not new; however, what *is* new are two essential concepts for making the old techniques really effective—vigor and combining. In Chapter 13, you will learn how to perfectly combine the 5 "S's" in the "Cuddle" Cure, but now I would like to share with you one of the least understood and most important elements of calming a screaming baby . . . the need for *vigor.*

Vigor: The Essential Tip for Calming Your Frantic Little Cave Baby

Many of our ideas about what babies need are based on a misunderstanding about their fragility. Of course, babies *are* quite fragile in many ways. They choke very easily and have weak immune systems. For this reason, being told to do *anything* vigorously may seem as counterintuitive to you as being told that adding a slimy, raw egg to a cake will make it delicious . . . yet, it's every bit as true!

That's because, in many other ways, your newborn is a tough little "cave" baby. He can snooze at the noisiest parties and scream at the top of his lungs much longer than you or I could. Parents are often amazed at how forcefully nurses handle babies when they bathe and burp them. Even breast-feeding may feel pushy when you first learn how. Yet experienced moms know they *must* be assertive when latching their baby on the breast or else they'll end up with sore nipples and a frustrated baby.

One mom in my practice, a psychologist, realized how impossible it was to gently guide her baby from screaming to serenity:

> *"Because of my professional training, I'm very good at remaining calm and reasonable even in the face of frantic and angry outbursts. I expected that this mild demeanor would also help me guide my one-month-old, Helene, out of her primitive*

screaming fits. What a joke! This little brawler needed me to take
control like police subduing a rowdy mob."

Parents often mistakenly believe that their job is to lead their unhappy baby into calmness by responding to his wails with soft whispers and gentle rocking. While that's a very reasonable, civilized approach, it rarely calms an infant in the middle of a meltdown.

Jessica tried to calm her frantic six-week-old by wrapping him up, turning on a tape recording of the vacuum, and putting him in the swing. But it backfired. Like a little Houdini, Jonathan freed himself from the swaddle in minutes and wailed longer and louder than ever. I suggested that Jessica try tightening the wrapping and turning on the real vacuum, not a tape. Jonathan's screaming bouts shortened from hours to minutes!

Most first-time parents don't feel instantly comfortable with their fussy baby's need for vigor. Let's face it, as a parent you're given so much contradictory advice. One minute, you're warned to handle your baby gently and the next you're told to deposit your shrieking child into a buzzing bouncy seat beside a roaring vacuum cleaner. Yet experienced baby "wranglers" know the more frantically a baby is crying the tighter his swaddling, the louder the shushing, and the more jiggly the swinging must be, *or else they simply won't work.*

The fastest way to succeed in stopping your baby's cycle of crying is to *meet his level of intensity.* Only after your screaming baby pauses for a few moments can you gradually slow your motion, soften your shushing, and guide him down from his frenzy to a soft landing.

The best colic-calmers say that soothing an infant is like dancing with him—*but they always let the baby lead!* These talented people pay close attention to the vigor of their infant's crying and mirror it with the vigor of their 5 "S's." If crying is frantic, the rocking and shushing are as spirited as a jitterbug. As cries turn into sobs, the response shifts to the fluid pace of a waltz. And once the baby slips into serenity, their actions slide into the gentle to-and-fro of a slow dance. Of course, any return to screaming is immediately met with renewed vigor and a bouncy tempo.

Three Reasons Your Baby May Have a Delayed Response to the 5 "S's"

You'll be able to soothe your baby quickly once you become skillful at using the 5 "S's." However, the first few times you use these methods you may notice something peculiar: Your baby may ignore you or even cry louder.

This is normal, so please don't worry. His brain may be having a little trouble getting your new message:

Augie was dozing angelically when I arrived at his hospital room to examine him. However, the moment I unwrapped him and the cool air touched his skin, he began to howl. I quieted him with some intense rocking and shushing, but as soon as I stopped and began probing his soft, marshmallow belly, he began to cry again. Were my hands too cold? Did I hurt him? No, he just hadn't fully recovered from his prior upset, and my touch rekindled his protests.

Augie bellowed and flailed, then suddenly he became stone silent. I looked down to see him staring out into space as if he were trying to ignore me. The calm was only momentary, however. In seconds, his frantic cry cycled through him once more.

I snared his hands and held them to his chest. Then I leaned over his struggling body, rocked him, and simultaneously made a harsh shhhh sound in his ear. Within seconds, Augie was again completely at ease.

Five seconds later, however, his cry surfaced one last time, like an exhausted boxer trying to get up off the mat. After just a few more seconds of vigorous shushing and rocking, Augie finally gave in and his little body relaxed for good.

As you can see, even if your "S's" are perfect, you may have to patiently wait a few minutes for your crying baby to fully respond. Three particular traits of an infant's nervous system can fool you into thinking the 5 "S's" aren't working:

1. Baby brains have a hard time shifting gears.

If *you* think your baby is screaming loudly, you should hear what's going on inside *his* head! Chaos so distracts and overloads your newborn's immature brain that he has a difficult time escaping his frenzy to pay attention to you. It's like when your good buddy is in a fight. You try to pull him out of it, but he struggles against you to keep slugging away. It's not until later, when he finally calms down, that he admits, "Thanks, you're a real friend. I just couldn't stop myself."

So expect your baby to resist the 5 "S's" until he calms down enough to realize that your shushing and jiggling are *exactly* what he needs from you.

2. Baby brains are very s-l-o-w.

When your baby is four months old, his eyes will quickly track you as you move around the room, but for now his brain is a little too undeveloped to do that. During these early months of life, it takes a couple of seconds for messages from his eyes ("I just saw mom move!") to travel to the part of his brain that gives out the commands ("Okay, so follow her!").

This dragged-out response time is even more pronounced in colicky babies. All the tumult going on inside their heads overwhelms their brains, making their processing time even slower.

3. Baby brains get into cycles of crying.

When your crying newborn does start responding to the 5 "S's," he may only settle for a minute before he bursts into crying all over again. That's because your baby's distress from crying is still cycling through his nervous system like a strong aftershock following his just ended "baby earthquake."

Your baby may need you to continue the 5 "S's" for five to ten minutes—or more—after he calms down. That's how long it may take for his upset to finish cycling through him and for the calming reflex to finally guide him into sleep.

These cycles can be confusing. They make it seem as if your baby has experienced a jolt of pain, but that's rarely the case. Instead, what's occurring is like what happens when you catch a fish. The fish struggles, gives up for a few moments, then suddenly fights again. With persistence you'll find that the 5 "S's" help your baby's cycles of crying gradually diminish and melt into a blissful peace.

> *Calming baby Frances reminded Suzanne of her job as a teacher. "It's like quieting a classroom of yelling five-year-olds. At first you raise your voice a little to get their attention. Then, as they begin to settle, kids who are still revved up from before have occasional outbursts. Gradually, the excitement cycles down and all the kids become still and focused."*

The next six chapters will teach you exactly how to switch your baby's crying reflex off and his calming reflex on. Once you have mastered these skills, crying will no longer be a cause of frustration. In fact, as odd as it sounds, you may even start appreciating your baby's wails as a great opportunity for you to help him feel loved—and to help you feel like a terrific parent.

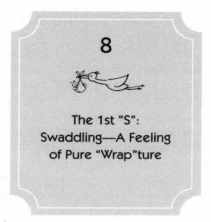

8

**The 1st "S":
Swaddling—A Feeling
of Pure "Wrap"ture**

Main Points:

- Swaddling is the cornerstone of calming. It gives nurturing touch, stops flailing, and focuses your baby's attention
- Swaddling by itself may not halt crying, rather it prepares babies for the other "S's" that *do* switch crying off
- The reasons our ancestors stopped swaddling centuries ago
- Six unnecessary concerns today's parents have about swaddling
- The perfect baby swaddle: The DUDU wrap

As my office was about to close one evening, Alex's mother called, in tears. Betsy said Alex had been having bouts of pain for more than two weeks. Here's how Betsy described it.

> *"When Alex was six weeks old, she began having terrible gas pains. At night she would wake up screaming almost hourly. I watched my diet, in case something I was eating was giving her gas. But that didn't alleviate her crying at all."*

Betsy asked me for some anti-gas medicine to help Alex with what she assumed were stomach cramps. She was surprised when I focused on how to calm her rather than curing the gas. I taught Betsy about the calming reflex and showed her how to swaddle, shhhh, and swing Alex to help her fall asleep. But, Betsy remained skeptical.

"I didn't use Dr. Karp's technique the first night. Swaddling Alex tight didn't feel natural. I was afraid she would be uncomfortable or have difficulty breathing. And I still believed the main issue was gas. That night Alex's 'pain' seemed severe, and I decided I would follow Dr. Karp's advice in the morning.

"The next day I swaddled Alex from morning till night, and surprisingly she seemed much more comfortable. At bedtime, even before I had finished wrapping her, Alex fell asleep—and she slept for seven hours. I could hear her stomach rumbling and knew that she was still having gas, but it was no longer waking her up.

"Tight bundling helped Alex become a much better sleeper. By the time she was four months old she slept well without needing any swaddling."

Swaddling: The Cornerstone of Calming

As Betsy discovered with Alex, soothing an irritable infant is one hundred times easier when her hands are snuggled straight at her sides. Why does this work so well? Here are three ways swaddling benefits fussy babies:

1. The Sweet Touch of Swaddling

Skin is the body's largest organ, and touch is the most calming of our senses. Swaddling envelops your baby's body with a continuous soft caress.

Every mother knows how delicious the touch of her baby's soft skin feels against her own, but for your baby, touch is more than a nice sensation—it's as lifesaving as milk! Babies given milk but never held or touched often wither and die. Of course, swaddling isn't as rich an experience for your baby as being cuddled, but it's a good substitute for those times she is not in your arms.

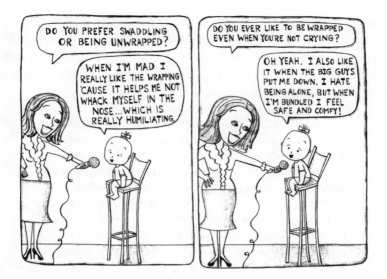

2. Swaddling Keeps Your Baby from Spiraling Out of Control

Not only does swaddling feel cozy, it also keeps your baby from whacking herself and inadvertently getting more upset. (You may have noticed how much calmer your baby is when she is "wrapped" in your arms.) Before birth, your uterus kept your baby's arms from spinning like a windmill. After her "eviction," this restriction disappears. Without the womb walls to prevent flailing, your baby's small upsets can quickly switch on her Moro reflex (the falling reflex) and start her thrashing and crying.

3. Wrapping Helps Your Baby Pay Attention to What You're Doing to Calm Her

When your baby is crying, she experiences a sensation similar to ten radios playing in her head—at the same time. Each jerk and startle shoots another alarm message to her brain, and together those signals make such a racket that your crying infant may hardly notice you're there!

Your little screamer desperately needs you to tell her, "That's it, I'm taking over now." And that's exactly what swaddling does. By

The Great Surprise About Swaddling

The biggest myth parents have about wrapping is that it's supposed to quiet their fussy baby. *Wrong!* Swaddling by itself doesn't turn on the calming reflex.

This point often confuses inexperienced parents. In fact, many new moms and dads lose patience with bundling because initially it makes their babies scream louder not less!

So why is swaddling the first step of calming? Because it prepares your baby for the soothing steps you will do next that *will* trigger her calming reflex.

Think of it this way: What's the first thing a mother does when her hungry toddler clamors for food? Set the table to serve the meal. Yet doing that often makes her scream louder, as if she's yelling, "Hey, just dump the spaghetti on the table!" Of course, *you* know she needs utensils and a plate before she can enjoy her delicious meal, so you buzz through your preparations despite her protests.

In essence, swaddling "sets the table" for the feast of calming you're about to serve. It's the critical step of preparation before the actual shhhhing and jiggling begin. So don't worry if your baby struggles more right after you've wrapped her snugly. Once you begin "feeding" her the other 4 "S's," you'll satisfy her needs completely.

restraining your baby's movements, you turn off most of the distracting "radio stations" so she can tune in and focus on all the wonderful things you're doing to soothe her. Wrapping also prevents new twitches from igniting the crying all over again.

Once upon a Time: How Parents Have Used Swaddling in Other Times and Cultures

I banish from you all tears, birthmarks, flaws, and the troubles of bed-wetting. Love your paternal and maternal uncles. Do not betray your origins. Be intelligent, learned, and discreet. Respect yourself, be brave.

Ritual instructions spoken when
swaddling a baby by the Berber people of Algeria,
Béatrice Fontanel and Claire d'Harcourt, *Babies Celebrated*

*After Elena emigrated from Russia to Los Angeles, she gave
birth to a healthy baby girl named Olga. As I examined Olga,
I described to her proud mother all of her daughter's wonderful
abilities. Elena concentrated intensely as I spoke, struggling to
understand my words.*

*When I placed her precious infant on a blanket to demon-
strate swaddling, she smiled. Gently touching my arm, she said
with a Slavic accent, "Doctor, you don't have to show me <u>dat.</u> In
my <u>willage</u> we wrap <u>dem</u> and put BELT around. It holds <u>dem</u>
<u>wery</u> good!"*

For tens of thousands of years, mothers living in cool climates have
swaddled their babies. While those in very hot climates hardly ever swaddle, they do hold their infants in their arms or in slings almost twenty-four
hours a day. Parents all over the globe wrap their infants because:

- *It's safe*—Babies are less likely to suddenly wiggle out of
  their parent's arms.
- *It's easy*—Babies can be strapped on a parent's back or slung
  on their hips.

Great Swaddling Moments in History

- History has recorded that Alexander the Great, Julius
  Caesar, and Jesus were all swaddled as babies.
- In Tibet, babies have always been swaddled tightly in blankets. Tradi-
  tionally, the wrapping was secured with rope and the baby was tied to
  the side of a yak to be carried as the family hiked through the valleys.
- On the high plains of Algeria, babies were swaddled to protect them
  from drafts and evil spirits.
- During the Middle Ages, European parents kept their babies immobi-
  lized in a tight, bulky swaddle for the first four to nine months.
- The American Academy of Pediatrics insignia features a swaddled
  fifteenth-century Italian baby.
- Many Native American tribes carried their papoose—young baby—
  tightly packaged and slung onto their backs. (The 2000 U.S. one-dollar
  coin displays an image of the Native American guide Sacajawea with
  her tiny baby snugly bundled on her back.)

■ *It's calming*—Babies get less upset because they can't flail about.

These parents envelop their babies in blankets and then usually secure the wrapping with strings and belts. And now, our nation has also rediscovered that babies like being wrapped as snug as a bug in a rug. In most U.S. hospitals, new moms are taught how to swaddle their babies, and I've even seen some nurses use masking tape to keep the blanket from unraveling.

Swaddling Gets Unraveled: How Our Ancestors Did the *Wrong* Thing for All the *Right* Reasons

Even in the Middle Ages, the top fashion ideas originated in Paris. However, about three hundred years ago, these trendsetters goofed when they declared, "*Le swaddling* is passé."

Before the 1700s, all Europeans wrapped their babies. Swaddling made babies easy to carry and kept them warm and quiet. Parents also believed wrapping prevented their infants from accidentally plucking out their own eyes or dislocating their arms.

Then two revolutionary trends became popular: science and democracy. As wonderful as these movements were, they led to two unfortunate misunderstandings that contributed to the abandonment of swaddling:

Science makes mistake #1: In the 1700s scientists proved that unwrapped infants *never* plucked out their eyes or dislocated their arms. From these observations they wrongly assumed that swaddling was a waste of time.

Democracy makes mistake #2: In the years leading up to the Declaration of Independence, our founding fathers (and mothers) wanted their children to live in freedom, but this attitude led them to reject swaddling as a form of "baby prison."

Within one hundred years, the combined pressures of science and democracy convinced most parents in the Western world to stop swaddling. While these great thinkers were right that unwrapped babies didn't hurt themselves and that adults would feel enslaved by such tight bindings, they were absolutely wrong to recommend parents stop bundling their infants. They didn't realize that swaddling had continued throughout the centuries because it truly helped babies stay happier. As parents stopped wrapping their newborns, the unexpected happened: The number of babies suffering from uncontrollable crying dramatically *increased!*

In their eagerness to stop this tidal wave of colic, scientists made yet another colossal mistake. They concluded that babies were crying because of pain, and encouraged parents to give their shrieking infants the two most effective anesthetics of the time—gin and opium. Of course, as soon as the serious side effects of those colic treatments were realized, they fell out of favor.

A Parent's Hesitations—Six Unnecessary Wrapping Worries

In the U.S. today, many parents and grandparents still hesitate to swaddle their babies. They worry that tight wrapping may deprive their babies of some unwritten constitutional right. But I'm afraid they are confusing the right to *bear* arms with the right to *flail* arms.

Through the years, I have asked many parents to tell me their secret prejudices against swaddling. Here are their six most common concerns:

1. *Swaddling seems primitive and old-fashioned.*
Well, it is. But what's wrong with primitive and old-fashioned? Eating and sex are both primitive and old-fashioned, and who wants to abandon them? Besides, swaddling may be a prehistoric practice, but it really works.

2. *Babies might be uncomfortable with their arms tightly down at their sides.*
Many new parents think their crying babies want their arms up. If that was why these infants cried, calming them would be a snap: Just never wrap them! Of course, as you've probably noticed, releasing your baby's arms usually only makes her scream even more.
It is true that your baby's arms have tightened into the bent-arm position by the end of your pregnancy. And, as a result, if you place

them at her sides, they tend to *boing* right back up, like curly hair pulled straight then released. However, the arms-down position is not at all uncomfortable, which is why babies sleep extra-long when they're bundled that way.

3. *Wrapping may make a baby feel trapped.*

Personally, I would hate to be swaddled. Without revealing too much about my married life, let me say that the first thing my wife and I do when we get into bed is untuck the blanket and give our feet some breathing room.

Of course, most of us would hate living in a womb. However, it's a mistake to think our babies want the same things we do. She's not struggling against the wrapping because she hates it. She looks like she wants her hands free, but the opposite is true. Newborns love being confined, and when they're frantic and out of control they need your help to restrain their frantic arms and legs.

4. *Babies will get spoiled or dependent on swaddling.*

Fortunately, this worry is totally unfounded. Holding your baby twelve hours a day is not an overindulgence; it's a fifty percent cutback from what she got in your womb! Once your baby is four months old she'll be able to push up, roll over, and grab, and she no longer will need to be wrapped. Until then, swaddling can be a great comfort.

5. *Wrapping frustrates an infant's attempts to suck her fingers.*

It was easy for your baby to suck her fingers before she was born: The walls of your uterus kept her hands right next to her face. After birth, however, it's much harder for her to get her fingers in that position. Even though she tries, they often jerk away as if yanked on by some practical joker. (Pacifiers were invented exactly because babies have such a hard time keeping their hands in their mouths.)

Please, don't misunderstand me, it's fine to let your infant have her hands out so she can suck on her fingers—*as long as she's happy.* Unfortunately, most babies aren't able to keep their hands there, especially when upset. So rather than calming a baby, loose hands usually fly by their owner's mouth, frustrating her and increasing her screams!

It will take three to four months for your baby to coordinate her lips, tongue, shoulder, and arm—all at the same time—to keep her fingers in her mouth. However, once your baby is able to manage all that, swaddling becomes unnecessary (although it may still help her sleep longer).

6. *Tight bundling might interfere with a baby's ability to learn about the world.*

Of course, your baby does need her hands unwrapped sometimes so she can get some practice using them. However, when she's crying your job isn't teaching, it's calming. In fact, even when your infant is calm, bundling may actually *help* her learn about the world, because she can pay attention better when her arms aren't constantly in motion.

It's Time for Swaddling to Make a Comeback

For centuries, parents have been hesitant about swaddling their babies. Critics have claimed swaddling was just a fad—and some continue to do so:

> About ten years ago, I visited a nursery for newborns in northern Italy. I shared with the nursery director the concept of the missing fourth trimester and my belief that the time had come for a worldwide "renaissance of wrapping."
>
> The director listened politely, but his face wore an amazed and amused expression. After I finished my impassioned speech, he patted my shoulder in a grandfatherly way and said discreetly, "We haven't done that in Italy for generations. We believe that babies must have their hands free to encourage their muscle development."
>
> At that moment, his secretary summoned him to take a phone call. No sooner had he left the room than a nurse shyly came up to me and whispered, "You know, <u>Il Directore</u> likes to keep the babies unwrapped, but as soon as he leaves for the day, we always bundle them all back up again!" She winked at me, adding, "They really are happier that way."

You probably already know that the number-one way to calm your fussy baby is to pick her up and hold her tightly in your arms. That's exactly what swaddling does, except it has the extra benefit of giving you a few minutes to cook a meal or go to the bathroom!

Swaddling is easy to do, but it does require precise technique and some practice. Many books recommend wrapping, but they rarely teach how to do it, which is problematic because incorrect swaddling can make your baby's crying worse.

Here's everything you need to know to become the happiest (and best) swaddler on the block. Don't worry if it feels weird at first; after five to ten tries swaddling will become as automatic for you as changing a diaper.

There are as many ways to swaddle babies as there are to fold napkins for a dinner party. But one method that a wonderful midwife taught me many years ago is clearly the best. I call it the DUDU wrap (pronounced "doo doo," standing for Down-Up-Down-Up).

Getting Started

You'll need a large *square* blanket. These are easier to use than rectangular blankets because their symmetry allows for an even, balanced wrap. Blanket fabric is your choice. Some like flannel, while others prefer stretchy, waffle-type fabrics. (You may find it's easiest to learn to wrap if you first practice it on a doll or when your baby is calm.)

1) Place the blanket on your bed and position it like a diamond, with a point at the top.

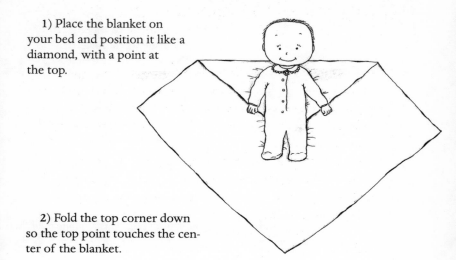

2) Fold the top corner down so the top point touches the center of the blanket.

3) Place your baby on the blanket so her neck lies on the top edge.

4) Hold your baby's right arm down straight at her side. If she resists, be patient. The arm will straighten after a moment or two of gentle pressure.

You now have your baby in the starting position for the DUDU wrap. An easy way to remember what to do next is to sing this little song as you do it:

> DOWN . . . tuck . . . snug
> UP . . . tuck . . . snug
> DOWN . . . a smidge . . . hold
> UP . . . across . . . snug

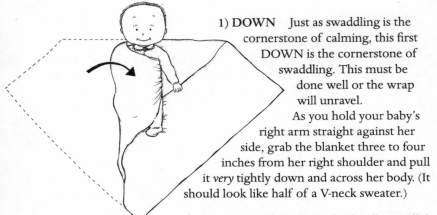

1) DOWN   Just as swaddling is the cornerstone of calming, this first DOWN is the cornerstone of swaddling. This must be done well or the wrap will unravel.

As you hold your baby's right arm straight against her side, grab the blanket three to four inches from her right shoulder and pull it *very* tightly down and across her body. (It should look like half of a V-neck sweater.)

Tuck—*Keeping the blanket taut, finish pulling it all the way down and* **tuck** *it under her left buttock and lower back. This anchors the wrap.*

Snug—*Hold the blanket against her left hip (with your left hand), grab the blanket right next to her left shoulder and tug it very, very snug. This will remove any slack around your baby's right arm and stretch the fabric tight.*

After this first "DOWN . . . tuck . . . snug," her right arm should be held so securely against her side that she can't bend it up, even if you let go of the blanket. (More on the critical importance of straight arms on page 118.)

Please don't be surprised or lose confidence if your baby suddenly cries louder when you pull the blanket tight. You're not hurting her! Her cry means she's still out of control and unaware that she's just seconds away from happiness.

2) UP   Now straighten her left arm against her side and bring the bottom corner straight up to cover her arm. The bottom blanket corner should reach just over her left shoulder. It's okay if her legs are bent (that's how they were in the womb), but be sure her arms are straight. If her arms are bent, she'll wiggle out of the wrap as fast as you can say, "Oops, she did it again!" And she'll cry even more.

Tuck—*Hold her covered left arm against her body, and tuck the blanket edge under it.*

Snug—*While your left hand holds her left arm down, use your right hand to grab the blanket three inches from her left shoulder and snug it (stretch it as much as possible). This again removes any slack from around her arms.*

3) DOWN   Still holding the blanket very taut, three inches from her left shoulder, pull the blanket *down* a smidge.

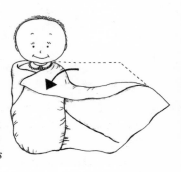

A smidge—*This DOWN should bring only a tiny bit of fabric over her shoulder to her upper chest, like the second half of the V-neck sweater. (Don't bring this fold all the way down to your baby's feet. Remember, it's just a smidge.)*

Hold—*Hold that tiny smidge of blanket against her breastbone with your left hand, like you are holding down a ribbon while making a bow.*

4) UP   Keeping that smidge in place, grab the last free blanket corner with your right hand and pull it straight out to your right. This will remove every last bit of stretch and slack from the wrap. Then, without releasing the tension, lift that corner in one smooth motion, up and across her body.

Across—*Bring it **tightly** across her waist and then all around her body like a belt. The belt should go right over her forearms, holding them down against her sides.*

Snug—*Finish the DUDU wrap by snugging the belt **tightly** to remove any slack. If the wrap is tight (and your blanket is big enough), the end of the belt will reach around her body and back to the front, where you can tuck it into the beginning of the belt. This last tight snug and tuck is crucial to keep the whole swaddle from popping open.*

The ancient tradition of bundling babies isn't a fad. It's the *end* of a fad—an anti-swaddling fad! Televisions and computers may become forgotten novelties a thousand years from today, but swaddling is as old as the trees and it's time for it to become part of our babies' lives once again.

Ironing Out the Wrinkles: Fixing the Most Common Swaddling Mistakes

Swaddling is simple, but watch for these common mistakes:

- *Wrapping too loosely*

  The key to wrapping is to keep it snug . . . snug . . . snug. Make sure you pull the blanket tight, removing any slack with every step of the DUDU wrap.

  Denise discovered the tightness of the wrap was the secret ingredient for her six-week-old son. "Our running joke was we swaddled Augie so tightly we were scared his eyes would pop out! But swaddling helped him enormously, and tight was exactly the way he needed it to be!"

- *Swaddling a baby with bent arms*

  Even with tight swaddling, it's easy for your crying baby to wiggle her hands out if she was wrapped with her arms bent. While it's true that new babies are comforted by having their bodies flexed into the fetal position, and preemies do best with bent arms at least until they reach their due date, babies swaddled with their arms down still have lots of flexion in their legs, fingers, and neck to keep them happy.

  Swaddling helped Ted and Shele's two-month-old daughter, Dylan, sleep through the night. To keep her arms straight, Ted tucked Dylan's hands under the waistband of her tiny sweatpants before wrapping her. He said, "I have to do this because every time she gets her arms bent, she pops them out and gets even madder."

- *Letting the blanket touch your baby's cheek*

  If your baby is hungry and the blanket touches her cheek, it may fool her into thinking it's your breast, accidentally setting off the powerful rooting reflex and making her cry out of confusion and frustration. To keep the blanket off the face, make it look more like a V-neck sweater.

- *Allowing the finished swaddle to pop back open*
   Another basic rule of wrapping is: "Whoever gets loose loses!" It's no use wrapping your baby tightly if she can pop out in seconds. That's why experienced parents in other cultures swaddle their infants and then secure the wrap by tightly tying it with ribbons, strings, or belts.

> *Ken and Kristie said, "Whenever Henry sneaks out of his blanket, he cries as if to say, 'What have you done for me lately?' We've found that securing the wrap with duct tape gives us an extra forty-five minutes of sleep between feedings!"*

Dads—The Swaddlers Supreme

I was surprised! I thought my baby girl, Valerie, wouldn't like to be wrapped, but once swaddled, she calmed within seconds. I even taught a guy in the barbershop how to do it.

                                          Pedro, father of Valerie

If women are from Venus and men are from Mars, then mothers are from Cuddleland and fathers are from Jiggleland! That is to say, men usually handle children much more vigorously than women do. We throw our older kids on the bed, have pillow fights, and hoist them into the air above our heads—but what about tiny babies? How do men handle them?

At first, we are often more intimidated by infants than our wives are; babies seem so tiny and fragile. When we *do* carry our little ones around, we often hot-potato them back to our wives the moment they cry.

Swaddling, however, is a great way for dads to build confidence. Fathers often have a natural talent for doing the tight wrapping. In my experience, their strength, vigor, and dexterity make them swaddlers supreme!

Mark said, "I can wrap Eli pretty easily. But my wife, Fran, has a hard time swaddling him. I think she's too timid to do it tightly enough."

The Whys About the "S's": Questions Parents Ask About Swaddling

1. *When should I start wrapping my baby?*
   Babies can be swaddled as soon as they're born. It makes them feel cozy and warm, like they're "back home."

2. *Are there babies who don't need to be swaddled?*
   Many calm babies do well with no swaddling at all. But the fussier your baby is, the more she'll need it. Tight bundling is so successful at soothing infants that some even have to be *un*swaddled in order to wake them up for their feedings.

3. *Can swaddling help a baby sleep?*
   Yes! Even easy babies who don't need wrapping to keep calm often sleep more when swaddled. Bundling keeps them from startling themselves awake. But make sure the wrapping is tight. It's not safe to put babies in bed with loose blankets.

   When Wendy and Brent swaddled Brandon, their two-month-old increased his night sleeping from a four-hour stretch to five to seven hours!

4. *If a baby has never been swaddled, when is it too late to start?*
   You can start wrapping your baby at any time during her first three months. But be patient. You may have to practice a few times before she gets used to it. Try swaddling when she's already sleepy and in her most receptive frame of mind.

5. *When is a baby too old for swaddling?*
   The age for weaning off swaddling varies from baby to baby. Many parents think they should stop after a few weeks or when their baby resists wrapping. But that's actually when bundling becomes the *most* valuable.
   To decide if your infant no longer needs to be wrapped, try this: After she reaches two to three months of age, swaddle her with one arm out. If she gets fussier, she's telling you to continue wrapping for

a few more weeks. However, if she stays happy without the swaddling, she doesn't need it anymore.

With few exceptions, babies are ready to be weaned off wrapping by three to four months of age, although some sleep better wrapped—even up to one year of age. (For more on using swaddling to prolong sleep, see Chapter 15.)

Twins Ari and Grace benefited from swaddling until they were eight months old. Unwrapped they would wake every three hours, but bundled they slept for a glorious ten hours.

6. *How many hours a day should a baby be wrapped?*

All babies need some time to stretch, be bathed, and get a massage. But you'll probably notice your baby is calmer if she's swaddled twelve to twenty hours a day to start with. (Remember, as a fetus, she was snuggled twenty-four hours a day.) After one to two months, you can reduce the wrap time according to how calm she is without it.

7. *How can I tell if I'm swaddling my baby too tightly?*

In traditional cultures, parents swaddle their babies tightly because loose wraps invariably pop back open. Although some Americans worry about snug swaddling, I've never heard of it being done too tightly. On the other hand, I've worked with hundreds of parents whose bundling failed because it was done too loosely. That's because no matter how snugly you do it initially, your baby's wiggling will loosen the blanket a little.

However, for your peace of mind, here's an easy way for you to make sure your wrapping is not too tight: Slide your hand between the blanket and your baby's chest. It should feel as snug as sneaking your hand between your pregnant belly and your pant's elastic waistband—at the end of your ninth month.

8. *How can I tell if my baby is overheated or overwrapped?*

Hillary thought her new son, Rob, needed the room temperature to be the same tropical 98.6°F he loved inside her body! But, she was taking the idea of the fourth trimester a bit too far. In 1994, doctors at UCLA tested babies to see if they could get overheated by heavy bundling. They put thirty-six babies (two to fourteen weeks old) in a room heated to about 74°F and wrapped them in terry coveralls, a cap, a receiving blanket, *and* a thermal blanket. Unexpectedly, their study showed the babies' skin got warmer but their rectal temperatures barely increased.

Preemies often need incubators to keep them toasty, but full-term babies just need a little clothing, a blanket, and a 65–70°F room. If the temperature in your home is warmer than that, just skip some clothing and wrap your baby in only her diaper in a light cotton blanket. (Parents living in warm climates often put cornstarch powder on their babies' skin to absorb sweat and prevent rashes.)

It's easy to check if your baby is overheated—feel her ears and fingers. If they're hot, red, and sweaty, she's overwrapped. However, if they're only slightly warm and she's not sweaty, her temperature is probably perfect.

9. How can I tell when my baby needs to be swaddled and when she needs to eat?

Your baby will give you several hints when she's hungry:

- When you touch her lips, her mouth will open like a baby bird waiting for food from the mother bird.

- She'll only suck on a pacifier for a minute or two before getting frustrated with it.

- If given the breast or bottle, she'll suck and swallow vigorously.

Please don't worry that swaddling might make your baby forget to eat. It may help calm a baby who's mildly hungry, but it won't satisfy one who's famished.

10. My baby often seems jumpy and nervous. Will swaddling help this?

Some babies can sleep through a hurricane, yet others startle every time the phone rings. These babies aren't nervous; they're just sensitive. Swaddling helps by muffling their startle reactions and keeping them from upsetting themselves.

11. Is there any risk to putting my baby to sleep wrapped in a blanket?

As mentioned earlier, doctors recommend that babies not sleep with loose bedding, such as pillows, soft toys, etc. Only use a blanket that is securely wrapped around your baby.

12. Shouldn't we be teaching our children to be free and not bound up?

Freedom is wonderful, but as we all know, with freedom comes responsibility. If a baby can calm herself, she has earned the right to be unwrapped. However, many newborns can't handle the great big world. They still need a few more months of cozy swaddling to keep from thrashing about uncontrollably.

13. *What happens if my baby gets an itch when her arms are swaddled?*
    Luckily, this is never a problem. Young babies don't get clear messages from their bodies, so they don't get an itchy feeling. Babies also have short attention spans. Unlike adults who go wild when they can't reach an itch, infants never give it a second "thought." (Besides, they couldn't really control their bodies well enough to scratch themselves even if they did get an itch.)

A Parent's Perspective: Testimonials from the Trenches

Swaddling helps the little one know where she is. Without it she has no sense of where her body ends and the universe begins.
Al, father of Marie-Claire, Esmé, and Didier

The vast majority of new babies stay calmer and sleep longer when they are swaddled. Here are some of their stories:

The day after Marie-Claire was born, she was crying. Not one of those newborn squeals that makes you go, "Ahhhh," but rather a really powerful bellow. I was shocked that a one-day-old could make such a sound!

Just then Dr. Karp came into our room. He casually walked over to the bassinet, picked our baby up, and wrapped her like a burrito. Then he put her on his lap with her feet toward his belly and her head at his knees and bending his face toward her ears, he made a loud "shhhh" noise. The swaddling and white noise worked together so well that she stopped crying almost instantly.

My husband and I were astonished. It was unlike anything we had ever witnessed. So we learned how to swaddle our baby tight, tight, tight in a receiving blanket, and she was the happiest, most content baby on the planet!

After she was three months old, people would often look askance when we wrapped her, as if we were resorting to barbaric measures. When curious onlookers asked, "Why have you wrapped your baby like that?" we'd proudly answer, "Because it makes her happy." And, as if on cue, Marie-Claire would smile ear-to-ear, and even the most skeptical person would be won over!

Renée, Al, Marie-Claire, Esmé, and Didier

Sophia had problems nursing when she was born. Our nurse practitioner advised me to use a special device to supplement her feedings. So, I taped this tiny tube to my breast and inserted it into her mouth, along with my nipple.

About that time, when she was three weeks old, she started becoming very fussy. During feedings, she would scream and flail, often accidentally knocking out both my nipple and the tube.

Despite my frustration, I stuck it out until the night before her two-month checkup. That night she was worse than ever. Sophia was thrashing, yanking on the tube, and mangling my nipple. I swore I would never feed her that way again, even if it meant I could no longer breast-feed.

The next day I told Dr. Karp about my struggles feeding Sophia, and he said four words that changed everything: "Don't forget the swaddling." We had swaddled Sophia initially but stopped after a few weeks because she fought it so much. However, Dr. Karp encouraged us to give it another go.

That afternoon, I tightly swaddled her and tried her on the breast (without the feeding tube). The most extraordinary thing happened: She breast-fed calmly and with focus. It was as though she never had a problem.

Sophia is now three months old, and feeding has been a breeze for the past month. We swaddle her now only if she has a bad day when she can't settle herself, and the cozy wrapping always works like a dream.

Colin, Beth, and Sophia

Starting at about one month of age, Jack began getting fussy each evening between six P.M. and midnight. I could comfort him but only by breast-feeding him nonstop.

Jack needed to be nursed to sleep and vehemently refused the pacifier, as if I were trying to swindle him out of his inheritance.

Then I discovered the greatest thing (besides breast-feeding) for calming him down: swaddling. He's not crazy about it while it's being done, but it settles him down within minutes. At a baby class I showed my friend how tightly we wrap him, and she was shocked when he went from screaming to complete calm right in front of our eyes! I was so proud of myself and of my great little boy.

Kelly, Adam, and Jack

In The Middle of the Night: Switch off

It's the middle of the night and you want to calm your baby! Can't remember exactly what to do? Here's a summary for those times when you want all the "S's" in one place to help you become the "Best Baby Calmer On The Block."

As you do the 5 "S's," remember these important points:

1) Calming your baby is like dancing with her...but you have to follow her lead. Do the 5 "S's" vigorously only lessening the intensity after she begins to settle.

2) The 5 "S's" must be done exactly right for them to work.

The 1st "S" – Swaddling

Don't worry if your baby's first reaction to wrapping is to struggle against it. Swaddling may not instantly calm her fussies but it will restrain her uncontrolled flailing so she can pay attention to the next "S" that will turn-on her calming reflex and guide her into sweet serenity!

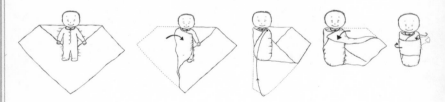

The 2nd "S" – Side/Stomach

The more upset your baby is, the unhappier she will be on her back. Rolling your infant onto her side or stomach will make her much more serene. Just this simple trick can sometimes activate a baby's calming reflex...within seconds.

The 3rd "S" – Shhhh

Shushing crying babies magically makes them feel at peace and back home, but you've got to do it about as loud as your baby's crying and close to her ear...or she won't even notice it. Use this super-effective "S" to keep her calm throughout her fussy period by using a radio tuned to loud static, a tape recording of your hair dryer, or a white noise machine.

The 4th "S" – Swinging

Like vigorous shushing, energetic jiggling can turn your baby from screams to sweet serenity in minutes...or less. As you support your baby's head and neck, wiggle her head with fast, tiny movements, sort of like you're shivering. Once she's entranced you can move her swaddled into a swing for continual, hypnotic motion. (Make sure the strap is between your baby's wrapped legs, the swing is fully reclined, and it's set on the fastest speed.)

The 5th "S" – Sucking

This last "S" usually works best after you have already led your little one into calmness with the other "S's." Offering her your breast, finger, or a pacifier will be the icing on the cake of soothing. You can teach your baby to keep the pacifier in her mouth by using "reverse psychology"—the moment she begins to suck on the pacifier, gently tug on it as if you're going to take it out. She'll suck it in harder and soon she'll learn to keep it in her mouth even when she's cooing.

9

The 2nd "S": Side (or Stomach)—Your Baby's Feel-Good Position

Main Points:

- How the side and stomach positions can calm your baby by switching his calming reflex on and his Moro (falling) reflex off
- Important information about SIDS and your baby's sleeping position
- The reverse-breast-feeding hold and other great ways to cuddle your baby and soothe his crying

Dugger's eyes opened wide when he saw how I handled his baby girl, Bobbie. The moment Bobbie cried, I placed her cheek in my palm and rolled her small body onto my sleeve, resting her chest and stomach against my forearm—Bobbie calmed in mid-scream! Then I jiggled her up and down like I was the most nervous person on the planet and she was asleep within two minutes.

Dugger later told me, "Football was my favorite sport when I was a boy, and I carried the ball as if it were a treasure. But I never would have felt okay handling Bobbie like that if I hadn't seen you do it first. Now I carry Bobbie like a football every day and I can usually make her fall right asleep."

In real estate, the most important rule is: location, location, location. In baby calming it's position, position, position!

There's no question that fussy newborns are easier to calm when they're lying on their side or stomach. Many babies are happy to lie on their backs when they're in a good mood, but it's a tough position to calm them in when they get cranky. Other babies feel insecure on their backs even when they're not fussy. These irritable infants often quiet as soon as they're put on their sides or have their tummies draped over their parent's shoulder or forearm.

Why Do the Side and Stomach Positions Make Your Baby Happy?

The side and stomach positions work so well because:

They trigger the calming reflex by imitating your baby's position in the uterus. Before birth, your fetus was never flat on his back. He spent most of his time on his side in the fetal position—head down, spine rounded, knees pressed against his belly. Over millions of years this position became a potent trigger for the calming reflex, keeping fetuses serene so they didn't accidentally move into a bad position or kink their umbilical cords.

Once out of the womb, bending your baby's neck down a bit, touching his stomach, and laying him on his side activate position sensors inside his head that trigger the calming reflex. Specialists in the care of premature infants place them flexed and on their sides as soon as these tiny newborns are healthy enough to be handled. (Even many adults find coiling up into the fetal position comforting.)

"Tummy touching" might also turn on calming as a reflex left over from our ape ancestors. For millions of years it has been crucial for ape babies to stay still when they were tummy-to-tummy, clutching their mama's fur. It's possible that those animals who were soothed by the sensation of tummy touching thrashed less, fell less, and therefore survived and passed their genes along to their own babies.

The side and stomach positions keep your baby from accidentally setting off his Moro (falling) reflex. Cuddling a fussy baby on his back is a little like calming and pinching him at the same time! The holding part feels great, but lying on the back can make some young infants feel insecure. In that position, any twitch or cry can trigger the brain's position sensors and unleash the Moro reflex, making your baby shriek and fling his arms out as if he's being dropped out of a tree.

On the other hand, putting your baby on his side or stomach makes the position sensors in his head send out a message that says, "Don't worry. Everything's fine!" (Once your baby's Moro has been turned on, it may take his brain a minute or two after he's rolled onto his side or stomach for an all-clear message to be recognized and the calming reflex turned on.) Some infants are so sensitive to position that just rolling them from their sides slightly over toward their stomachs calms them, and rolling them a tiny bit from their sides toward their backs makes them panic.

A Position for Life: Helping Babies Avoid SIDS

Babies love to lie on their sides and to be touched on their stomachs. These positions are like cookies and warm milk for them. However, while having your infant in these positions is great during his waking hours, your baby's back is the preferred position in which to put him to sleep.

In 1992, the American Academy of Pediatrics (AAP) recommended that babies never sleep on their stomachs. Research showed that infants who were put down in that position had an increased risk of dying from crib death, or what's known as Sudden Infant Death Syndrome (SIDS). In a giant victory for families, we were able to lower the death rate from SIDS from six thousand babies a year to three thousand five hundred, just by keeping sleeping babies off their stomachs.

In March 2000, the AAP issued its latest advice on protecting babies from SIDS. They stated that SIDS was rare under one month of age, peaking between two and four months. They also noted that babies with the highest risk of SIDS were those who slept on their stomachs, slept on a soft substance, had moms who smoked, were overheated, had no prenatal care, had teenage mothers, or were born prematurely. They went on to state that the back was the preferred sleeping position and that the side position was also acceptable, although it had a slightly higher risk of SIDS (probably due to babies accidentally rolling onto their stomachs during sleep).

To prevent SIDS, the AAP recommends that you don't smoke during pregnancy and eliminate all smoking from your house; don't take alcohol or sedative drugs, especially when you bed-share; never sleep with your baby on a sofa or waterbed; keep soft objects out of his bed (toys, pillows, sheepskins, loose blankets, comforters); and don't let your baby get hot and sweaty to the touch.

Once Upon a Time: How Parents Have Used the Side/Stomach Position in Other Times and Cultures

Among the Inuit (Alaskan natives), a very deep hood is used as a baby bag and serves as an extension of the womb. The newborn lives in a heated climate, completely buried inside the mother's clothing, and curled up like a half-moon.
Béatrice Fontanel and Claire d'Harcourt, *Babies Celebrated*

In most traditional cultures around the world, babies hang out—literally. Their mothers, sisters, aunts, and neighbors carry them in baskets and sheets on their fronts, backs, hips, and shoulders for up to twenty-four hours a day, seven days a week.

Few parents across the globe place their infants on their backs, but when they do, they usually put them on a *curved* surface, not a flat one. The arc of a small blanket suspended from a tree or tripod puts a baby back into the familiar and reassuring rounded fetal position, which allows him to sleep more restfully.

- The Lapp people of Greenland carry their babies curled up in cradles that hang on one side of a reindeer (counterbalanced on the animal's other side by a heavy sack of flour).

- The !Kung San people of the Kalahari Desert carry their infants in leather slings all day long. They keep them in a semi-sitting position, because they believe that posture encourages a baby's development.

- In parts of Indonesia, loving mothers never let their babies stretch out completely; in their culture that is the feared position of the dead. Infants are compactly bundled in a seated position and suspended from the ceiling to sleep like little floating Buddhas. (Even new mothers must sleep sitting up for forty days after the delivery to evade evil spirits who are attracted to people weakened by illness or injury.)

- The Efé tribe of pygmies in Zaire hate putting their babies down—even for a moment. They keep their tiny tots happy by holding them upright or curled up in their arms all day long, and even while they are sleeping. However, since it's such a big effort for one person to do all this carrying, the Efé believe in teamwork. For the first several months, tribal members pass newborns back and forth among up to twenty people, an average of eight times an hour!

Even when women in different cultures take their infants out of their arms, they hang them over their laps or chests, which allows their babies' soft tummies to remain in constant contact with their mother's warm, comforting skin.

Go with the Winning Side: How to Use Position to Help Soothe Your Baby

Here's how you can treat your baby to the calming pleasure of being on his side or stomach. First, wrap your baby in a cozy swaddle, then try one of these positions used by countless experienced parents:

The Reverse-Breast-Feeding Hold

This hold is my favorite for carrying a crying baby while I'm walking or bouncing him into tranquillity. It's easy and comfortable to do, and it supports his head and neck perfectly.

1. Sit down and lay your baby on your lap; have him on his right side with his head on your knees and his feet on your left hip.

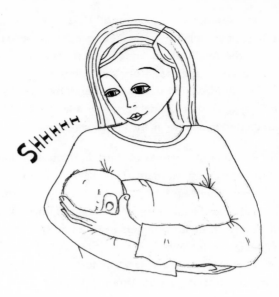

SHHHHH

2. Slide your left hand between your knee and his cheek so you support his head (or head and neck) in your palm and outstretched fingers.

3. Roll him onto your left forearm so his stomach rests against your arm and bring him in to your body, lightly pressing his back against your chest.

   In this position, your thumb will be right next to his face and you can even let him take it into his mouth for added pleasure. (Always wash your hands first.)

The Football Hold

Fathers love the football hold. This stomach-down position requires a little extra arm strength, but it's fun and effective. In fact, silencing babies, mid-squawk, with the football hold is one of the greatest baby "magic tricks" of all time.

1. Sit your swaddled baby on your lap, face him to your left, and place your left hand under his chin, supporting it like a chin strap.

2. Gently lean him forward and roll his hips over so his stomach is lying on your left forearm. His head rests in

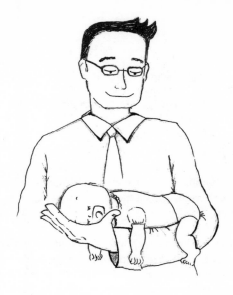

your palm, his chest and stomach are snugly cushioned against your forearm, and his legs are straddled over your arm, hanging limp.

The Over-the-Shoulder Hold

Hoisting your fussy baby up onto your shoulder can have a powerful, soothing effect. Often, simply lifting your baby into an upright position gets him to open his eyes and perk up.

When your baby is upright you can also let the weight of his body press his stomach against your shoulder to provide him with some extra tummy touching, making this hold doubly comforting. Be sure to swaddle your baby *before* you put him over your shoulder. It will help him stay asleep when you move him off your shoulder to his bassinet.

This is by no means an exhaustive list of calming baby holds. You can also try the cannonball position, where your baby is curled in a ball, knee to chest, across your lap, or the hot-water-bottle position, with your baby draped over a warm hot-water bottle so the heat and pressure are against his stomach. (Remember, don't let him sleep on his stomach.) Have fun discovering the position that makes your baby the happiest.

The Whys About the "S's":
Questions Parents Ask
About the Side/Stomach Position

1. *Where should I put my baby's hands when he's on his side?*

   Your baby's arms should be placed straight along his body. Even with the tightest wrap, there's enough wiggle room to allow your baby to move his bottom arm a little bit forward to get into a comfortable position.

2. *Can a baby's arm ever go to sleep when he's lying on his side?*

   No. Arms only fall asleep when there's firm pressure on the part of the elbow called the funny bone. That's why it happens when you snooze on a hard desk using your arm as a pillow. Since the arms of a swaddled baby move a little bit forward once wrapped, there's never enough pressure on the arm to cause it to fall asleep.

3. *If babies miss the womb sensations, wouldn't it make sense to position them upside-down?*

   Well, that's an interesting thought, but the answer is no. You might think babies who have spent months upside-down would like this position, but the womb is filled with fluid so the fetus actually floats almost weightlessly inside. Once outside of the uterus, the buoyancy is gone, and an upside-down baby would develop uncomfortable pressure as blood pools in his head.

A Parent's Perspective: Testimonials from the Trenches

These fussy babies were "be-side" themselves with joy when their parents put them in these feel-good positions:

Dina was confused. At the hospital, she was told to let Noah sleep on his back, but when her mom came to visit she told her the opposite. "We argued about the best position for my six-week-old baby to

sleep in. He had a really hard time settling himself when he was
flat on his back. I had to pat him for fifteen to twenty minutes
until he finally drifted off, and even then he'd still wake up every
three hours.

"My mom said I should let him sleep on his stomach. While he did
sleep more soundly in that position, I was terrified of doing anything
that might increase his risk of SIDS.

"I asked Dr. Karp his opinion. He showed me how to wrap Noah
tightly and put him down to sleep on his back. I was thrilled because
it worked as well as my mother's stomach-down position, but was
much safer."

Alfre said that when she was growing up she learned an easy
way to calm babies, which the women in her family had passed
down from generation to generation. It was called the "Big Mama"
technique.

The way it worked was to sit down with a pillow on your lap and
place the screaming baby stomach-down on top of it. Then you start
bouncing the heels of your feet up and down (hard), patting the baby
on the bottom (hard), and singing a lullaby right in the baby's ear.

Once the sun went down, two-month-old Ruby began her nightly
twist-and-fuss routine. Her parents, Steve and Sarah, worried she was
suffering from stomach pain, until they discovered that Ruby would
promptly fall asleep if they placed her over their shoulder with her
stomach pressing firmly against them as they marched around the
backyard, jiggling her body with every step.

Baby Michael's father was the family pro at soothing Michael's
screaming. He would sit in the rocker with a pillow on his lap, lay
Michael belly-down on top of the pillow, and rock him hard and
fast. Within five minutes Michael was always out in lullaby-land.

10

The 3rd "S":
Shhhh—Your Baby's
Favorite Soothing Sound

Main Points:

- Shhhh triggers your baby's calming reflex
- The whooshing sound your baby heard in your uterus was as loud as a vacuum cleaner
- Shhhhing only soothes screaming babies if it is loud
- Ten machines you can use to make a soothing white noise

My young husband walked our crying baby up and down, making that shshshshshing sound of comfort that parents know only too well.

Eliza Warren, *How I Managed My Children
from Infancy to Marriage*, 1865

As I was making my rounds at a local hospital, I saw Carol trying to calm a crying newborn in the nursery. Carol, a wonderful and experienced nurse, had wrapped the baby snugly, placed her on her side, and was softly whispering in her ear, "It's okay. It's okay." She even offered her a pacifier, but nothing helped.

I asked Carol if I could try soothing the baby. She describes what happened next:

"Sophia had been inconsolable for her first two days of life. After Dr. Karp offered to help he bent over Sophia's bassinet, with his face near her ear, and emitted a harsh, continuous 'shooshing' sound for about ten seconds. That was it! Sophia stopped crying within the first few seconds of this magical sound and remained silent for the next two hours."

Of course, one loud shhhh won't keep an infant calm forever, but it was exactly what Sophia needed to get her attention long enough for Carol's other calming methods to work.

Why Does Shhhhing Make Your Baby So Happy?

Did you ever notice how the sound of the wind or the rumble of the ocean makes you feel relaxed and at peace? Shhhhing is so deeply a part of who we are that it's even profoundly calming for adults.

For new babies, loud shhhhing is the "sound of silence," the anti-cry. Shushing may seem a strange way to help a crying baby; however, so is turning on a vacuum cleaner. Yet that's what many baby books suggest! What's so special about that sound?

The answer is, this loud white noise imitates your baby's experience inside the womb and switches on her calming reflex.

When I asked Nancy and Gary to guess what their baby, Natalie, heard inside the womb, Nancy said it was probably something like, "Hey, Gary, get over here!" Nancy was partly right. Fetuses do hear the muttering of voices and other "outside" noise. However, most of their daily entertainment is a continuous, rhythmic symphony of shhhh. Wave upon wave of blood surging through the arteries of your womb makes this harsh, whooshing sound, which is as loud and rough as a gale wind blowing through the trees.

How do we know this is what they hear? In the early 1970s, doctors placed tiny microphones into the wombs of women in labor and found the power of the sound was an incredible eighty to ninety decibels (even louder than a vacuum cleaner)! (You may have heard this womb noise

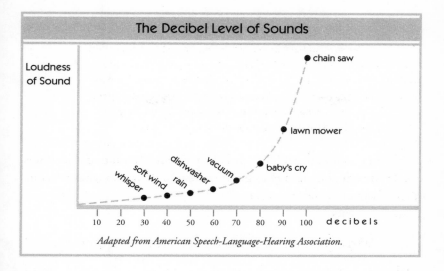

The Decibel Level of Sounds

Loudness of Sound

chain saw

lawn mower

vacuum

dishwasher

baby's cry

soft wind

rain

whisper

10 20 30 40 50 60 70 80 90 100   d e c i b e l s

Adapted from American Speech-Language-Hearing Association.

when your doctor or midwife checked your fetus with an abdominal microphone.) To get a good idea of what this sounds like to your baby, try dunking your head under the bathwater while the faucet is turned on—full blast.

Don't worry that your newborn baby might get overwhelmed by such a forceful noise. Although the sound inside the uterus is louder than a vacuum cleaner, *your baby doesn't hear it that loud.* That's because her middle ears are waterlogged with fluid, her ear canals absorb sound and are plugged with waxy vernix, and she has thick, inefficient eardrums.

These sound-damping factors last until a few months after birth. Gradually your baby's hearing will improve as her eardrum changes from being like a piece of thick paper to a tightly stretched piece of cellophane that vibrates with any distant noise. However, for a while, her reduced hearing reduces the intensity of your shhhhing, or vacuum cleaner, to a comforting din.

Imagine your baby's shock at birth when she emerges from that rich uterine world of loud quadraphonic whooshing into the quiet world of whispering and tiptoeing that parents create for their newborns. Sure, *we* may enjoy resting in a still room, but for your baby the silence can be deafening. And her muffled hearing will make your house seem even more stark and empty. New babies experience a type of sensory deprivation, and so it shouldn't surprise us that they cry from excessive quiet. It's as if they're saying, "Please, someone make a little noise!"

Once Upon a Time: How Parents Have Used Shhhhing in Other Times and Cultures

Do you remember when your grade-school librarian shushed you? All humans go "shhhh" (or "ssss") to say "Be quiet" to each other. This sound is one of the very few vocalizations understood by *all* humans, in every corner of the globe. And in many unrelated languages it's the root of the word asking for silence:

"chut" *(Urdu)*	"shuu" *(Vietnamese)*
"chutee" *(Serbian)*	"soos" *(Armenian)*
"chuu-chuu" *(Kahnada of So. India)*	"teeshina *(Slovenian)*
"hush," "silence" *(English)*	"toosst" *(Swedish)*
"hushket" *(Arabic)*	"chupraho" *(Hindi)*
"sheket" *(Hebrew)*	"shuh-shuh" *(Chinese)*
"stille" *(German)*	

Even the Japanese use shhhh as the root of their request for quiet: "shizukani" (although as a lover of Japanese food I might have guessed it would be "shu-shi").

As strange as it may seem, I believe that the calming effect of shhhh is something that babies taught *us*. If it were not for the immediate reaction cave babies had to shushing, parents would never have noticed its tremendous value. I'm sure that once a Stone Age mom learned this great trick, she couldn't wait to share it with her friends. And through the centuries, the discovery and teaching of this technique was probably repeated in every village and tribe around the world.

Unfortunately, most of us today haven't had much experience watching women with their babies. That's one of the reasons why so many parents and grandparents have forgotten this age-old, effective technique.

The Story of Shhhh: The Calming Sound That Babies Taught . . . Us

How did mothers from the Alaskan tundra to the swamps of Albania discover that this strange sound soothes screaming babies? No one is absolutely sure, but my guess is that it happened something like this:

About fifty thousand years ago, two Stone Age mothers were eating lunch together when one woman's baby started to shriek. Her mom immediately leaned over her "cave" baby's cradle and tried to calm her by squawking in her ear—the way she had seen a mother pterodactyl sucessfully calm her young. But the baby continued to cry.

When the poor child had just about wailed to the point of "Neanderthalmania," her mom's friend asked if she could try something she had once seen another mom do to soothe her frantic baby. The "cave" mother handed her wild little "infantasaurus rex" over and watched in amazement as her friend held her tightly and made a harsh, shhhhing sound right in her infant's ear. Like magic, the baby suddenly became calm!

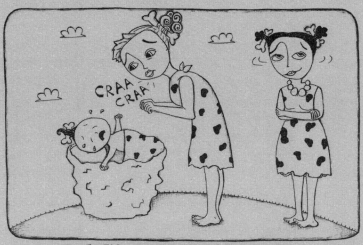

THERE'S GOTTA BE A BETTER WAY...

As a nurse walked by the room of a first-time mother, the door popped open and the father emerged, pushing a bassinet that was practically vibrating from the cries of his red-faced, screaming baby. In an attempt to help the poor little girl, the nurse lovingly leaned her face over the baby and let out a "Shhhh" as loud and harsh as a burst steam pipe!

I'm confident that had she continued her shushing for a few moments longer, the infant would have calmed. But she was stopped in her tracks when the baby's father yanked the bassinet away. Glowering at her, he said, "How dare you tell my daughter to shut up!"

Of course, this caring nurse was not telling the baby to shut up. But this father reacted as he did because he didn't understand that the nurse was speaking in a different "language."

In "adult-ese," shhhh is a rude way of telling someone to be quiet or to shut up. However, in this case the nurse was speaking "baby-ese," in which shhhh is a very polite infant greeting. All babies recognize the "word" *shhhh,* and they love it!

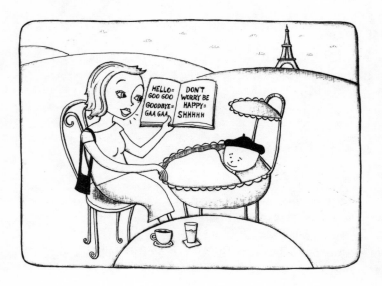

Mothers all around the world shush their babies in exactly the same way. Here's how to do it:

1. Place your mouth two to four inches away from your baby's ear.

2. With your lips pursed, start releasing a shhhh sound.

3. Quickly raise the volume of your shhhh until it *matches* the noise level of your baby's crying. Try to sound like the world's most irritated librarian! This is not a gentle or polite shush but a rough, harsh, insistent shhhh. But remember, your shushing will sound much louder to you than it will to your baby because her hearing is quite muffled. And besides, her own screaming gets broadcast at a jolting seventy to eighty decibels (louder than a vacuum cleaner)—and that's blasting right next to her ears!

Some parents feel it's callous and vulgar to shhhh their colicky baby or that it has an angry sound to their ears. However, to a baby's ears, shhhh is a sound of love and welcome.

4. As mentioned earlier, calming your baby is like a dance—but she is leading. You aren't guiding her into quiet, you're following her there. So, don't soften your shhhh until her decreasing cries show you she's ready for it.

When you first try shhhhing, your baby should quiet within a minute or two. And, after you get really good at it, you may find she calms in seconds. However, once your fussy baby settles, she will probably need continuing, moderate white noise to keep her from returning to crying. This shouldn't be a surprise to you. After all, she used to be serenaded by this loud sound 24/7, so needing it for a few hours, or even all night long, is a major compromise on her part.

(It's fun teaching your older children how to shhhh. It makes them more involved in baby care, and they feel so proud when *they* can calm the baby's cries just like daddy and mommy!)

Mary and Sigfried were delighted at how well shushing helped soothe their crying three-week-old baby, Eric:

"We never would have thought Eric could be quieted by such an annoying sound, but we've discovered the louder he cries, the louder our shushing needs to be. And, we can only lessen the intensity of our sound after he starts to quiet down.

"Shushing for two to three minutes can make us pretty dizzy. Yet Eric often seemed to need it for longer periods of time. Finally, after several days of taking turns shushing him, we realized that a sustained hiss from our music synthesizer was a perfect substitute for our flagging lung capacity. This sound works really well all by itself. And it's one hundred percent successful when combined with swaddling and motion."

Making a Shhhh-ound Investment for Your Baby

Continuous intense shhhhing can be hard to do, so parents have invented methods of making white noise to entrance their fussy babies. For example, some Amazonian Indians present new mothers with a baby sling decorated with monkey bones that make a rattling white noise with her every move.

However, if you and your family are out of monkey bones, I suggest you acquire a mechanical sound assistant. Some people feel strange using these, but if you can drive a machine to work every day, why not use one

Testing Out Your Baby's Shhhh Sensitivity

If your baby is fussy but not hungry, try this experiment to test her shhhh sensitivity:

Swaddle your baby and place her over your shoulder. Put your mouth right by her ear and shhhh softly for ten seconds. If she continues to cry, let your shhhh become louder and harsher.

When you have found the right sound she will quiet in seconds, as if suddenly entranced. Practice making the shhhh at different pitches and see what works best with your baby.

After your infant calms, gradually lower the volume of your sound. If she starts to wail again, just crank back up the intensity.

Weird Noises You Can Make at Home (But Don't Let Your Friends Hear You)

For soothing their newborn's cries, Alise says her husband swears by a deep, resonating hum that's a cross between shushing and the vibrations of a bouncy seat.

Tom and Karen discovered their son, Ben, quieted when they moaned. "He gets alert when I make a loud moan, like when I was in labor or like a bunch of Buddhist monks chanting together. Ben likes the sound to be deep and vibratory."

Several noises other than a simple shhhh can help your crying baby come down for a soft landing. Some parents I've worked with make a rhythmic chant like Native Americans doing a rain dance (*Hey . . . ho, ho, ho*); others sound more like foghorns or buzzing bees.

Pediatrician William Sears recommends what he calls the "neck nestle." You snuggle your baby's head into the groove between your chest and jaw, with your voice box pressed against her head, and make deep groaning sounds in the back of your throat.

to help make your baby happy? Here are ten useful shhhh substitutes that can help your baby in the throes of colic:

1. A noisy appliance, like a hair dryer or vacuum cleaner
2. A room fan or a microwave or bathroom exhaust fan
3. Running water
4. A white-noise machine
5. A CD with white-noise sounds
6. A toy bear with a recording of the sounds of the uterus
7. Static on the radio or baby monitor
8. The clothes dryer with sneakers or tennis balls inside (never leave the baby alone on a dryer . . . she can fall off)
9. A dishwasher
10. A car ride

The best way to know exactly the right level of sound your baby needs is to gradually increase the volume and see how she responds.

These final tips will help you use your shhhh-ound investment wisely:

- Harsh whooshing sounds work better than the patter of rain or the sound of a heartbeat.
- Tape-record the sound so you can start by playing it at the volume that works the best and then lower it after your baby is deeply asleep.
- Place the sound one to two feet away from your baby's ears to get the maximum effect with the lowest volume.
- Don't hesitate to use your white-noise sound machine all night if it helps your baby sleep longer and better. (See Chapter 15.)
- If the sound is driving you absolutely nuts, try some earplugs!

The Story of Tessa and the Vacuum Cleaner

Tessa, now five years old, is a "pistol"—smart, funny, and passionate. However, during her first weeks of life, she would get as frantic as a hurricane. Her parents, Eve and Todd, wrapped her, walked her, and even went for car rides, but nothing worked.

One afternoon, Tessa was really wailing but Eve couldn't hold her because she had to get the house ready for company. So she left her baby to cry and began to vacuum. The instant the vacuum was switched on, Tessa became stone silent!

Eve bolted over to check her. Tessa was sleeping sweetly, her body relaxed. She wasn't sleeping despite the ruckus but because of it! Amazingly, the womb experience that Tessa was missing most was "channeled" to her through the sound of Eve's seven-year-old upright vacuum.

From that moment on, whenever Tessa went ballistic, her parents used the vacuum cleaner to soothe her. Eve and Todd began to joke that Tessa was receiving secret messages from the planet Hoover. This calming trick was so predictable that they began inviting their friends over during Tessa's fussy time to watch the show.

Over the next six months, whenever Eve had to take Tessa to work with her, she always brought along a little portable vacuum to help Tessa settle in for a good long nap!

The Whys About the "S's":
Questions Parents Ask About Shhhhing

1. *Which sound will calm my cranky baby the best: a heartbeat, lullaby, or shhhh?*

   When your baby is resting peacefully, all of these can lull her into a deeper level of relaxation. However, if she's really upset, the most effective calming sound is a white noise that imitates the turbulent "shhhh" of your womb.

2. *How many hours a day can I use these sounds? Is all night too much?*

   Many babies sleep better, and longer, when their parents use calming white noise all night long. Even if you use it twelve hours a day, that's a fifty percent cutback from what you gave her in your womb.

   You don't have to worry about making your baby dependent on the sound, because—if you want to know the truth—she already is! She's dependent on it because, for her nine months inside you, she was surrounded by loud shushing every minute of the day.

   > *Jane's six-week-old son, Josh, woke up fussing every two to three hours during the night until she began using white noise. "The first night I used a white-noise machine, Josh calmed down quickly and slept five hours. Then he fed and slept for another three hours!"*

3. *When should I wean my baby off white noise?*

   Most parents who use these soothing sounds to help their babies sleep begin to gradually lower the volume after their babies turn three months old. Some parents, however, find that white noise continues to be a great sleeping aid for many more months. (See the discussion on weaning off the 5 "S's" in Chapter 15.)

4. *Does shushing lose its effectiveness if you do it too much?*

   You would think babies would eventually get bored with this

sound, but they don't. Just like milk, it continues to be comforting for infants for months and months.

5. I worry that white noise is too strong for my baby. Is it possible that, rather than calming her, it overwhelms her?

Please remember three things:

1. Your baby is accustomed to the loud noise of your womb, not the silence of your home.

2. You will always be right if you follow your baby's lead. Only use loud sounds when she is screaming, and gradually lower the intensity once she calms.

3. All new babies have muffled hearing. So the noise that sounds loud to us sounds much quieter to them.

A Parent's Perspective: Testimonials from the Trenches

The different types of shhhhing noises moms and dads come up with are inspired examples of parental ingenuity. Here's how some parents I know used sound to guide their babies to happiness:

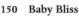
Patrick noticed that his son, Chance, was calmed by the sounds of aquarium pumps. So he mounted one on each side of his little boy's crib. The noise and vibration helped Chance settle himself and fall asleep.

When Talia began screaming in the supermarket, I put my face right next to her ear and uttered a rough "shhhh" until she calmed. While this seemed rude to the people watching me, it soothed her in seconds.

Once, when Talia had a mini-meltdown at the local Federal Express office, I quieted her with this same technique. The shushing worked so well that a clerk asked me for a repeat demonstration. She told me her daughter had twins and was searching for an effective tool to relieve their crying.

Sandra, Eric, Talia, and Daniel

We turned on the radio for our fussy daughter, Camille, but instead of putting on soft music we tuned it between stations to get loud hissing static. We discovered Camille didn't like the popping, crackly sound of static on the AM radio—she was an FM static aficionado only! Within a few minutes of tuning in to her favorite "non-station," her face would soften and then she would close her eyes and drift into a peaceful sleep.

Hylda, Hugo, and Camille

Steve and Nancy's six-week-old, Charlie, stayed calm in the car only if they played a tape of the hair dryer while they were driving. After he was four months old he no longer needed the tape to help him tolerate car rides.

Not only did two-month-old William have serious fussy periods, but he slept so lightly that he heard every squeak in the house. His parents, Fern and Robert, discovered that the white noise of their room fan muffled the outside sounds and helped him sleep longer.

Annette calmed her baby, Sean, by calling him "Shhhh-ean." It worked so well, the family joke became that when he was four years old, the little boy thought his name was pronounced "On"!

11

The 4th "S": Swinging—Moving in Rhythm with Your Baby's Needs

Main Points:

- Vigorous jiggly movement can switch on your baby's calming reflex
- The three key points to successful swinging
- Lullabies: What swinging sounds like when it's put to music
- The "Windshield Wiper": A great way to calm your fussy baby when you're tired
- Eight tricks for turning a swing into your baby's best friend

Life was so rich within the womb. Rich in noises and sounds. But mostly there was movement. Continuous movement. When the mother sits, stands, walks, turns—movement, movement, movement.

Frederick Leboyer, *Loving Hands*

Every night, Ellyn and Harold put their son Zachary in his stroller and rolled him repeatedly over an elevated threshold on the floor. Each time, Zack got jolted like a car racing over a *speed bump. Harold sometimes bounced Zach this way one hundred times in a row to get him to stop crying. And if his son was still fussing after that—he did it one hundred times more!*

Zachary's brother, Ezra, preferred another type of motion to snap him out of his yelping. Ellyn and Harold held him while "bopping" to the Rolling Stones. Ellyn said over four months they almost wore out their living-room carpeting from dancing Ezra around for hours each night!

Why Does Swinging Make a Baby So Happy?

When we think of the five senses—touch, hearing, vision, smell, taste—we often forget we have a powerful sixth sense. No, not ESP; I'm referring to our ancient and deeply satisfying sense of movement in space. This wonderful sense is exactly what gets stimulated when you sway side-to-side to settle your fussing infant (and it also explains why rocking chairs are such a favorite of grandparents).

Rhythmic movement, or what I call swinging, is a powerful tool for soothing our babies—and ourselves. Most of us can remember being lulled by the hypnotic motion of a porch swing, hammock, or train.

Why do these movements cause such profound relaxation? Swinging motions that mimic the jiggling your baby felt inside you turns on "motion sensors" in his ears, which then activate the calming reflex.

Once Upon a Time: How Parents Have Used Swinging in Other Times and Cultures

There was something so natural as well as pleasant in the wavy motion of the cradle . . . and so like what children had been used to before they were born.
Michael Underwood, *Treatise on the Diseases of Children*, 1789

Since the dawn of time, perceptive parents have recognized the wonderful effect movement has on babies. For our ancestors, soothing their infants with continuous motion was easy, because they spent all day long walking and working with their infants on their hips.

As every parent knows, it's impossible to keep still while you're holding a baby. You constantly shift your weight, pat your baby's bottom, touch her head, and kiss her ears. Imagine how foreign the stillness of a bassinet must feel to your baby compared to the gentle strokes and movements she's pampered with while she's in your arms.

Of course, all moms have to put their babies down every once in a while. But in many cultures it's dangerous to place a baby on the ground, so a mother will hand her infant to a relative or put her in a homemade moving device, like a cradle.

In *Gynecology,* one of the world's oldest medical books, a 200 A.D. physician named Soranus instructed women on how to keep their babies healthy. Some tips from this "Dr. Spock" of ancient Rome have not stood the test of time, such as warning parents that carrying their son on their shoulders could injure his testicles and turn him into a eunuch! However, some of his advice has proved priceless, like his recommendation to jiggle babies by "balancing the crib upon diagonally opposed rocks" and teetering it back and forth. This idea inspired the invention of the cradle (a crib placed upon rockers instead of rocks), which rewards babies with an equally hypnotic, albeit much less jolting, motion.

In many countries today, babies are still kept in constant motion. Their bodies are bounced and wiggled all day while strapped to the backs of their mothers or sisters or family yak. Thai parents rock their babies in baskets fastened to the ceiling. Eastern European women swing their infants in blankets that they hold like a hammock. Iranian women sit on the floor, with their babies placed in the grooves between their outstretched legs, and pivot their heels side-to-side, swishing their tiny children like metronomes.

In the United States, however, parents have long been warned not to handle their babies too much. In the early 1900s, Dr. Emmett Holt, America's leading pediatrician at that time, wrote in *Care and Feeding of Children:* "Babies less than six months old should never be played with at all. To avoid overstimulation, babies need peaceful and quiet surroundings." He worried parents would jar their babies' fragile nervous systems.

By the 1920s, the question "to rock or not to rock" a baby was no longer open to discussion. Quite frankly, no one dared admit doing it anymore.

Of course, it goes without saying that one has to be gentle with babies. You must always hold and support your baby's head when she's in your arms or when you're moving her from one place to another. But remember your baby was constantly bounced and jiggled inside your uterus as you walked, or hustled up and down stairs. Savvy mothers know that when their baby is fussy, vigorous rocking calms them much faster than slow, gentle movements.

Putting the Moves On:
Using Motion to Calm Your Fussy Baby

Jeannie drove Jordan around to quiet her fiery outbursts and was shocked to discover that her little red-haired "tornado" settled best when her mom hit every pothole she could find.

When Ruby was in the middle of a scream-fest, Jean Marie would pick her four-week-old up, sit on the bed with her feet on the ground, and bounce up and down in quick, jerky little motions like a child on a pogo stick.

Babies love to bounce. Why else do we call our infants bouncing baby girls and boys? Over the centuries, parents have perfected countless innovative ways to jiggle their unhappy tots into tranquillity. Here are the Top Ten:

1. Rocking in a rocking chair
2. Dancing (with quick little moves up and down)
3. Infant swings
4. Rhythmic pats on the back or bottom
5. Hammocks
6. Baby carriers
7. Car rides
8. Vibrating bouncy seats
9. Bouncing on an exercise ball
10. Brisk walks

A Bonus Eleventh Technique— The Milk Shake

This method may sound odd, but you'll be amazed how well it works:

1. Sit your baby on your lap (facing to your left) and place your left hand under his chin like a chin strap. Lean him forward a little so his chin rests solidly in your hand.

2. Slip your right hand directly underneath his buttocks.

3. Lift him straight up into the air with your right hand; he'll be leaning forward a tiny bit so his head will be cradled in your left hand a few inches in front of his body.

4. Now, with your right hand, bounce him with *fast* (two to three times a second) but *tiny* (one to two inches) up-and-down movements, like you're making a milk shake.

The Milk Shake is also a great way to burp your baby—and build your biceps.

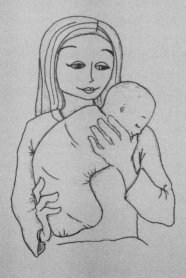

*Those who find that rhythmic rocking doesn't work are almost
certainly rocking too slowly.*

Penelope Leach, *Your Baby and Child*

For really fussy babies, the swaddle must be tight, the shhhh must be harsh, and the swinging must be fast and jiggly. Remember, swinging refers to all manner of rhythmic actions, from patting to car rides to bouncing.

The three rules of successful swinging are:

1. Start Out Fast and Jiggly

Calming most frantic infants requires small, trembly movements, like someone with the world's biggest case of shivers. This type of motion switches on the calming reflex and makes your baby think, *Wow . . . that feels really good!*

Some babies also like the free-fall feeling their parents give them when they suddenly dip or bend over. But be careful. If your baby is sensitive, that motion may startle him and set off his Moro reflex, upsetting him even more.

2. The Head Jiggles More Than the Body

Jiggling triggers your baby's calming reflex by switching on motion detectors in his head. So, it is the jiggling of the head (the site of these sensors), *not* the motion of the body, that really turns the reflex on.

As you jiggle your baby, don't cup your hands firmly around his head. It's critical that you allow your hands to be a little open and relaxed so his head makes tiny wiggles, *like Jell-O quivering on a plate.* If you hold his head too snugly, it won't wiggle and you probably won't activate the reflex.

3. Follow Your Baby's Lead

How forceful should your jiggling be? The vigor of your motion should reflect the level of your baby's crying. Gentle movements are fine for relaxed, sleepy infants, but the more agitated your baby is, the faster and more jiggly you need to be. Wait for his cries to lessen before you reduce your pace. Then, the calmer he gets, the slower your swinging can become.

Tamar and Dan realized they had to play "follow the leader" with their baby:

> *The most effective technique we've found to quiet Damian is putting him up on our shoulders and thumping his back quickly and firmly. As he calms, we downshift the intensity of the patting, bit by bit.*
>
> *Vigorous movement also works, either in a rocking chair or dancing from side to side. And, combining rocking and patting is a winning combination for us that never fails to settle him as long as he's not hungry or wet.*

Although thumping your baby's back may sound harsh, he'll probably love it, and it will also help him burp! As a rule, thumping should sound like a drum, loud enough to hear across the room—but not in the *next* room.

Is Jiggling Ever Bad for Babies?

> *Ken and Lisa were hesitant to jiggle baby Emily. Like many other parents, they feared it would make her spit up, get overstimulated, or even harm her. But when they tried it, they were amazed: "We worried it would be too strong for her, but it worked like a charm!"*

Almost any mother with more than three kids has learned that fussy babies settle fastest when they're energetically bounced. And jiggling is certainly much safer for infants than driving them around town with a weary parent behind the wheel. However, for many first-time moms and dads, jiggling may seem counterintuitive and wrong. When I teach new parents my technique, they often ask in a concerned voice, "I know it's been done for millions of years, but are you sure jiggling can't accidentally cause Shaken Baby Syndrome?"

Fortunately, the answer is . . . No! No! No!

Shaken Baby Syndrome: The Big Difference Between a Jiggle and a Shake

The act of shaking leading to Shaken Baby Syndrome is so violent that individuals observing it would recognize it as dangerous and likely to kill the child.

American Academy of Pediatrics, Report on
Shaken Baby Syndrome, July 2001

Shaken Baby Syndrome is a horrific type of child abuse that requires a force even greater than falling off a bed or out of your arms. It occurs when a baby's head is whipped back and forth, an extreme movement that has also been referred to as Baby Whiplash Syndrome. Why whiplash? Because it involves the forceful snapping of his head, side to side, like cracking a whip. That aggressive shaking can tear open tiny veins under the skull, causing bleeding and brain damage.

Jiggling, on the other hand, differs from the violent whipping motion that causes Shaken Baby Syndrome in two important and fundamental ways:

1. With jiggling, your motions are fast but *tiny*. Your baby's head does not dramatically flail about. Instead, it moves—at most— one to two inches from side to side.
2. With jiggling, your baby's head always stays in line with his body. There is no whipping action with the body going in one direction and the head moving abruptly in the opposite one.

It is my firm belief that jiggling can actually help prevent Shaken Baby Syndrome. Because it calms babies so quickly and successfully, it can keep parents from reaching the point of desperation that might drive them to a violent response.

Nevertheless, even with all the very best tips and advice, parenting can sometimes make anyone feel frustrated, edgy, and inadequate. That's why it's crucial that you *never shake—or even jiggle—your baby when you're angry!*

Please—if you're at the end of your patience, put your baby down (even if he is crying) and give yourself a break. Don't hesitate to call for help from your spouse, your family, a friend, or a crisis hotline.

Kristi Discovers How to Calm Kyle's Colic with the "Jell-O Head" Jiggle

Kristi and John's son, Kyle, was a big, apple-cheeked baby with a wave of copper hair. He would be fine one night but scream for three hours the next! Kristi called for help after her five-week-old baby had been shrieking at the top of his lungs for hours. I made a house call.

Kristi describes what happened that Sunday night:

> "As luck would have it, Kyle finally fell asleep moments before Dr. Karp arrived. I didn't really want Dr. Karp to wake him up or even touch him. Sure enough, when he placed his stethoscope on Kyle's chest, he started shrieking.
>
> "Dr. Karp apologized for waking him, but reassured us that Kyle seemed healthy and his biggest problem was that he was having trouble calming. Then he deftly swaddled and jiggled our frantic baby, and we were stunned that within a minute Dr. Karp had Kyle resting angelically on his lap as if his last explosion had never happened.
>
> "John and I practiced the technique and did okay, but we wimped out and asked Dr. Karp to put Kyle back to sleep before he left. Our boy did great that night, but the next day he was unbelievably fussy. And we just didn't feel comfortable trying the tricks we had learned the night before.
>
> "Finally, my mom came to the rescue. She wrapped Kyle tightly, placed him on her lap (laying him on his side with his head cradled in her hands), shhhhed loudly, and did what I like to call the 'Jell-O head.' She wiggled her knees back and forth, making his head quiver between her loosely cupped hands, like Jell-O on a plate. At first, Kyle resisted her efforts. He strained against the blanket and cried even harder. However, after three or four minutes he quieted, and after fifteen minutes he was fast asleep!
>
> "My mother repeated this miracle many times throughout her stay with us and I began to view <u>her</u> as the expert on Dr. Karp's method. I found that I had a hard time doing the Jell-O-head part, but I kept working at it and eventually began to feel more confident.
>
> "At first it took almost twenty minutes for this trick to settle Kyle into sleep. But soon I got it down to ten minutes, and by the

time he was seven weeks old I could take him from shriek to smile in two minutes flat.

"The more I practiced, the more I learned that the crucial steps for Kyle were tight swaddling and the Jell-O head. Gentle rhythms helped him when he was already quiet, but to calm screaming he needed almost an earthquake. Then, after a short time, he would heave a huge sigh and tension seemed to leave his body. I felt like a great mom! By four months of age, Kyle was adorable, happy, and doing fine without swaddling, the swing— or the Jell-O-head jiggle."

Kristi, John, Kyle, and Cassandra

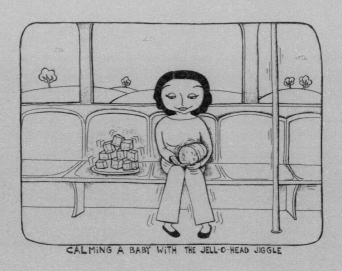

CALMING A BABY WITH THE JELL-O-HEAD JIGGLE

Lullabies: What Swinging Sounds Like When Put to Music

The word *lullaby* means *to sing to sleep,* and the tempo of these tunes is usually one beat per second—approximately the same as a heartbeat. The slow, rhythmic pace of lullabies is perfect for your baby after he has been fed and is drifting into the land of Winken, Blinken, and Nod.

However, these tranquil songs are usually powerless to stop babies in the midst of a crying frenzy. By that point, they're so lost in screams they can't hear you, even though you may be singing their favorite song. Just as adults can be "blind with rage," babies can become "deaf with distress."

Fortunately, you can rescue your baby from crying by switching to a tune with a zippy rhythm of two to three beats per second. These fast songs work especially well after your baby is swaddled. They're the original "Wrap" music! If you're a Beatles fan, try calming your baby with a fast jiggle like "It's Been a Hard Day's Night." As he begins to settle, slow down to "We Can Work It Out" or "All You Need Is Love." And when he's putty in your hands, shift to a slow song like "Golden Slumbers" or the number-one favorite of all new parents, "I'm So Tired."

Lullabies work better and better with repetition, as your baby gradually learns to associate the music with the sweet cuddling you give him every time you sing.

Lullabies Help Parents Too!

Lullabies calm babies—and parents. These songs gently soothe *our* jangled nerves and lull us into a more peaceful state of mind. Lullabies also often contain a dash of black humor to help sleep-deprived parents vent their feelings and laugh a little. Consider, for example, the lyrics of the classic lullaby, "Rock-a-Bye Baby":

> Rock-a-bye baby on the treetop,
> when the wind blows the cradle will rock,
> when the bough breaks the cradle will fall,
> *and down will come baby, cradle and all.*

The rhythms may be for sleepy babies, but the words are definitely for frazzled grown-ups!

The Windshield Wiper and Infant Swings: Two Great Ways to Move Your Baby in the Right Direction

Deborah's two-month-old son, Max, loved being lifted up and down, over and over again, using his mother like a carnival ride.

Genevieve's mom found she had to walk her baby, lap after lap, around the block to keep her happy.

Dancing, bouncing, and carrying your baby all day is hard work, especially when you're exhausted. Is there a way to jiggle your baby that doesn't wear out your back, your carpet, your tires, or your sense of humor?

I suggest these two user-friendly and highly successful calming motions: the Windshield Wiper, which is great for calming frantic babies, and the infant swing, which keeps babies quiet after they've been calmed.

The Windshield Wiper: How to Use Your Lap to Quiet Your Colicky Baby

The Windshield Wiper perfectly combines the 5 "S's" for a very powerful soothing experience. It's my favorite method for switching on a baby's calming reflex.

Don't get discouraged if the movement seems a little complicated the first time you try it. After five to ten practices, you'll see it's one of the easiest ways for pooped parents to soothe upset infants. (It's best to practice the Windshield Wiper with a doll or when your baby is quiet and alert.)

Here's what to do:

1. Swaddle your baby tightly (the 1st "S").
2. Find a comfortable chair to sit in with your feet resting flat on the floor. (Most parents find that sitting forward in the chair works best.)
3. Sit with your knees together and your feet a few inches apart (approximately the same distance as your shoulders).
4. Nestle your baby on his right side in the groove between your legs (the 2nd "S"), allowing his cheek and head to rest in your left hand (on top of your knees). If your baby is long, or your arms are short, pull him closer to you and let his ankles rest on your left hip.
5. Slide your *right* hand under his head so your two hands overlap a bit and his head is cradled in an open, *loose* grasp.
6. Soften your shoulders, take a deep breath, and let your body relax.
7. Roll your baby partly, or totally, onto his stomach. His tummy

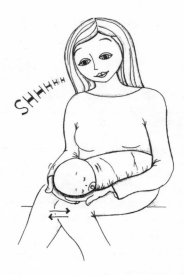

should press against your left arm or legs. *Make sure he's not at all rolled toward his back.*

8. Lean forward over his body, and make a rough shhhh right next to his ear (the 3rd "S"). Your shhhh should be as loud as his crying.

9. Now swing (the 4th "S") your knees side-to-side—like a windshield wiper. If he's crying hard, move faster *but* make your moves smaller and smaller. In seconds you'll be making quick, tiny movements—two to three beats per second and one inch from side to side. The louder your little one cries, the faster and smaller your swinging should be. Then, as he calms, gradually slow your motion down. (Remember, his head must jiggle like Jell-O back and forth between your hands to turn on the calming reflex.) Some parents prefer bouncing their baby up and down on their knees, but this often doesn't work as well as swinging.

10. Finally, if your hands are well positioned, your left thumb should be in front of his mouth. Offer him your clean thumb to suck on (the 5th "S"). Don't worry about your thumb being too big to fit; remember how big he can open his mouth when he cries! Or, if

you prefer, your hand is also in position to hold a pacifier for him to suck on.

A Beginner's Version of the Windshield Wiper

Until you master the Windshield Wiper, try this easier version:

1. Swaddle your baby and securely wedge him on his side (as described in Chapter 9) in the bassinet or crib.
2. Grab the bassinet on the side, near his head.
3. Jiggle it quickly, like you're shivering, making his head wiggle like Jell-O.
4. Shhhh loudly or turn on some harsh white noise.

Your baby should calm after twenty to thirty seconds of this method. Then roll him on his back and let him sleep.

Infant Swings: Get Your Fussy Baby into the Swing of Things

Many of you probably live far from your families, and the burden of baby care falls on your shoulders twenty-four hours a day. No wonder you need some help! That's why it was inevitable that the inventors of labor-saving devices like washing machines and garbage disposals would create some baby-calming devices like swings, bouncy seats, and . . . cars. (Of course, cars weren't invented for this reason, but that's how many parents use them.)

Many weary parents find products that vibrate or swing are even better than car rides. When used properly, these devices are more effective, don't cause accidents or pollution, and they let you stay in your PJ's!

Unfortunately, some parents hesitate to use swings because they believe myths like: "It moves too fast." "It can hurt a baby's back." "It makes them vomit." "Babies get dependent on them." "It's meant for older infants."

Betsy found the swing helpful, but she was so afraid it would hurt Hannah that she put two pounds of bananas in it with her just to slow the thing down!

Lisanne felt torn. The swing helped Sasha, but she worried, "I don't want him to become hooked on it."

Of course, the last thing any parent would ever want to do is hurt her child or impair his development. But, don't forget, babies are jiggled and rocked for months in the womb. That's why, far from spoiling Sasha, his eight hours in the swing were a small compensation for his having been evicted from the uterus. Once Sasha reached three months, he was old enough to soothe himself without any help from a swing. Like Sasha, most babies by three to four months of life find the swing isolating and boring. I've never seen a baby who couldn't be easily weaned from the swing by five months of age. (See Chapter 15 on weaning babies from the swing.)

Occasionally, your friends and families may also have worries about infant swings. Some comment disapprovingly: "Babies should be in their mother's arms, not in a machine." Or, "It shouldn't be called a swing, it's really a 'neglectomatic'!"

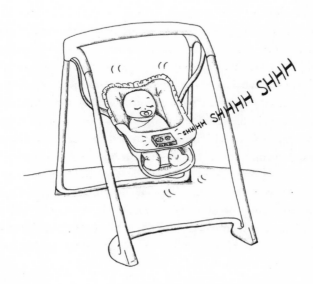

All this is silly. Thinking you're a better parent because you never use a swing is like thinking you're a better cook because you never use an electric can opener. Remember, throughout time, parents have had kith and kin to lend hands of support. In today's mini-families, a swing can help replace that missing extra pair of hands you need to comfort your baby while you shower, go to the bathroom, or just sit and rest for a moment. Your swing is like the substitute of a helpful next-door neighbor—only it's battery-operated and there are no loud parties.

Eight Tricks for Getting the Most Out of Your Swing

> Fern boasted, "The swing was magic for our son William. The motion and the noise worked great to get him into a peaceful sleep. It became my third hand."

Like all baby-calming techniques, there are tricks to using swings that can improve your success with them.

1. Start swinging early. Three weeks of age is not too young for a baby to be in the swing; they've been rocking and rolling in your belly for months. (Always consult your doctor before using a swing if you have a sick or premature baby.)

2. Never put your baby into the swing when he's screaming. Karp's Law of Swings states: If you put a screaming baby in a swing, what you'll get is a swinging screaming baby!

A little-known fact about swings (and bouncy seats too) is that they're not very good for *making* frantic babies calm. However, once your baby's crying has been temporarily quieted, they're great for *keeping* him calm and lulling him into sleep. So, always settle your baby for several minutes before you put him in the swing.

3. Keep your baby's arms wrapped. Swaddling helps swinging babies quiet faster and stay quiet longer. However, you still need to strap him securely into the swing's seat by putting the bar or belt between his wrapped legs.

4. Recline the seat back as much as possible. If the seat is too upright, it can be hard for your baby to support his head. Recline it back as far as it can go or use a swing with a cradle attachment.

5. Do a twenty-second jiggle whenever crying starts up again. After your baby is in the swing, he may start to fuss again. Remember, only *vigorous* motion turns on the calming reflex. So if his crying flares up, grab the back of the swing seat and start jiggling it forward and back an inch, two to three moves a second. Within twenty seconds he should relax again.

6. Use the fastest speed. Unless your baby is soundly asleep, the slow speed will probably be too mild to keep him into a deep state of relaxation. Cranky kids settle best on the fast speed and many sleep best that way all night long. See what works best for your baby.

7. Use loud white noise at the same time. Play a loud white noise one to two feet from your baby's head until he is so deeply asleep you can lower it a bit (to a strong rumble) without waking him up.

8. Practice makes perfect. As with all of the 5 "S's," after a few pleasant experiences in the swing, your baby may start getting happy as soon as you put him in it.

> Sandy could calm Harriet in her lap, but when she moved the baby to the swing, little Harriet roared all over again. Sandy, warned not to overstimulate her already frantic child, would set the swing on the slowest speed. But this was too gentle to keep her little firecracker "zoned."
>
> Sandy changed her approach by wrapping Harriet's arms snugly and turning on the hair dryer to quiet her momentarily. Then she hustled her into the swing and jiggled it by hand for a few seconds. Once her baby looked peaceful, Sandy set the swing at the maximum speed. Immediately, everything came together. Soothing Harriet became a snap, and suddenly the swing worked every time.

The Whys About the "S's":
Questions Parents Ask About Swinging

1. *Are swings ever bad for a baby's legs, hips, or back?*

   No. Inside the womb, your baby was twisted like a pretzel. His supple body is incredibly flexible, which is why he can be placed in a swing without any concern for his legs, hips, or back.

2. *I sometimes worry my baby's neck is too doubled over in the swing. Is that possible?*

   In the swing, your baby should be reclined back as much as possible. His neck should not be doubled over. That could make it hard to breathe especially if he is premature or sick.

3. *Should I avoid rocking my baby vigorously right after he has eaten?*

   Believe it or not, jiggling doesn't make babies spit up more. In fact, keeping him from crying may even make your baby less likely to throw up. Bouncing can also loosen a gas bubble and help your baby burp.

4. *Can a baby get dizzy or nauseous from the swing or the Windshield Wiper?*

   No. Jiggling motion does not set off the nausea center of the brain. Dizziness and nausea are triggered by big *wide* movements like driving down a curvy mountain road. Swinging makes fussy babies feel more comfortable, not less.

5. *If I put my baby in the swing too much, will it lose its effectiveness?*

   Some babies love to suck, some need white noise to stay calm, and others are only happy when they're swinging all day. Luckily, what babies love, they love all the time! That's why they never tire of milk, cuddling, or swings.

6. *What should I do if my baby cries more when I rock him fast?*

Your infant may keep yelling for a few minutes after you begin jiggling him, since it can take a little time for him to realize you're doing something he likes. If, however, your baby continues crying despite vigorous jiggling, check your technique. Make sure your moves are fast and tiny, you're using loud white noise, he's tightly wrapped, and, when he's in your lap or arms, that he's on his side or stomach.

A Parent's Perspective: Odes to Swings and Other Things

Everyone knows that people can be moved to tears, but many parents are learning that their babies can also be moved to happiness. Here are a few babies who calmed once their parents got a little mojo happening:

When baby Noah began to cry, David tried burping him by hoisting Noah onto his shoulder and lightly patting his back. Despite David's loving attempts to get a burp out, Noah continued to wail.

Perhaps out of frustration or from some ancient instinct, David started patting Noah harder. He thumped him like a tom-tom drum, with a cupped hand, at about two pats per second.

Almost instantly, Noah quieted. His body melted into his dad's arms and a few minutes later he fell asleep. "I was surprised to see how firmly he liked to be patted. But he relaxed so fast and so deeply that I knew it was right."

When Margie and Barbara's son, Michael, was six weeks old, he screamed so loudly at night that their downstairs neighbor would often bang on the ceiling.

Margie tried to placate him with gentle rocking and soothing songs, but nothing worked until she discovered what she called the "Native war dance." She clutched Michael to her chest, his stomach pressed against her and her arms around him like a straitjacket, and shouted, "HA-ja ja ja, HA-ja ja ja." With each loud "HA" she doubled over and bent at the knees, making Michael feel as if he'd fallen through a trapdoor. With each "ja" she thumped him on the back and ratcheted her body partway back up. By the third "ja" she was standing straight again, ready for the next "HA."

Margie said that at three A.M., the vigor of the rhythm and the loudness of the chant were essential. Usually, within ten minutes or so Michael was snoozing again.

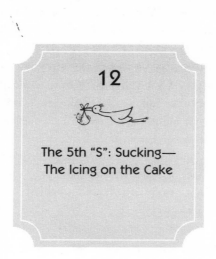

12

The 5th "S": Sucking—
The Icing on the Cake

Main Points:

- Sucking calms babies by satisfying their hunger and by turning on their calming reflex
- Three ways to help your baby succeed with pacifiers
- How to sidestep six common pacifier problems

Suck, and be satisfied.
Isaiah 66:11

If mixing all the "S's" together is like baking a cake, then sucking is the icing on the cake. This last sweet nudge allows babies to settle down, let go, and fall asleep.

A baby's survival outside the womb depends on her ability to suck. Like an actor rehearsing for a starring role, your baby began practicing sucking on her fingers long before birth. (Ultrasound photos of fetuses show them sucking on their hands as early as three months before their due date.) It was easy for your fetus to suck her fingers, because the soft walls of your womb kept her hands conveniently right in front of her mouth. Likewise, once she reaches four months of age and has enough muscle control to park her thumb in her mouth anytime she wants, it will again become a breeze for her to suck her fingers.

However, during your baby's fourth trimester she'll spend very little time sucking her fingers. It's not that she doesn't want to—she'd probably slurp on them twenty-four hours a day if she could. But for a newborn, getting a finger into the mouth and keeping it there is almost a Herculean feat. Even when your baby concentrates hard, drooling in anticipation of her success, her poor coordination usually causes her hands to fly right by their target, like cookies narrowly missing a hungry toddler's mouth!

Why is sucking such a sweet experience for babies? What does it do that gives them so much pleasure?

Why Does Sucking Make Babies So Happy?

Sucking makes babies feel extraordinarily good for two reasons:

1. It satisfies their hunger—of course. Who doesn't love to eat? Well, new babies love it so much that they pack away a milky meal eight to twelve times a day! For babies, all this eating means hours of pleasure from sucking, sucking, sucking.

Some people say that babies eat like "little pigs," but even piggies have a hard time holding a candle to a baby. Every day, young infants "snort down" about three ounces of milk for every pound of their body weight. That's equivalent to an adult drinking five gallons of whole milk a day, seven days a week. No wonder they need to eat so often.

2. It turns on their calming reflex. Babies suck to eat, but sucking is yet one more way prehistoric fetuses used to turn on their protective calming reflex and improve their chances of survival.

Sucking for food is called eating, and sucking for soothing is called non-nutritive sucking. If your baby is hungry she'll probably only suck a pacifier for a minute before crying, as if to complain, "Hey, I ordered milk—not rubber!" However, if she just wants some comfort, she'll happily suck on the pacifier for a good long while.

Can a Young Baby Suck Too Much?

Some authors warn parents not to let their babies suck "too much," cautioning that sucking is habit-forming. (I wonder if, given the option, these experts would reach into your womb and pull your baby's thumb right out of her mouth!) Fortunately, it's impossible for young babies to suck too much. Sucking isn't candy or an addiction; it's a highly sophisticated, self-calming tool. It's an integral part of the fourth trimester and one of your baby's first steps toward self-reliance.

The same deep calm that's activated in your baby's brain by sucking can also be switched on in the brains of older kids and adults by other "sucking" experiences, such as lollipop licking, cigarette smoking, and nail biting. (No wonder psychologists compare cigar smoking to thumb sucking!)

Many studies have shown that non-nutritive sucking is healthy for babies. It's like vitamin S! It lessens stress (blood pressure, heart rate, etc.) and can stimulate the release of natural pain-relieving chemicals in a baby's brain that decrease suffering from shots, blood tests, or circumcisions. Scientists have also found that premature babies who suck pacifiers grow faster, and full-term babies who are "paci" suckers have a lower risk of SIDS.

Once Upon a Time: How Parents Have Used Sucking in Other Times and Cultures

Have you ever noticed how nicely your baby falls asleep while sucking? Most babies just soften like melted butter. Of course, mothers throughout time have traditionally satisfied their infants' need to suck the old-fashioned way, with the breast. Mother's milk is the center of an infant's world—which is why some people even refer to breast-feeding moms as Earth Mothers.

But, rather than Earth Mother, I think a breast-feeding mom should be called Galactic Goddess! That's because the ancient Greeks invented the words *galaxy* and *galactic* out of their word *gala,* meaning *milk.* Legend said that the stars in the heavens came from milk spraying out of the breasts of the goddess Juno, which is also why we call our galaxy the Milky Way.

For mothers from tribes like the Efé of Zaire and the !Kung San of Botswana, sucking is usually the first solution they try to calm their babies. At the least little squawk, these moms plunk their babies onto the boob thirty, forty, one hundred times a day!

In past centuries, it was common in some cultures to put sugar inside a rag for babies to suck on. Sometimes this "sugar teat" was dunked in brandy if a baby was particularly fussy. My friend Celia, raised in Russia in the 1920s, remembers that her neighbors, unable to afford sugar, instead offered colicky babies a small piece of chewed-up bread wrapped in a thin cloth.

As rubber nipples for bottles became popular in the early 1900s, so did rubber pacifiers for sucking on. The English called these "dummies," choosing this name not because a baby looked dumb with a pacifier in the mouth, but because these little rubber teats silenced cries so well.

Helping Your Baby "Suck"ceed with Pacifiers

For most babies, sucking their thumb is like picking up ice with chopsticks—it slips away despite the best efforts. That's why they usually need a little sucking assistance.

You can satisfy your baby's sucking needs one of two ways:

1. *You* as a pacifier
2. *Use* a pacifier

For thousands of years, mothers have offered their breasts to their babies as pacifiers. That arrangement may be fine for some moms, but it's a burden for others. Luckily, parents today have a very effective alternative—pacifiers.

As with other aspects of baby calming, there are certain tricks to using pacifiers well. These tips increase your baby's chances for pacifier "suck"cess:

- *Try different nipples*—In my experience, no pacifier shape is superior to another. Some babies like orthodontic pacifiers, with their long stems and tips that are flattened on one side. Others prefer nubbier pacifiers with short stems. Ultimately, the perfect pacifier shape for your baby is the one she likes the best.

■ *Don't try the hard sell*—You can try putting the pacifier in your baby's mouth when she's crying, but don't force it if she refuses. You'll be most successful if you calm her first with the other "S's" and then offer the pacifier.

■ *Use reverse psychology to keep the pacifier from falling out*—This is the best trick I've ever seen for teaching a baby to keep the pacifier in her mouth. When your baby is calm, offer her the pacifier. The moment she starts to suck, tug it lightly as if you were starting to take it out of her mouth (but don't tug so hard that it actually comes out).

Your baby will respond by resisting your tug and automatically sucking on the pacifier a little harder. Wait a moment and then give a little pull again. Repeat this process ten to twenty times, whenever you give your newborn the pacifier. Her natural tendency to resist you will train her mouth to keep a firm grip on the pacifier. Many two- to three-month-old infants can be trained to keep the pacifier in their mouths even while smiling—and crying.

This reverse psychology technique is based on a simple principle of human nature: We all believe that what is in our mouth belongs to us! That's why trying to pull your nipple out of your baby's mouth is like prying a toy from the arms of a two-year-old; the harder you pull, the more she resists, and thus develops the coordination and strength to keep hold of it.

Pacifier Pitfalls

Some parents and grandparents worry that pacifier use may teach a baby bad habits. But truthfully, a pacifier is just a tool to help calm your baby until she can do it herself. There are, however, six potential pacifier problems you'll want to steer clear of:

1. Nipple confusion—Before nursing is well-established, some breast-feeding babies get confused when they're given rubber nipples to suck on. A baby sucking on a rubber nipple often uses a lazy, biting motion, which requires much less effort and coordination than sucking on the breast. Unfortunately, this also sometimes teaches a baby an improper way to use her mouth muscles.

You may offer your baby a pacifier on Day 1, but be prepared to stop using it for a while if your baby is having any trouble breastfeeding. I recommend you not offer your baby a bottle until she's two weeks old and the feeding is going really well. Then a bottle every day is fine. Most moms fill the bottle with breast milk, water, glucose water, or non-caffeinated peppermint or chamomile tea.

Don't wait one to two months before introducing the bottle. Parents who do this are often rudely surprised by their baby's emphatic rejection of the synthetic nipple.

2. Chemical contamination—Buy clear silicone pacifiers instead of yellow rubber ones. The yellow rubber gets sticky and deteriorates after a while and may release tiny amounts of unwanted chemical residue.

3. Keep sweets away—Don't dip a pacifier into syrup to make your baby suck on it more eagerly. Sweeteners like honey and maple or corn syrup run a risk of giving your baby botulism (a disease causing temporary paralysis, and even death).

4. Keep it clean—When you buy a pacifier, wash it well with soap and hot water. Rinse it when it falls on the floor—and several times a day even if it doesn't. Don't suck your baby's pacifier to clean it in your mouth, since your saliva may spread colds, herpes, or other illness.

5. No strings attached—Never hang a pacifier around your baby's neck. Strings or ribbons may get caught around her fingers, cutting off the circulation, or wrap around the throat and choke her.

6. Enough is enough—Once a baby reaches four to five months of age, I usually get rid of pacifiers. By that time, your infant can suck on her own fingers and do many other things to calm herself. Stopping the pacifier after six months is more difficult, because by then your baby has already started to develop a close emotional relationship with her "paci," much like a teddy bear or security blanket.

The Whys About the "S's":
Questions Parents Ask About Sucking

1. *How can I tell if my baby needs milk or just wants to suck?*
   These signs indicate your baby is crying for food:

   - When you touch her face, she turns her head and opens her mouth in search of the nipple.
   - A pacifier may initially calm her, but within minutes she'll start fussing again.
   - When you offer her milk she takes it eagerly and afterwards becomes sweet and calm.

2. *Does sucking on a pacifier shorten breast-feeding?*
   Since how a baby sucks on a pacifier differs from how she sucks on a breast, wait a week or two, until breast-feeding is going well, before introducing the pacifier. At that point, pacifiers can occasionally make breast-feeding *more* successful by lessening a baby's crying and helping her mom get a break from nonstop sucking.

3. *Can pacifiers cause ear infections?*
   A few studies have reported that babies using pacifiers get more ear infections. This probably happens because sucking hard on a pacifier disturbs the pressure in the ears (the same way pressure changes on airplane flights can give kids ear infections). Fortunately, young infants can't suck a pacifier hard enough to cause much pressure to build up. So you don't have to worry about this for the first four months.

4. *Can pacifiers protect babies from SIDS?*
   Scientific studies consistently report a lower incidence of SIDS among infants who use pacifiers. However, since it's not clear how they might protect babies, the American Academy of Pediatrics

cautions parents not to conclude from these studies that pacifiers actually prevent SIDS.

5. *Can my baby become addicted to the pacifier if she always sleeps with one?*

No! This is one old wives' tale you can put to bed. When Hannah was five months old, it took her mother a mere three days to wean her pacifier use down from all night and several hours a day to just two minutes a day.

However, as mentioned, a baby over five to six months may begin to develop an emotional attachment to her binkie. Although you can still wean her from the pacifier after that age, it's often more traumatic.

6. *If sucking is so important, should I wrap my baby with her hands out so she can get to them?*

Calm babies may do fine with their hands unwrapped, but fussy babies have a hard time sucking their fingers without accidentally whacking themselves in the face. For these kids, having their hands free is a frustrating tease. It's much easier on agitated babies to swaddle them and give them pacifiers, because they can control their bodies and suck better when their arms are not flailing and disturbing them.

7. *Will frequent feeding spoil my baby or make her tummy more colicky?*

Many parents, like Valerie and David, are warned that "overfeeding" can give their baby tummy pain:

> *"Our baby, Christina, was screaming and would calm only on my breast. My husband said I was making her colicky by feeding her every time she cried. My friends warned me I would spoil her by feeding her so often. What should I do?"*

When Valerie asked me this, I told her, first, thank goodness she had a method that worked to calm her baby. Second, it's impossible to spoil a fetus—and all babies are "fetuses" for the first three months. Third, she needed to call her doctor to make sure her baby was getting enough milk.

However, those three points notwithstanding, it sounded to me as if Valerie was making one important error. Do you know the saying, "When the only tool you have is a hammer . . . everything looks like a nail"? Well, it sounded like the only "tool" Valerie had for calming Christina was her breast.

I don't worry about young babies picking up bad habits or that too much milk will upset their tummies, but I did think Valerie was ignoring some other excellent calming tools. So I recommended she and David learn the other 4 "S's."

Dads are especially eager to master other calming tricks, because they often feel left out when the only method that calms their baby is a milky breast. Once fathers learn how to quickly soothe their babies, they feel much more confident caring for them.

8. *If I let my baby suckle on my breasts all night, I sleep well and it feels very cozy. Is there anything harmful in doing this?*

Spending the night with your baby at your side is how most people have slept throughout the ages. I think one of the most blessed feelings a woman can have is the sweet sleep that she shares with her nursing child. When you are together like that, it's natural that she may want to nibble a little on and off. However, it's your choice. You can go along with your baby's wishes or keep your shirt on and try to pacify her another way. There's no right or wrong about this—the decision is yours. (See Chapter 15 for a discussion of the pros and cons about co-sleeping.)

However, if you're sleeping with your baby, please be aware of the following:

- Keep pillows and blankets away, avoid waterbeds, and make sure she can't fall off or get stuck under the headboard or against the wall. (Swaddling will help keep her from scooting into dangerous places.)

- Make sure you're getting enough rest. You're no good to your baby if you get sick or become a menace when you are driving.
- Once your baby's teeth begin to come in, be aware that feedings lasting more than a half hour may cause tooth decay.

9. *There are a lot of thumb suckers in my family. Will giving my baby a pacifier prevent her from sucking her thumb later . . . or encourage it?*

Some babies are just incredibly driven to suck. Their strong desire is not a sign of being overly immature, dependent, or insecure (or of your being too lax as a parent). In my experience, the vast majority of cases of prolonged thumb and pacifier sucking is simply an inherited trait, no different from eye color or dimples. Or, to put it another way, it's one thing you really *can* blame on your parents!

There is little doubt that pacifiers prevent thumb sucking; it's just too hard to get both into the mouth at the same time. But in my experience it doesn't affect the length of time a baby demands to suck on something (finger or paci).

A Parent's Perspective: Testimonials from the Trenches

Some babies are interested in sucking only when they want to eat. For other babies sucking is like a massage, tranquilizer, and hot bath all rolled into one!

Here are stories of some babies who were "suckers for sucking":

> *Annie and Michael were especially worried when their little boy screamed; Rylan's heart problem made extreme exertion dangerous. So Ann carried him around the apartment for hours, until her back was in such pain that she couldn't stand it any longer.*
>
> *She resisted giving Rylan a pacifier because she "didn't want to start teaching him bad habits that he would have trouble stopping later on." Finally, however, driven to desperation, Ann reluctantly gave it a try and "Bingo! Giving Rylan the pacifier was a godsend! We still had to entertain him, but the binkie let me walk away and take a break, especially when he was in his vibrating seat."*

Stanley began to struggle with his feedings when he was seven weeks old. He had always begun his meals with gusto, but now after ten minutes he was pulling away and licking at the nipple as if he had forgotten how to eat. Seconds later he would arch back and wail as if he wanted to jump out of his mother's arms. But that wasn't what he wanted either, because as soon as Stanley was put down, he cried even harder.

Stanley's parents, Maria and Bill, tried rocking and wrapping him, but when he was really agitated he could free his hands in seconds. Maria, confused and frustrated, wondered if her milk had turned bad or dried up.

Fortunately, the problem was much less complicated than that. Maria had plenty of milk—in fact, too much. When Stanley tried extra suckling for fun at the end of his feeding, Maria's breasts continued releasing a stream of milk into his throat. Stanley had to pull away to avoid choking, but he was in a pickle because he still wanted to suck.

Once Maria and Bill began offering the pacifier at the end of his feedings, he became an angel again.

Steven and Kelly said their one-month-old bruiser, Ian, loved sucking on his paci. But if it fell out of his mouth he started to scream. Kelly lamented, "It works great, but we feel like we're becoming his pacifier slaves. My mom joked that we should just tape it in his mouth. I knew that even kidding about that was terrible, but we were going out of our minds."

When Steven and Kelly called, I taught them about "reverse psychology." One week later Kelly called back, amazed at how quickly the paci problem was solved. Within a week Ian's mouth muscles were so well trained he could hold the pacifier for one to two hours without dropping it.

Kelly said, "It's weird. I thought the best way to keep Ian's pacifier in his mouth was to keep pushing it back in. But what worked was to do exactly the opposite!"

Some babies will suck on anything you put in their mouths, but some are like miniature gourmets. Take Liam, who as a two-month-old refused to suck on anything—not pacifiers, not his fingers, not even a bottle, with <u>one</u> exception: He loved to suck on his mother's second finger!

13

The Cuddle Cure:
Combining the 5 "S's"
into a Perfect Recipe
for Your Baby's Bliss

Main Points:

- Some babies can be calmed with just one "S" but most need several "S's" to settle well
- The Cuddle Cure is the powerful combination of all 5 "S's" at the same time
- Two essential steps for perfecting the Cuddle Cure:
    Precision—A review of the most important points of each of the "S's"
    Practice—Why you must practice to excel at the Cuddle

As you know by now, the most successful baby-calming techniques handed down for centuries are based on the 5 "S's." However, if you haven't yet been successful at soothing your baby in minutes using the 5 "S's," don't lose heart. You can still learn how to guide your unhappy baby from tears to baby bliss using these methods.

What If the Crying Continues—
Even When You're Doing Everything Right?

To make no mistake is not in the power of man; but from their errors and mistakes the wise and good learn wisdom for the future.

Plutarch

Any one of the 5 "S's" can have a comforting effect on mildly fussy babies. However, for real explosive, colicky kids, a little swaddling or shushing may not make a dent. Here are reasons why your "S's" might not have succeeded in calming your crying baby:

1. She's having a little problem—Your baby may be hungry or struggling with a poop. Fortunately, these problems are usually obvious and easy to resolve without the "S's."

2. She's having a big problem—Approximately ten to fifteen percent of colicky babies have a medical explanation for their irritability, such as food intolerance or stomach acid reflux. (See Appendix A to review the medical causes of colic and Chapter 14 to review the treatment for many of those problems.)

3. The "S's" are being done one at a time—The more powerfully a baby is wailing the more she will need the help of several "S's" simultaneously.

4. The "S's" aren't being done correctly—As with any reflex, if it's not triggered in exactly the right way it just won't happen.

This chapter focuses on perfectly combining the 5 "S's" into the Cuddle Cure and reviews the common mistakes parents make as they begin to learn the "S's."

If One Is Good, Two Are Better:
Calming Babies with Multiple "S's"

Nina and Dimitri were dismayed that their champion cryer, Lexi, got more enraged when they tried to calm her with the sounds of

*the hair dryer or the infant swing. However, when they used the
hair dryer and swing <u>together,</u> they worked like a charm.*

Someone once said, "There's a sucker born every minute." Well, when it comes to babies that's especially true. In fact, thousands of suckers, swingers, and even shhhhers come into the world every day! Just as babies have different hair color and temperament, each infant differs slightly in the way he needs to be calmed. Some settle best with rocking, others quiet instantly with white noise, and some surrender as soon as they're put on their stomachs. These easy babies require the help of only one of the "S's" to make them feel calm and serene.

Cranky infants, however, need more help. They often require two, three, or four of the "S's" done together to cease their cycle of screaming. And the fussiest, most colicky babies demand all 5 "S's" simultaneously.

Getting Acquainted: An Experiment in Soothing Your Baby

To find your baby's favorite calming technique, place him on his back when he's a little bit fussy. One by one, add another "S" and see how many it takes to settle him down.

1. Shhhh him softly. If that doesn't work, do it louder, right in his ear.
2. Swaddle his arms to keep them from flailing. Do that while shhhhing.
3. Place your wrapped baby on his side or stomach and shush him again.
4. Now add a quick, jiggly motion.
5. Finally, on top of all of these, offer a pacifier or your finger to suck on.

By this time, most fussy babies will usually be calmed.

The Cuddle Cure: Combining All 5 "S's" into a Recipe for Baby Bliss

*On a plane from New York to Los Angeles, I watched an elderly
woman calm a baby with such precise, elegant moves that I
imagined I was witnessing an ancient ballet.
In mid-flight, this infant suddenly erupted into crying. After*

a few piercing wails, the frail grandmother picked up her frantic traveling companion and began a symphony of responses. She nestled the little girl's stomach against her shoulder, made a continuous shhhh sound in the baby's ear, rhythmically thumped her bottom, and swayed her torso side to side like a snake working its way uphill.

In less than a minute her tiny bundle was sound asleep.

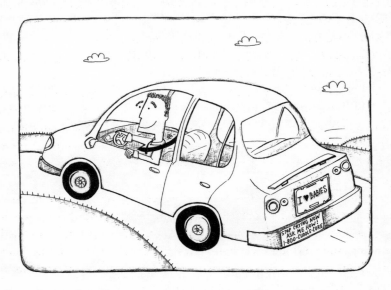

It's tempting to believe that someone who's good at calming babies has "the gift," but that's not the case. Soothing young infants has nothing to do with special talents. It has everything to do with understanding why babies cry and learning and practicing the skills to soothe them.

Most parents automatically rock and embrace their crying babies, but sometimes that's not enough. The Cuddle Cure combines all 5 "S's" into a technique so powerful it turns on the calming reflex in even the fussiest babies.

Mothers in many cultures around the world use variations of the Cuddle. In Tanzania, some women soothe crying babies by cuddling them while they pretend to grind corn! They vigorously bend and straighten and hum rough, grinding noises until the baby settles.

If the Cuddle is like an ancient cake recipe, with the ingredients being the 5 "S's," most baby books are unfortunately like incomplete cookbooks. They list the 5 "S's" but don't mention exactly how to do them or how to mix them together.

Without instructions on how to mix the ingredients for a cake, you're more likely to end up with warm goop than a wonderful dessert. And, without instructions detailing how to do each "S" and how to mix them together, it's easy for parents to end up with a *more* fussy baby rather than a perfectly calmed one!

And, once the Cuddle has helped you stop your baby's screams, that's not the end of it. The Cuddle is also a valuable tool for keeping your baby calm *after* you soothe his crying.

After your little one falls asleep in your arms, you may not be able to put him down and walk away. He may be very relaxed, but he's not in a coma. Deep within their brains, snoozing babies are still aware of the world around them. That's why abruptly stopping the hypnotic rhythms of the Cuddle may make a baby explode back into tears even from what appears to be a sound sleep.

Fortunately, the Cuddle is perfect for keeping your baby calm after you've quelled his cries. Your colicky baby may stay happy for hours as long as he feels like he's still safely packaged in the womb (swaddled, swinging, and with loud white noise playing close by). If your baby suddenly starts thrashing again, simply picking up the tempo should help regain his attention so you can lead him back to serenity.

How to Be the Best Cuddler on the Block

Although the Cuddle works better than anything else for calming colic, it may not feel natural at first. Many new parents find it's like riding a bicycle; it initially seems complicated and intimidating. Some parents give up after a few tries, thinking, *This may work for some kids but our baby hates it.*

I certainly understand this frustration. It's excruciating to try to quiet your baby's shrieking when everything you do seems to make it worse. But, like riding a bicycle, once you get the hang of doing the Cuddle it's really a lot of fun. Soon you'll feel like you've been doing it your entire life.

And if the Cuddle isn't working perfectly, it's probably just because you need a little technique tuneup. The most common reason this ancient method fails is because it's not being done properly. In fact, incorrect swaddling, swinging, and shushing may even make your crying baby *more* upset! So, like the song says, "If you're gonna do it, do it right, right."

Let's recap the important pointers to get each of your "S's" in gear:

Swaddling

Parents often abandon swaddling because their babies strain against it. They misinterpret this struggling to mean, "Let me out. I hate this. It's unfair!" But please don't give up on this crucial first step. To be successful with wrapping, you must:

- Keep your baby's arms straight down at his sides.
- With each fold of the swaddle, tuck and snug the blanket as tightly as possible.
- After swaddling, don't allow the blanket to loosen and pop back open.

Remember, *swaddling is not meant to calm your baby!* Its purpose is to stop his flailing and to help him pay attention to the other "S's," which *will* soothe him.

Side/Stomach Position

Lying on the back is fine when your baby is calm. But if he's sensitive, being rolled toward the back may upset the position sensors in his head and trigger a "red alert," making his crying even worse.

- When your baby is on his side, keep him rolled at least a bit toward his stomach. Some babies are so sensitive they will have difficulty getting calm if they're rolled even slightly toward their backs.

- Make sure your baby is not hungry. If he's eager to eat, holding him in a way that touches his cheek may trigger his rooting reflex and make him think you're offering food. You can imagine how this could confuse and frustrate a famished baby.

Shhhhing

The shhhh sound is easy to make, and most parents find it natural to do—softly. Therein lies the problem: Most parents shhhh too quietly and too far from their baby's ear.

- Crank up the volume of your shhhh until it's a bit louder than your baby's screams. Remember, the sounds in the womb are louder than a vacuum cleaner and your infant's ears naturally muffle sound for the first few months.

- If you're using a machine to make white noise, place it one to two feet from your baby's head so it's loud enough to trigger the calming reflex.

Swinging

Gentle swinging may keep a quiet baby content, but it's much too mild for screaming babies. The most important tips for successful swinging are:

- Move your fussy baby in quick, teensy, shiverlike wiggles. Slow, wide moves may keep a baby asleep, but they're not vigorous enough to calm a crying infant.

- Support your baby's head and neck, but hold his head a little loosely so it can jiggle a little like Jell-O in your hands.

> *Jake's father, Jimmy, told me he tried the Cuddle, but it wouldn't work. I reviewed each step of his technique and discovered he was doing almost everything right, except his swinging was too wide. Rather than sliding his knees an inch from side to side, he was going twelve inches with each move. These wide swings didn't get Jake's head jiggling enough. Once he made the motion fast and short, the swinging calmed Jake almost every time.*

Sucking

Sucking is usually the easiest "S" to get right. But if your baby rejects the pacifier, here's how to change his mind:

- Calm him first. Most babies can't take a pacifier while they're screaming.

- Try different brands. Some babies prefer a particular pacifier shape.

- Use reverse psychology. Gently tug on the pacifier as soon as he begins to suck it. He'll resist you, and the more you play this game, the sooner you'll train his mouth to keep a good long grip on the binkie.

Becoming a Cuddle Expert: Practice Makes Perfect

If at first you don't succeed—you're running about average.
M. H. Alderson

Remember, this technique has worked for millions of years, so even if it doesn't work perfectly the first few times you try it, you'll definitely get the hang of it if you keep practicing. (In the beginning, it's best to practice this technique with a doll or when you and your baby are calm. It's harder to learn when you're exhausted and your little angel is making noises that could shatter glass.)

Parents aren't the only ones who improve with practice. As you get better, your baby is getting better too. Bit by bit, he'll learn to recognize what you're doing—and that he likes it.

Patience is especially important if you're starting these techniques when your baby is already six to eight weeks old. It may take several tries for you to learn them and then several more tries for your baby to unlearn his prior experiences and begin to get used to the 5 "S's." However, if you persevere you can still be one hundred percent successful!

14

Other Colic Remedies: From Massage and Feeding Problem Cures to Old Wives' Tales

Main Points:

- ◼ Three ancient colic cures proven to be true paths: massage, fresh air, and extra warmth
- ◼ Effective remedies for four medical causes of infant crying: allergies, constipation, feeding problems, reflux
- ◼ A look at four unproved colic treatments

Put cotton in your ears and gin in your stomach!

19th-century colic advice

Through the centuries, experts continually thought up colic treatments to fix whatever they believed to be causing their baby's unhappiness. These false assumptions led them to champion many different types of therapies that have proven to be total dead ends: alcohol, sugar water, sedation, anti-cramp medicine, and burp drops. There are, however, besides the 5 "S's" a few other ways of helping crying babies that are true paths.

Three True Path Colic Cures:
A Grandmother's Bag of Tricks

When you want a break from the 5 "S's," here are three time-honored tricks for colicky babies that work well: massage, walks outside, and a little extra warming.

Massage: The Miracle of Touch

Massage is love which is one unique breath, breathing in two.
Frederick Leboyer, *Loving Hands*

Massage is a very ancient treatment for colic. Its extraordinarily soothing effects are based upon our oldest and most profound sense—touch.

Touch and the Fourth Trimester

There's an old saying, "A *child* is fed with milk and praise," and I would say a *baby* is fed with milk and caresses. Your baby's loving caresses began inside your womb, where she enjoyed a feast of velvety cuddling twenty-four hours a day. Once born, your baby still loves to be touched and stroked. Your skin-to-skin embrace of her is the touch equivalent of calming, hypnotic movement or sound.

Cuddling Builds Brains

A recent study from McGill University asked, "Does extra cuddling make animals smarter?" The researchers looked at two groups of little rat pups. The first group had very "loving" mothers who licked and stroked their babies a lot. The second group received much less affection from their moms.

When the rats became old enough to be taught mazes and puzzles, scientists noticed that the cuddled animals were extrasmart. They had developed an abundance of connections in a part of the brain crucially important in rats (and people) for learning.

The moral of the story is clear: Cuddling your baby feels good, and it may even boost her IQ!

Touch is not only a wonderful reminder of a baby's time as a fetus; like milk, it's an essential "nutrient" for her growth. In fact, in some ways it's even more beneficial than milk. While stuffing your baby with extra milk won't make her any healthier, the more tickles and hugs she gets, the stronger and happier she'll become.

In 1986, a brilliant baby-watcher named Tiffany Field confirmed the benefits of touching in a study on the effects of massage on premature babies. She had nurses massage a group of preemies for fifteen minutes, three times a day, for ten days. The results were astounding. Massaged babies gained forty-seven percent more weight than expected and were able to go home almost a full week earlier than babies who didn't get massaged. In an equally stunning follow-up study, when the massaged babies were examined one year later, their IQ's were higher than the babies' who were handled routinely. Dr. Field also discovered that when healthy full-term babies were massaged for fifteen minutes a day, they cried less, were more alert and socially engaged, gained weight faster, and had lower levels of stress hormones.

Infant Massage: Rubbing Your Baby the Right Way

Beautiful, big-eyed Mica was so sensitive and vigilant that she often had difficulty shutting out the world, even when she was exhausted. When Mica was one month old, I recommended that her parents, Lori and Michael, try using massage to help their daughter wind down:

> *At first Mica seemed leery of this type of touching. She accepted some foot massage, but that was as far as I could get before she became unhappy. I stuck with it, though, and after a week, Mica began to enjoy the touching. She even became excited when she heard me rub massage oil into my hands. I was delighted! Massage time soon became our special bonding time. Mica would deeply relax and sometimes fall asleep. I loved doing this for our daughter. And best of all, it helped her become calmer in general and to get over her evening fussies.*

Lori, Michael, and Mica

Here are the five steps for giving your baby a perfect massage:

1. **Prepare for pleasure**—About an hour after your baby has eaten, remove your jewelry, warm the room, dim the lights, take the phone off the hook and, if you like, you may turn on some soft music. Have

some slightly heated vegetable oil (almond oil is great) within easy reach, and some wipes and diapers too, just in case.

2. Bring yourself to the moment—Sit comfortably with your naked baby right next to you or on your bare, outstretched legs. Place a towel around her body to keep her warm. Now take five slow, deep breaths to allow yourself to be fully present for this wonderful experience. Massage is not a mechanical routine, it's an exchange of love in one fleeting and tender moment of time.

The first few times you massage your baby, you may notice that you're "in your head," thinking about how to do the massage. Don't worry: Once you become more familiar with the routine, your attention will naturally begin to focus on your fingertips, your baby's soft skin, and your loving heart.

3. Speak to your baby with your hands—Rub some oil between your hands and start by touching your baby's feet. Always try to keep one hand in contact with her skin and softly talk to her about what you are doing and what your hopes are for her life to come or sing a lullaby. Uncover one limb at a time and massage it with a touch that is fluid but *firm.* Let your massage strokes move slowly along her body, in synchronicity with your calm breathing.

Use smooth, repetitious strokes over her feet, legs, stomach, chest, arms, hands, back, face, and ears, gently rotating, pulling, stretching, and squeezing. Twist her arms and legs as if you were lightly wringing a wet sponge. Feel free to experiment with using your fingers and different parts of your hands, wrists, and forearms.

4. Reward your baby's tummy—Thank your baby's tummy for doing such a good job. Bicycle her legs and then firmly push both knees to the belly and hold them there for ten to twenty seconds to give a nice, satisfying stretch. Then massage the tummy in firm, clockwise, circular strokes, starting at her right lower belly, up and across the top of her tummy, and ending at the lower left side. (This sometimes helps babies release gas or poop.)

5. Follow your baby's signals—If your baby begins to get restless, it's a sign to change your pace or end the massage. Wipe the excess oil from her body, letting a bit remain to nourish her skin. Bathe her with soap and warm water later that day or the next morning.

Giving your baby a massage is also wonderful for moms and dads because it can lower your stress and boost your self-esteem.

If you would like to learn more about the technique of baby massage, an excellent resource is Vimala McClure's *Infant Massage*.

Walks Outside:
Calming Some Babies Is Just a Stroll in the Park

If our babies could talk, they would probably bug us, "Why can't we live outside like all the other Stone Age families?" Our ancient relatives lived outside, and perhaps that's one reason why some of our little cave babies get deadly bored sitting at home. For them, nothing is more fun than hearing the wind in the trees, feeling the air on their faces, and watching the continually moving shadows.

Some parents ask me how calming by being outside fits with the idea of the fourth trimester. For babies, a walk outside is a parade of calming out-of-focus images and jiggly, soothing rhythms. I believe they are lulled by this hypnotic flow of gentle sensations, like a constant, multisensory white noise.

So, when your baby is crying, try giving her a breath of fresh air. Going for a walk will also help lift your spirits and fill you with a sense of peace.

Warming Your Baby Up to the Idea of Calming Down

In the uterus, infants are constantly in "hot water"! That may be why so many babies love warm things. To help you soothe your baby when she's fussing, try these "hot tips":

■ *A warm bath*

> Every time their six-week-old son, Jack, was fussy, Kim and John calmed him by submersing him in warm water. "Jack always gets super relaxed when he is put into a hot bath. He goes into a Zen-like state and is mellow and ready for bed afterward."

■ *A warm blanket*

> When her niece, Erica, was very fussy one day, Barbara heated the baby blanket in the clothes dryer for a few minutes, <u>thoroughly checked it for hot spots,</u> and then bundled Erica in it. Erica calmed so quickly that from then on, whenever she became fussy she got swaddled in warm wraps. (Barbara was always very careful to avoid overheating or burning her.)

■ *A warm hat*

Covering your baby's head makes her feel cozy and comfortable. Newborns lose twenty-five percent of their body heat through their heads, so a baby with an exposed head is like an adult walking around on a chilly night in underwear.

■ *A warm hot-water bottle*

Dr. Spock loved to tell parents to lay their colicky babies tummy-down on a warm hot-water bottle. He thought it helped relieve stomach pain, the way warmth can help menstrual cramps, but more likely it works by putting soothing

Warning: Keep Your Baby from Becoming a Red-Hot Pepper

Keeping your baby warm can be helpful, but overheating her is not good. It may make her restless, cause a heat rash, and there is a slight chance it can increase a baby's risk of SIDS.

Pay attention to the following to avoid the pitfalls of overheating:

■ If your baby's ears or toes are red and hot and her armpits are sweaty, she's probably too warm and needs to be dressed more lightly.

■ You can warm towels, blankets, socks, and hats in the clothes dryer, with a hair dryer, or in a microwave oven for thirty seconds. But before you put any heated item on your baby, always open it up and hold it against your forearm to make sure it isn't too hot.

■ Never microwave any clothing with metallic thread.

■ Never use an electric blanket or heating pad. These can overheat babies and expose them to unnecessary electromagnetic radiation.

■ In hot weather, swaddle your baby in light wraps.

pressure on your baby's stomach and turning on the calming reflex.

■ *Warm socks*

As with a blanket, you can warm up your baby's socks to make her feel extra toasty. Just check for hot spots before putting them on.

Four Modern True Path Colic Cures: A Doctor's Bag of Tricks

Although medical problems are not commonly the cause of colic, I estimate that ten to fifteen percent of extremely fussy babies cry because of one of four tummy troubles: food allergy, constipation, feeding problems, or stomach acid reflux.

Children who suffer from these treatable conditions may get some relief from the 5 "S's" and the grandmother's tips discussed earlier; however, what many of these infants truly need is a medical solution for their particular difficulty.

Here are a few hints on how to soothe these unhappy infants.

Preventing Food Allergies: Getting Tummies Back on Track

It's believed that approximately ten percent of colicky babies cry due to food sensitivities. Unfortunately, doctors have no accurate test to check babies for this problem. To discover if your child has a food allergy, you must play Sherlock Holmes and eliminate foods from your diet or switch your baby's formula to see what happens. (Always consult your doctor before doing so.) It usually only takes two to four days to see if the crying gets better.

If your baby improves when you eliminate foods from your diet, she may have a food allergy. However, sometimes this improvement is just a coincidence. To be sure your child truly has to avoid those foods, I advise you to wait for the fussiness to be gone for two weeks and then to eat a spoonful of the suspected food, or feed your baby a half ounce of the suspected formula. Try this over four to five days; if there's an allergy the crying will return.

Most babies with food allergies are allergic to only one or two foods, with the most common, by far, being cow's milk and dairy products.

Calcium Rules

If you're breast-feeding and you stop eating dairy products because your baby is sensitive to them, rest assured there are many other ways to get adequate calcium in your diet. Besides calcium supplements, you can also get calcium from green vegetables (broccoli, leafy vegetables), sesame-seed butter, dark molasses, fortified orange juice or soy milk, corn tortillas, etc.

Eliminating dairy foods from your diet is not a risk to your child. However, if you stop dairy products for more than a few weeks, speak to your doctor to make sure you're meeting *your* body's calcium needs.

That's why doctors often recommend bottle-fed babies switch from cow's milk formula to soy. Many babies improve by doing this, but as I noted earlier, at least ten percent of milk-allergic babies are soy-allergic too. These babies require a special, hypoallergenic formula; ask your doctor about these.

Constipation: Interesting Ideas on a Dry Subject

Like grandma always said, "It's important to stay regular," and that's especially true for babies! Fortunately, breast-fed babies are almost never constipated. They may skip a few days between poops, but even then the consistency is pasty to loose. Bottle-fed babies, on the other hand, do get constipated, but several commonsense approaches can usually help rectify the problem:

- *Change the formula*—Sometimes changing your baby's formula can help resolve her constipation. Some infants have softer stools when they drink concentrated formula versus powder (or vice versa); others do better with cow's milk formula versus soy; and, rarely, some may improve with a switch to a low-iron formula.
- *Dilute the mix*—Your baby's poops may improve when you add one ounce of water or half an ounce of adult prune juice (organic is best), once or twice a day, directly to the formula. (Never give babies under one year of age honey or corn syrup as a laxative.)
- *Open the door*—One last way to relieve constipation is to get your baby to relax her anus. Infants who strain to poop often accidentally tighten their anus. Like adults who can't pat their heads and rub their tummies at the same time, many babies have trouble tightening their stomach muscles and relaxing their rectums simultaneously.

  Try getting your baby's anus to "loosen up" by bicycling her legs and massaging her bottom. If this fails, insert a Vaseline-greased thermometer or Q-tip one inch into the anus. Babies usually respond by trying to push it out, and they often push the poop out at the same time.

A Poop Advisory: Sometimes Constipation Signals a More Serious Problem

Healthy babies may skip a day or two between poops. However, less frequent BM's may signal a more worrisome problem. If your baby goes more than two or three days without a stool, you should check in with your doctor. He may want to evaluate her for three rare, serious, but curable diseases that can masquerade as constipation:

1. *Hypothyroidism*—This easily treated condition is caused by an underactive thyroid gland and may slow mental development if allowed to continue untreated.

2. *Hirschsprung's disease*—This rare intestinal blockage happens when the rectal muscles can't relax to let the poop out. Surgery can correct it.

3. *Infantile botulism*—This very rare disease temporarily paralyzes babies. It's brought on by botulism spores that live in the ground and in liquidy sweets like honey or corn syrup (which should never be given to babies).

Feeding Problems—Babies Who Cry from Too Much (or Too Little) of a Good Thing

Fortunately, 99.9 percent of the time, your baby and your milk are perfect together. However, getting too little or too much milk may trigger severe crying.

"Got Milk?"—Babies Who Cry Because They Don't Get Enough Milk

It's usually easy to tell if a bottle-fed baby is getting her fair share of milk: Count the number of ounces she eats. With breast-feeders, however, it's trickier. If you are nursing, answer the following questions to figure out if your baby is crying because she's not getting enough milk:

Are your breasts making enough milk? If your breasts feel heavy when you wake up, if they occasionally leak, and if you can hear your baby gulping when she's feeding, it's likely that your breasts are making plenty of milk.

Is your baby happy to suck on your finger or pacifier? Just because your fussy baby wants to suck doesn't mean she's hungry. Offer her your finger to suck on. If she sucks happily for a few minutes, she probably wants recreation, not nutrition.

Does your baby become serene after a feeding? Well-fed babies are usually blissful, calm, and relaxed after a feeding.

Is your baby peeing enough? During the first few days of life, infants don't urinate very often, but once your milk comes in, your baby should pee five to eight times a day.

Is your baby gaining weight normally? Many moms and grandmoms are always worried that theirs is the only skinny baby in town while all the other infants are little sumo wrestlers! To know if your baby is gaining enough weight, you need to put her on a scale. For the most accurate weighing, check her on the scale at your doctor's office. Remember, babies lose eight to twelve ounces over the first few days of life, but thereafter they gain four to seven ounces per week.

If you answered no to any of these questions, you should call your baby's doctor to discuss her feedings because it is possible her cries are a sign of hunger.

Rebuilding Your Milk Supply

If extra milk calms your baby's crying and you want to rebuild your milk supply, you probably can. Speak to your doctor, a lactation consultant, or a La Leche League leader for advice. You can try some of these remedies too:

1. **Diagnose the Problem**
   - Sometimes poor feeding is caused by a "mommy problem." You may be trying to put your baby on the breast incorrectly. Or you may have flat nipples, a thyroid problem, fatigue, pain, poor nutrition, and—rarely—insufficient breast tissue. If your nipples are cracked or sore, let a little of your milk dry on them after each feeding. Breast milk contains special factors that speed the healing of irritated skin.
   - Poor feeding may also be caused by a "baby problem." Some babies have a hard time getting the hang of nursing.

Some are weak, some are "lazy," some suck their tongue instead of your nipple, a few are tongue-tied, and others are just plain confused and try to bite instead of suckle.

Regardless of the cause, if you are having a nursing problem, get help as soon as possible.

2. **Increase Your Supply.** Once you know your breasts are fine and your baby is sucking well, the next step is increasing your milk supply. Here's how:

- Eat well and get as much rest as you can.
- Empty your breasts frequently. Nurse your baby every two to three hours (during your waking hours). Some lactation consultants recommend that moms use only one breast per feeding; however, especially when you want to build up your milk supply, I think it's best to switch breasts frequently (move her from one breast to the other every seven to ten minutes until she stops wanting to suck).

  If you are not too tired or overwhelmed, you may build up your milk supply further by pumping or expressing milk once or twice a day. I recommend pumping for five to ten minutes *before* the first feeding of the morning, or whenever your breasts feel the fullest. Don't worry about depriving your baby of milk. You'll remove some foremilk, but that still leaves the rich hindmilk for her to enjoy. After a few days you should notice your supply increasing.

- Use imagery while you're nursing or pumping to increase milk production. Get comfortable and imagine your favorite safe, relaxing place and visualize your breasts making lots of milk. One mother I know imagined lying in the sun on a tropical island, with rivers of milk flowing out of her breasts to the ocean, turning the seas white—it worked!

- Try some fenugreek tea or a product called Mother's Milk tea made of fennel, anise, mint, and fenugreek to stimulate your breasts' milk glands.

- Ask your doctor about prescription medications that help increase your milk supply or the letting down of the milk you already have. Also ask if you need your thyroid checked.

3. **Supplement Your Baby's Breast Milk with Some Formula.** You could also help your hungry baby by giving her pumped milk or formula. These can be given to her in a bottle or with a device called a Supplemental Nursing System (SNS). The SNS is a bag of milk connected to a soft, strawlike tube, which allows the baby to drink from the bag and the breast simultaneously. This method helps a woman rebuild her milk supply without teaching her baby the wrong way to suckle, a problem that may occur when nursing babies are given too many bottles.

"My D Cup Runneth Over!"—Babies Who Cry Because There Is Too Much Milk

Some babies love milk so much, they overeat. These kids guzzle down four to eight ounces each feeding and then vomit it all up because, as the saying goes, "their eyes were bigger than their stomachs." Other babies, however, guzzle not out of gluttony but out of self-protection. Their mom's milk is pouring out of her breast so quickly that they're trying not to choke.

Flooding can also occur in bottle-fed babies. Rubber nipples that are too soft or have holes that are too big can make a baby with a strong suck feel like she's drinking from a running faucet.

If you think your milk flow may be too much for your baby to handle, look for these signs:

- Does your milk quickly drip out of one breast when your baby is sucking on the other?
- Does she gulp and guzzle loudly?
- Does she struggle, cough, or pull away as soon as the milk starts to flow into her mouth?

If you answer yes to these questions, try expressing one to two ounces from your breasts immediately before the next feeding. Also, during the feed, hold your nipple between your second and third fingers, like a cigarette, and press against the breast to slow the flow of milk and see if the meal goes better.

Stomach Acid Reflux: Calming the Cry by Soothing the Burn

Bitter crying during or just after a feeding may indicate insufficient or excessive milk flow, a strange taste in your milk, a strong gastro-colic reflex in your baby (see Chapter 4), or that your baby is one of about three percent of colicky babies who suffers from stomach acid reflux.

If you suspect acid reflux as the cause of your baby's misery you should review the telltale signs of reflux mentioned in Chapter 4. Of course, if you think your baby may be suffering from this problem, you should consult your baby's doctor.

Through the years, several remedies have been recommended to alleviate reflux. A few are dead ends, but many are true paths to success.

Dead-End Stomach Acid Treatments

- *Position*—Parents of refluxing babies have long been told to keep their baby sitting up in a swing or infant seat after eating so gravity can help keep the milk in the stomach. However, studies show this position does not lessen the frequency or severity of reflux (although some parents still swear by it).
- *Rice-cereal-thickened feeds*—Some doctors recommend thickening a feeding with rice cereal to "weigh" the milk down and keep it in the stomach. But studies have also failed to show that this causes any real improvement in reflux.

True-Path Stomach Acid Treatments

- *Position*—Although sitting up may not help, two positions *have* been proved effective for lessening reflux: lying on the stomach or lying on the *left* side.

   Both positions are great while your baby is awake. The left-side position is also fine for sleep, as long as your baby is swaddled and wedged to keep her from rolling onto her stomach. The back is the preferred position for all babies to sleep in; however, some doctors recommend the side position for babies with severe reflux and nighttime vomiting. Ask your child's doctor for her opinion.

- *Burping*—Burp your baby every five to ten minutes during a feeding. Otherwise a big burp at meal's end may accidentally bring up the burning, acidic contents from your baby's stomach.

- *Feeding tips*—Make sure your infant isn't overeating. Try feeding a little less and see if the spitting stops and the crying improves. You can continue giving her shorter feeds as long as she's gaining four to seven ounces per week and she's satisfied for a few hours after a feeding.

- *Eliminate cow's milk products*—For some babies, reflux indicates a milk allergy. Discuss this possibility with your doctor to decide if the elimination of cow's milk is warranted.

- *Antacids*—Your doctor may suggest over-the-counter antacids or prescription acid-reducing medicines like famotidine (Pepcid), ranitidine (Zantac), omeprazole (Prilosec), and lansoperazole (Prevacid) in the hope of lessening her "heartburn" pain. (Never give your baby antacids without consulting a physician.)

- *Stomach-emptying aids*—During the 1990s doctors discovered that certain medicines caused the stomach to quickly empty its acidic contents into the intestines as well as "shut the door" at the top of the stomach so acid couldn't squirt up toward the mouth. Medicines such as metoclopramide (Reglan) and erythromycin are now occasionally used for babies with stomach acid reflux who continue to scream despite all the other approaches.

Herbal Teas, Homeopathics, Chiropractic, and Osteopathy: Dead Ends or True Paths?

Herbal Teas: A Cuppa Comfort?

Through the ages, herbal teas that aid digestion have been recommended for unhappy babies. Traditionally, mothers brewed either chamomile, peppermint, fennel, or dill for their babies' upset tummies.

The ancient "roots" of this practice are reflected in the names chosen for these herbs. In Spanish, the word for peppermint is *yerba buena,* meaning the *good grass;* in Serbian it's *nana,* meaning *grandmother.* Dill has settled stomachs in ancient Egypt, Greece, and in Viking times. Its English name derives from the Old Norse word *dilla,* meaning *to soothe or calm.*

Chamomile is said to have calming properties; peppermint eases intestinal spasms; dill helps soothe gas; and fennel dilates the intestinal blood vessels, facilitating digestion and producing a warming effect.

As much as I love herbal teas, I'm sorry to say that little proof exists that they offer any real benefit for colicky babies. However, they do no harm, so if you would like to give some to your baby, here's how:

To make dill or fennel tea, steep two teaspoons of mashed seeds in a cup of boiling water for ten minutes. A teaspoon of this may be given to a fussy baby several times a day. If your baby refuses the tea, you may sweeten it by adding a little baby apple juice or sugar (do not use honey or corn syrup).

Additionally, dill can be given in the form of a tonic called "gripe water," a popular folk remedy for colicky babies in Great Britain and the Commonwealth countries (although its effectiveness has never been proved).

Homeopathy, Chiropractic, Osteopathy: Are They Worth a Try?

Homeopathy is a philosophy of healing that teaches "like cures like." In other words, the body can be made to heal itself by giving a tiny dose of something that would actually *cause* the very same problem if given in a large dose. For example, a homeopath might recommend minuscule amounts of poison ivy extract to stop an itchy rash.

Do homeopathic remedies work? Some parents swear by them; however, hard evidence is difficult to find. Hopefully, this will change over the next five to ten years as the National Institutes of Health gets results from studies they are conducting on the subject.

There are four main recommended homeopathic remedies for colic: chamomila, colocynthis, magnesium phosphorica, and pulsatilla. These may be given singly or in combination; however, in general the correct homeopathic remedy is chosen according to the specific characteristics of a patient's symptoms—in this case, a baby's fussiness.

As with Western medicine, it's best to use homeopathics in consultation with an experienced practitioner.

The same uncertainty that surrounds homeopathy surrounds the claims that chiropractic or osteopathy can help calm crying babies. While there are some studies reported by these practitioners about the treatment of colic through the manipulation of the spine or skull bones, I have seen several colicky babies whose frustrated parents sought out chiropractic or osteopathic help with little or no success.

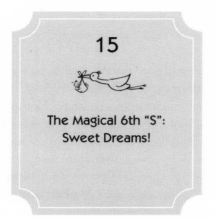

15

**The Magical 6th "S":
Sweet Dreams!**

Main Points:

- What a baby's normal sleep pattern should be
- How to use the 5 "S's" to help your baby sleep longer and better
- Weaning your sleeping baby off the 5 "S's"
- The truth about putting your baby on a schedule
- A few more helpful sleep hints, from extra feedings to darkened rooms
- Co-sleeping: The natural way to sleep (but it's not for everyone)

At Allison's two-month checkup, her mother told me Ally slept only for three-hour stretches at night. Shaya confided that getting up so often was wearing her down and making it hard for her to be patient with her other two young children.

I asked Shaya if she was still swaddling Ally at night. She wasn't. "I stopped about a month ago because the nights have been so warm and she always gets out of it!" I suggested she dress Ally in just a diaper, wrap her tightly in a larger blanket that could be securely tucked around her, and play some loud

white noise in her room. The next week Shaya reported the good
news. Allison, now tightly swaddled, was sleeping for an eight-
hour stretch every night, without interruption.

Ahhh . . . sleep!

For most new parents, a good night's sleep is the pot of gold at the end of the rainbow, shimmering in your sleep-deprived mind like a mirage. Newborns sleep in such short dribs and drabs that we should never brag we're "sleeping like a baby." It makes much more sense to say we're sleeping like a bear, or a ditch digger, or, better yet, like a new parent.

Why don't babies sleep more? Your baby actually sleeps quite a bit; however, nature could have been a teensy bit more considerate about helping your baby choose when to enjoy his sweet dreams. Most newborns distribute their snooze time pretty evenly throughout the night (and day).

Mothers around the world usually take the erratic timing of these sleep periods in stride. Many years ago, Dr. T. Berry Brazelton reported that babies in rural Mexico also had evening fussy periods, just like our babies. However, their mothers were amused rather than upset by this, joking that since adults gab all day long, nighttime was a baby's turn to talk.

Anthropologists observing the !Kung San of southern Africa found their babies woke as often as every fifteen minutes. Their moms responded by pulling them to the breast for a little snack. Usually, they would fall back asleep in seconds.

In the U.S., most parents prefer to let their newborn sleep in a bassinet by their bed. For the first few months of life, your baby will likely request the pleasure of your company for a meal every two to four hours throughout the night. Bottle-fed babies often sleep a bit longer, because formula turns into big curds that sit in the stomach longer than the easily digested, tinier curds of breast milk.

I'm sure it's hard to believe right now, but your baby's early-morning feedings may turn into some of your sweetest memories. Those beautiful moments—when all noise and commotion are stilled—may make you feel like you're floating in a cloud suspended in time. Gretchen, mother of three, said, "Our two-month-old, Julian, will be our last baby, and as crazy as it sounds, I look forward to nursing him in the middle of the night! It's the only time when we can really be alone, and I get to enjoy my delicious little boy in peace and quiet."

Baby Sleep: Your Infant's Normal Patterns

All babies have sleeping and waking cycles. If you're like most new parents, your goal is to get your baby to do his longest sleeping at night and be most awake during the day.

But, exactly how long should your baby sleep? On average, babies snooze fourteen to eighteen hours in a twenty-four-hour period. That might sound like a lot but it's broken up into little snippets, slipped between short stretches of wakefulness. In effect, it's like being given a thousand dollars—*in pennies!*

As you can see in the sleep pattern graph, during your baby's first weeks of life two-thirds of each day will be spent asleep (gray areas). The average infant takes naps lasting two to three hours alternating with hour-long awake-breaks (white areas) for feeding, fussing, and some alert time. Initially, your baby's longest stretch of sleep will probably be about four hours.

By three months, your baby will still sleep fourteen to eighteen hours a day, but the awake time (white areas) will join into longer periods of wakefulness, and sleeping (gray areas) may extend for up to six to eight hours.

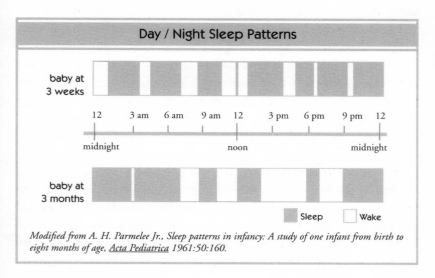

Modified from A. H. Parmelee Jr., Sleep patterns in infancy: A study of one infant from birth to eight months of age, Acta Pediatrica 1961:50:160.

During these initial months, your baby's brain gets better and better at dividing the twenty-four hours of the day into three main activities:

- *Awake time*—to eat and learn about the world
- *Active (REM) sleep*—to dream and "file away" the day's lessons
- *Quiet sleep*—to rest and recover from all the day's efforts

Both babies and adults have two different types of sleep (and I don't mean too little and none). Quiet sleep makes up fifty percent of your baby's slumber. It's when he's out like a log, his breathing easy and regular, his face still and angelic. During quiet sleep your baby's muscles are actually a little tensed; he's not floppy like a rag doll.

The other fifty percent of your baby's snoozing consists of active sleep. This sleep is characterized by sudden bursts of brain activity called REM (Rapid Eye Movement), and it occurs between periods of quiet sleep. REM sleep is when your baby's dreams are spun and his deep memory centers organize all his new experiences of the day. In active sleep, your baby has irregular breathing, sudden twitches, limp dangling limbs that feel like overcooked spaghetti, and, most spectacularly, he makes tiny heart-melting smiles. Contrary to myth, these grins are not caused by gas; rather, your baby is practicing what will soon become his most charming and powerful social tool—his smile.

Adults enjoy a full two hours of REM when we sleep. By comparison, your new baby revels in almost eight hours of REM every day. Why do babies have so much more REM than we do? No one knows for sure, but one theory posits that they need much more time to review the day because so many experiences are new to them. It's as if their brains are saying, "Wow! So much new stuff today, and I want to remember *everything!*" By comparison, most of an adult's day is so routine that our brains fast-forward through this period of review, as if to say, "I can skip all that. I know it already."

Sleeping obviously is not a time of alertness, but it's not "coma" time either. You are aware of many things around you while you snooze. For example, you probably have no trouble hearing the phone ring in the middle of the night and even when you sleep on the edge of the bed you rarely fall out of it.

Babies, too, receive a constant flow of information from the world around them while they slumber. That's why your baby may experience their still bed and the extreme quiet of your home as disturbing understimulation.

The waves of quiet and active sleep that your infant moves through take place within larger cycles of deep and light sleep. These repeat, like the tides, over and over again, all night long. Your baby cycles between deep and light sleep about every sixty minutes. Infants with good state control and mellow temperaments can often stay asleep during their lightest sleep, and even if they wake up, they usually fall right back to sleep. However, babies with poor self-calming abilities and challenging temperaments often have trouble staying asleep when they enter their light-sleep periods. During this phase of sleep, they may be so close to wakefulness that the added stimulation of hunger, gas, noise, or startle may be enough to rouse them to alertness or even agitated crying.

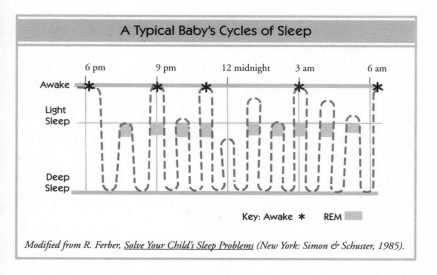

A Typical Baby's Cycles of Sleep

Key: Awake ✳ REM

Modified from R. Ferber, <u>Solve Your Child's Sleep Problems</u> (New York: Simon & Schuster, 1985).

Rest Easy: Helping Your Baby Stay Asleep with the 5 "S's"

When it comes to sleeping, you and your baby are a team, and you will both have to be flexible to make it work. However, as every mother knows, for the first four to six months, you will be the team member who bends the most. You will rearrange your priorities, put off chores, and try to sleep in synch with your baby's schedule.

But don't despair. There are five specific ways you can nudge your baby into a better sleeping schedule during these early months: the 5 "S's." These womb sensations will keep your infant's calming reflex turned on and, when they're used at night, they may even keep him soothed until daybreak.

1. Swaddle—

Tight wrapping prevents your baby's accidental whacks and disturbing startles. Just by swaddling your baby, you may increase his sleeping periods from three to four or even six hours at a stretch. Remember, his blanket must stay tight for it to work all through the night.

Karen's son, Connor, was three months old (and seventeen pounds!), but he still had trouble sleeping more than three hours at a stretch:

> "When I put Connor down after nursing, he would struggle and squirm for over half an hour until he finally settled down to sleep. He hadn't been swaddled since he was a newborn, but Dr. Karp suggested I try again.
>
> "I was surprised that he not only accepted the swaddling (after a little struggling) but settled down immediately and slept one hour more than usual. Wrapping also extended his daytime sleeping from fifteen-minute catnaps to one-to-two-hour luxurious naps, morning and afternoon.
>
> "I was delighted with this improvement, until a friend came by the next week and showed me that I was still swaddling Connor too loosely. She taught me how to do it tighter and he began sleeping eight hours straight at night!"

2. Side—

The back is clearly the safest sleep position for your baby. The side should ONLY be used if your baby is a terrible sleeper and even then you MUST make sure that he's tightly swaddled and wedged into position by placing receiving blankets (tightly rolled and taped) securely at his waist and lower back to keep him from accidentally scooting onto his stomach. Please consult with your physician if you have further questions.

3. Shhhh—

Most babies sleep better when a harsh, continuous white noise plays near their bassinet. These womb-like sounds drown out other distracting noises and have a profoundly lulling effect. As with swaddling, the mere addition of white noise to your baby's nursery may extend his sleep by an hour or two.

4. Swing—

The movement of a swing (and to a lesser extent, a vibrating seat) can help your baby nap better and sleep longer at night. Not all babies need to swing to sleep well, but I know many parents whose babies sleep well only when they are allowed to swing all night during their first four months of life.

5. Suck—

Sucking on a breast or pacifier may help your baby fall asleep, but it won't really help him stay in deep sleep.

Even babies who have never experienced the 5 "S's" can benefit from their sleep-enhancing effects. Don't be concerned if your baby initially resists them. If you patiently persist, you'll be surprised by your success.

Weaning Your Sleeping Baby Off the 5 "S's"

All children eventually must learn to fall asleep on their own and to put themselves back to sleep when they wake during the night. In my experience, by three months most babies are ready to learn how to do this and should be placed in the crib sleepy but semi-awake.

I know that the parents of infants under three months are warned by some baby book authors that using nighttime sleep aids like the 5 "S's" will spoil their babies and make them abnormally dependent. I couldn't disagree more! For nine months before your baby was born, your womb surrounded him with sensations like the 5 "S's" every second of every day. That's why all babies sleep better and longer with a couple of "S's" to keep them company during the long night. But don't worry—by the time your baby is three to four months old, you will be able to wean him off them without difficulty.

The first "S" I advise you to wean is sucking. I like babies to get used to falling asleep without something in their mouths as early as one month of age. Don't misunderstand me: I think it's fine for your baby to fall asleep sucking your breast, bottle, or pacifier, but a minute or two after he conks out I recommend you wake him up—just a tiny bit—as you put him down. This lets him start learning how to put himself to sleep. (If he begins to cry, just soothe him with shushing and rocking.)

Another good reason for weaning your baby from a bedtime pacifier is because they fall out so often they aren't a reliable sleep tool. You're in control of the wrapping and can easily keep your baby wrapped till morning, but you have no control over the paci, which he can spit out anytime he wants.

The next "S" I phase out is swinging. At two to three months you can reduce the swing speed to the slowest setting. A few days later, if your baby is still sleeping well, let him sleep in the nonmoving swing. Finally, a few days later, if he still is sleeping soundly, move him to the bassinet.

Next, many parents wean the swaddling. After four months, try wrapping your baby tightly—with one arm out. He should be able to suck his fingers and soothe himself. If he sleeps just as well that way, try putting him to bed with no bundling. However, if he starts waking up more, take a step back and return to the wrapping.

Lastly, wean the shhhhing sound. Over a period of two weeks you can gradually lower the white-noise volume until it is so low you can turn it off.

In general, my little patients are out of their swings by three to four months, out of the swaddle by three to six months (a handful have continued until nine months), and sleeping in a quiet room by three to twelve months. (The shhhh noise is the last "S" to be dropped because it is so easy, effective, and simple to control.)

When your sweet baby goes all night without any of the "S's," give him a diploma. He's now graduated from the fourth trimester and is ready to start his life adventure!

The Truth About Putting Your Baby on a Schedule

New parents are often confused about the importance of putting their baby on a schedule. Should schedules be avoided or embraced? Like so many other child-rearing issues, there's more than one right answer.

Toddlers and young children love routines. They feel secure and safe when they know what's going to happen. In another year or two, you'll probably have a bedtime ritual: "blankie," warm milk, and *Goodnight Moon* to guide your sweet child into peaceful sleep—every night.

Similarly, flexible eating/sleeping schedules can be a great help to young babies and their parents. That's especially true if you have twins, older children, if you're working out of the house, and/or you're a single parent.

But before you try to put your new baby on a schedule, you should know that scheduling is a fairly new parenting concept. Mothers in the past didn't feed their babies according to the time on the sundial. And many moms today don't feel right trying to fit their baby into a preset mold.

I am not saying it is wrong to try to put your one-month-old baby on a schedule. Just as long as you understand that babies have only been "asked" to bend themselves to our clock-driven schedules over the past hundred years, and many babies are simply too immature to do it.

Your baby's receptiveness to being put on a schedule depends upon his ability to handle delayed gratification. In other words, how good is he at holding off his need for food or sleep? Some newborns are easily dis-

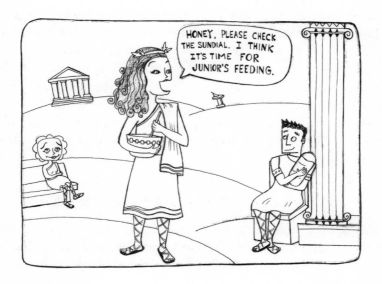

tracted, but others take months before they can ignore their brain's demands for milk or rest. The parents of these babies must patiently delay their desire to get their infants on a schedule until their babies are ready for one.

That said, if you want to try your baby on a schedule after one to two months, the best way to begin is by increasing the time between his daytime feedings to three hours. Of course, if he's hungry before two hours are up (and you can't soothe him any other way) forget the schedule and feed him. Also, wake him up and feed him if he goes more than four hours without crying for food. Babies who go too long without food during the day often wake up and feed more at night.

The next step in scheduling is to train your infant to fall asleep without a nipple in his mouth. After his feeding, play with him for a little while before you put him to sleep. That will begin to teach him he can put himself to sleep. If he immediately passes out after you fill his belly with warm milk, that's okay, just jostle him until he opens his eyes. Then lay him down and let him float back into sleep. With patience over the next month or two, this will help your baby develop the ability to put himself to sleep.

Most infants automatically fall into a regular pattern after a month or

It's easier to establish a schedule if you follow the same pattern every day. After your baby is a month old, start this reassuring nighttime routine:

low lights
toasty bath
loving massage with heated oil
some warm milk
cozy swaddle
a lullaby . . . softly sung
and
gentle white noise playing in the background

Within a short period of time, the constant association of these experiences to your baby's sleep time will work almost like hypnosis. As soon as you start the routine he'll say to himself, "Wow, I feel sleepy already!"

two; however, if you can't wait to establish a more predictable routine, feel free to give scheduling a try.

If, on the other hand, he seems to resist being molded to your schedule, I encourage you to respond to your tiny baby's needs with promptness and love; you can always try the schedule again in a week. The bottom line is that your job as a parent is to adapt to the needs of your newborn, not the other way around.

A Few More Helpful Sleep Tips

Here are a few more tips to help your baby sleep longer:

Feed Your Baby More During the Day

These steps can increase your baby's daytime eating and nighttime sleeping as he reaches the end of the fourth trimester:

- Wake him for a feeding if he naps for more than four hours.
- Feed him in a quiet room so he doesn't get distracted and refuse to eat.
- Give him "cluster feedings" (several meals given every two hours in the late afternoon and early evening to load him up with calories).
- "Top off the tank" by waking him for a midnight feeding.

One thing that will not help your baby sleep better is feeding him rice cereal at bedtime. While it is true that some nighttime formula can help a breast-fed baby sleep longer, repeated scientific studies have proved that rice cereal does not prolong a baby's sleep. And why should it? From a nutritional point of view, it makes no sense that four to six ounces of milk (with all its fat and protein) would leave a baby hungry but a few spoons of rice starch would keep him satisfied all night.

If you have any doubts at all that your infant is getting enough to eat, ask your doctor to weigh him to make sure that he's thriving.

Hold and Rock Your Baby During the Day

Parents are often told to keep their baby awake during the day in the hope of getting him tired and making him want to sleep longer at night.

Although this sounds logical, keeping a tired baby awake often makes him miserable, overtired, and thus *worsens* his sleep at night. In fact, not only should you let your newborn sleep during the day but you should give him motion while he naps (in a swing, a bouncy chair, or on you in a baby sling). In my experience, babies who are carried ("fed" with nourishing touch and motion) throughout the day are often calmer (less "hungry" for that stimulation) at night.

Turn the Lights Down

Reducing the lights in your house as evening comes also gives your baby the signal it's time for sleep. Low lights quiet a baby's nervous system and prepare him to relax. Many hospital nurseries have an evening routine of dimming the lights and covering the incubators of premature babies to block the light and help them get into their parents' day/night rhythm.

> *Mabel, the mother of four daughters, piqued my curiosity when she mentioned that her pet theory about the cause of colic was <u>electricity!</u> She said, "I noticed my kids are more stimulated and have a harder time falling asleep when we keep the house well lit in the evening. I think the artificially long 'daytime' we create with electric lights tricks them into believing it's still time to play. Our kids consistently sleep better when we dim the lights at night or use candles."*

Co-sleeping: "I Just Got Evicted— Can I Sleep at Your Place?"

Thou shalt sleep with thy fathers.
Deuteronomy 31:16

Since mankind's earliest days, parents and babies have slept together for mutual protection, warmth, and to make nighttime feedings convenient. Japanese parents traditionally sleep with their baby between them, safe as a valley protected by two great mountain ranges. They don't question whether a mother and infant should be together all night; they consider themselves to be two parts of one person and therefore they should be sep-

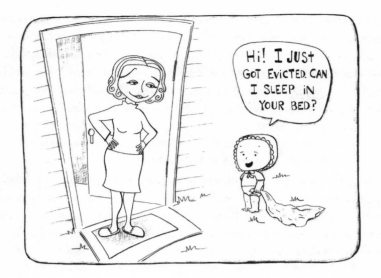

arated as little as possible. Mayan families are very social and for them the shared bed is a time to be together. These parents believe making their baby sleep alone is an unfair hardship.

Until the late 1800s, American children also slept in bed with their parents. However, at the turn of the century, U.S. parents were frightened away from co-sleeping. They were warned it could spread illness, spoil children, or cause them to suffocate. So we moved our babies to their own cribs and eventually to their own rooms. Today, we Americans see our children's sleep as a time for privacy and to begin learning about self-reliance. Many now view sharing the bed as a sacrifice or a bad habit. (Oddly, many of these same parents nap with their babies during the day without harboring similar concerns.)

This resistance to co-sleeping is slowly changing. As breast-feeding continues its rise in popularity, nursing mothers are realizing the cozy convenience of having their baby nearby. In addition, the immigration of non-Europeans into the U.S. has introduced a potpourri of cultural traditions—most of which encourage the intimacy of co-sleeping.

However, like so many other prehistoric customs, co-sleeping doesn't always fit the needs and lifestyles of contemporary parents. One mother in my practice said, "I can't sleep in bed with my four-week-old baby. I just keep worrying about him." Other parents get frustrated because co-sleeping babies wake up more during the night. My nurse practitioner, Dana Entin, explains the frequent night feedings that co-sleeping babies request as a case of temptation. "If I had a piece of chocolate cake in bed next to me, I would wake up all night and want a little nibble too!"

If you decide not to co-sleep, don't feel guilty! As Shakespeare wrote, "To thine own self be true." You certainly don't need to co-sleep to be a good parent. You have the wonderful alternative of keeping your baby all swaddled and cuddly in a cradle or bassinet.

On the other hand, if bringing your baby into bed with you feels right, trust your instincts. Sleeping with your baby is a natural continuation of the womb experience. Your baby enjoys your body's companionship and its help in molding his breathing, temperature stability, and sleep pattern. Additionally, after the rigors of pregnancy it's an abrupt change for *you* to be all the way down the hall from your infant, connected to him by an intercom only. One mother who worked long hours shared, "Sleeping with my baby lets me make up some time I couldn't spend with her during the day."

As long as you and your baby are happy with co-sleeping, enjoy this sweet, fleeting opportunity. If you are planning to move your baby out of your bed, it's easiest to do so by four to five months of age, before he gets used to this bedtime routine. You can still end co-sleeping after that time, but in general, the longer you wait the tougher it is for your baby to make the switch.

One additional bonus of co-sleeping may be prevention of SIDS. Researchers like James McKenna of Notre Dame University believe the lighter level of sleep of co-sleeping babies may lessen their risk of SIDS.

Is Co-sleeping Dangerous to Your Baby's Health?

In 1999, the U.S. Consumer Product Safety Commission (CPSC) issued a disturbing warning to parents about the possible dangers of co-sleeping. They reported an average of sixty-four infant deaths (children less than two years old) each year related to a baby being in an adult's bed. Their conclusion? Parents should never place infants in their beds.

Unfortunately, their recommendation was as off-target as someone suggesting we try to prevent the fifty thousand fatal car accidents each year *by not driving*. Obviously, a more constructive answer to traffic deaths is for all of us to drive better. Likewise, the vast majority of infant deaths in bed are preventable by taking a few reasonable precautions. For example, eighty percent of the deaths noted by the CPSC could have been avoided by filling the spaces around the bed to keep babies from getting wedged in and by never sleeping on waterbeds. Most of the remaining twenty percent of deaths could have been prevented by using a co-sleeper attachment (a small baby bed with raised rails that fits right next to a parent's bed).

Nine Ways to Keep Your Baby Safe in Bed With You

Any parent co-sleeping with their infant *must* protect him in the following ways:

1. Avoid pillows, toys, or loose bedding that could smother your baby.
2. Never put your baby to sleep on a waterbed.
3. Eliminate spaces between the mattress and the wall, or the mattress and the headboard, where your baby's head might get trapped.
4. Use a co-sleeper attachment on your bed so your baby can't fall off or get rolled on.
5. Don't sleep on the sofa with your baby.
6. Keep your baby swaddled tightly all night long so that he doesn't move into a dangerous position during the night.
7. Let your baby sleep only on his back.
8. Give up smoking! Babies are more likely to die of SIDS if their mom is a smoker.
9. Always go to bed sober.

The Whys About the "S's":
Questions Parents Ask
About Sleeping

1. *Every time I put my sleeping baby down, he's up and yelling in min-utes. Why?*

    Even though your baby is asleep when you put him down, he still has some awareness of his surroundings. To him there's too big a difference between your arms and a quiet, still bassinet.

    Try using the 5 "S's" to help your baby make the transition to his crib. Swaddling, white noise, and swinging lessen the abrupt change from your cuddle to his cradle and can eliminate one or two night wakings.

2. *When my baby falls asleep after a feeding, should I burp him and risk waking him up?*

    Yes. You should burp him, to keep him from spitting up in his sleep, and change his diaper too, to prevent a diaper rash. After a feeding, most babies feel a little "drunk" and usually go back to sleep quickly, especially if you're using the 5 "S's."

    By the way, it is also a good idea to put ointment on your baby's bottom at night to protect his skin from any pee or poop that comes out while he's asleep.

3. *I worry about overbundling my baby in the warm weather. How can I tell if he's getting overheated at night?*

    It's quite easy to know if your baby is overbundled: feel his ears and toes. If they are red, sweaty, or very warm, he's too hot; if they are cold and bluish, he's too chilly; and if they feel "fresh" (not hot, not cold, but a tiny bit on the cool side), his body temperature is just right.

    Even on the hottest summer days, your baby will benefit from swaddling. Dress him in a diaper only and wrap him in a very light cotton blanket.

For summertime, Talia's grandmother made some ultralight
blankets by cutting a sheet in quarters and hemming the edges.

4. Can a baby have trouble sleeping because he's going through a growth spurt?

Yes. Babies grow tremendously fast during the first few months, doubling their weight in about six months. Some babies do all this growing at an even, steady pace, but many babies grow in fits and starts (growth spurts and plateaus). In the midst of a growth spurt, your baby may wake up more frequently and yell for a meal. (That's really *demand* feeding!)

5. Will my baby sleep better if he takes both breasts or just one, so he gets the hindmilk?

Unlike formula, which doesn't change from the first drop to the last, breast milk changes greatly during the course of a feeding. The milk that spurts out for the first five minutes is loaded with protein and antibodies, and it's more watery to satisfy your baby's thirst. By the time the breast is almost empty (after ten to fifteen minutes) the milk slowly dripping out is as rich as half and half. This creamy, sweet dessert is called the hindmilk.

Some experts tell mothers not to switch their breasts during a feeding. They worry that feeding just a few minutes on each side will deprive a baby of the hindmilk, which they consider nature's way of making babies satisfied and sleepy (like the drowsiness we feel after a heavy meal).

Other experts believe babies get more milk if their moms switch breasts during a meal. They advise mothers to feed for about seven minutes on one side and then, after that breast has released its quick, easy milk, switch to the other side, which is full and waiting to be emptied.

I recommend this to my patients: Experiment to find what's best for you and your baby. If one breast keeps him happy for two hours in the day and sleeping four hours at night, then there is no need for switching. However, if he feeds too often or is gaining weight too slowly, try giving him seven minutes on one side and then let him suck for ten to fifteen minutes, or longer, on the second side (that's enough for him to fill up with the early milk from both breasts and still get the hindmilk from the second side).

6. *Why does my baby always get up at the crack of dawn?*

Even when babies are asleep they still feel, hear—and see! For many babies, the early-morning light filters through their closed eyes and thin skull and acts like an alarm clock. Fortunately, many of these babies can be coaxed to sleep a little longer by using black-out curtains to shut out the sun's first rays; white-noise machines to help obscure the early-morning sounds of birds, dogs, traffic, and neighbors; or, by bringing them into bed with you for some cozy time.

Parents who can't charm their infants back to sleep are often forced to wave good-bye to their warm beds and take their little "rooster babies" out for an early-morning constitutional. (Believe it or not, these strolls may become some of your most treasured memories of when your baby was little.)

7. *Is it wrong to let my baby get used to sleeping in his infant carrier?*

It's almost impossible to *keep* your baby from falling asleep when you tote him around outside in an infant carrier. That's because putting your baby in a carrier or a sling and taking him for a walk gives him three of his favorite sensations: jiggly motion, cuddling, and the rhythmic, soothing sound of your breathing. These devices are great ways to treat our babies to a sweet reminder of the fourth trimester.

So, don't worry about accidentally teaching him bad habits. After the fourth trimester ends, your four-month-old baby will be able to entertain himself and it will be relatively easy to get him used to less contact—if that's what you really want. (Truthfully, by then many parents love their carrier so much they want to "wear" their baby more and more.)

8. *Is it okay to let my baby sleep on my chest?*

In general, I don't recommend this position. I once had a couple call me in the middle of the night when their four-week-old baby fell off his father's chest and hit the wall next to the bed. (The exhausted duo had slipped into a sound sleep.) Fortunately, he wasn't hurt, but a fall like that could have caused a serious injury.

We went through fire and water almost in trying to procure for him a natural sleep. We swung him in blankets, wheeled him in little carts, walked the room with him by the hour, etc., etc., but it was wonderful how little sleep he obtained after all. He always looked wide awake and as if he did not need sleep.

G. L. Prentiss, *The Life and Letters of Elizabeth Prentiss*, 1822

Poor Elizabeth Prentiss could have learned a thing or two from the parents whose stories below reveal how they transformed their nighttime experience with their babies from getting "nickel and dimed" to money in the bank:

Debra and Andrew swaddled their twins, Audrey and Sophia, from the very first days in their lives. Swaddling prolonged their children's nighttime sleep. Even at four months old, the twins still preferred being swaddled. It helped them sleep a full eight hours every night.

Debra, Andrew, Audrey, and Sophia

As she reached the four-week mark, our daughter Eve became more wakeful and more distressed with the world around her. When she wasn't eating or sleeping, she was fussing—and at times she screamed inconsolably. One night she yelled so much her nose got stuffed and she began to snort. I called Dr. Karp's office for advice. As I spoke with his nurse, Louise, I cradled Eve in my arms and rested them on top of the dryer. The noise, vibration, and warmth of the dryer calmed her, allowing me to talk for a few minutes.

Over the next couple of weeks, as I became skilled at using the "S's" Nurse Louise had described that night, Eve rewarded us with six-to-eight-hour periods of uninterrupted sleep every night. At six months, we were still swaddling Eve at night but by then we would let one of her arms stay out so she could suck her fingers.

Shari, Michael, Hillary, Noah, and Eve

Didi and Richard were exhausted from Cameron's hourly wak-ing—all night long. They tried keeping their six-week-old up more during the day in the hope he would sleep better at night, but that

just seemed to get him overtired and make him cry even more. At night, they tried to calm him with a bath, the vacuum, or a ride in the car, all of which worked for a while but Cameron would get upset again as soon as the "entertainment" stopped.

Then, they discovered their son liked to sleep tightly wrapped and seated in the swing next to a white-noise machine with the sound cranked up loud. However, they worried about leaving him in there, so after he fell asleep they would put him back into his bassinet. Cameron slept better that way, but still awoke every three or four hours.

Finally, Didi and Richard stumbled onto the secret for getting Cameron to sleep longer. One night when he was in the swing his exhausted parents fell asleep and let him stay in the swing, with white noise, all night long. It made a huge difference. With that nighttime assistance he began to sleep a six-hour stretch, eat, and then go back down for another three hours!

When Wyatt was two months old, his parents—Lise, a nurse, and Aaron, a physician—noticed he would sleep five hours at night when wrapped and serenaded by white noise but only three hours when his arms were free and the room was quiet.

Lise said, "I was happy to see how well our son did with swaddling. But I still worried he would get 'addicted' to it and have trouble sleeping unwrapped when he got older. So as soon as he turned three months, I began putting him to bed unwrapped.

"Everything seemed fine, until a month later when Wyatt turned four months. Out of the blue, he began waking every two hours through the night—screaming! One friend told me he was teething, but Tylenol didn't help. My husband guessed he was going through a growth spurt, but rice cereal didn't help either. At Wyatt's four-month checkup, I told Dr. Karp about my frustration and fatigue. He suggested I stop the medicine and cereal and try the wrapping and white noise again. To be honest, I thought Wyatt was too old for swaddling, but I was desperate.

"Within two nights, he went from waking up and shrieking five times a night to waking once, chowing down his milk, and then immediately sacking out again until 6 AM! He loved the waterfall sound of our sound machine. I played it loud for him for the first hour and then kept it turned on medium all night long. (It helped me to sleep, too!)

Everything worked so well that I continued the routine until one night, when Wyatt was six months old, I skipped putting him in his cocoon and still enjoyed a deep, beautiful sleep."

Lise, Aaron, Wyatt, and Rachel

I never would have believed it, but wrapping was the key to everything! Our first son, Eli, never resisted being bundled up, but Benji fought it with all his strength. However, only after he was tightly swaddled did the rocking, pacifier, and shushing calm him.

After a few days of practicing the 5 "S's," I could put Benji down for hours at a time with no problem. Now at six weeks of age, and at the peak of what should be his worst time, he's a pretty easy baby. He takes long naps and sleeps for seven to nine hours at night (with one very brief feeding).

For naps, I let him sleep in the swing on the fast speed and keep the noise machine on pretty loud.

I let him nap frequently because I've noticed that Ben gets overstimulated and has a hard time settling himself if I let him have long awake periods during the day. So, when he starts getting cranky, I take that as my cue to put him back in the swing and do my womb imitation.

I recommend this method for anyone with a "difficult" baby. I can't imagine what my mental state would be if I were still carrying him all day and rocking him all night. It has made an enormous difference for both me and Benji, as well as my first guys, Steve and Eli!

Wendy, Steve, Eli, and Benji

Conclusion

The Rainbow at the End of the Tunnel:
Finally Your Baby Is Ready to Be Born!

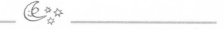

He's starting to love us back a little.

Francie about four-month-old Jackson

At birth, Esmé was a pudgy, sweet-smelling baby who needed to use all her concentration to gaze into her mother's eyes. Yet, by four months, she could shoot broad grins out at anyone in the room, as if to say, "Ain't I great!"

Hooray! After months of fuzzy stares and long sleeps, your four-month-old's laugh and gurgle announce to the world: "Dress rehearsals are over . . . I'm ready for my Grand Premiere!"

It has been three long months since you cut the umbilical cord, but finally your baby is *really* ready to be born. He has weathered the challenging transition from your womb to the world and is no longer trapped inside his immature body. Now the rapidly increasing control he has over his actions offers him many new ways to handle his upsets without having to resort to crying.

Please don't underestimate what your baby has achieved during his brief lifetime. It truly is amazing. In essence, he has zipped through millions of years of evolution in a mere ninety days. He may have started out as helpless as a mouse yet now he's well on his way to mastering the most important skills of our species—the ability to reach out both manually and socially. His relaxed and open hands now allow him to latch on to his rattle (or your nose) and, like Esmé, he's already learning how to use his adorable, toothless grin to make everyone he meets fall in love with him!

Like a child on the first day of school, your scrubbed-cheeked, four-month-old baby's happy jabberings bubble forth energetically. Now, there's no question he's ready to learn and start making friends. And, as a direct consequence of your baby's increasing curiosity, you'll probably notice his sudden dislike for being put on his stomach. While newborns enjoy "tummy time" because it's calming and helps them ignore the chaos of the world, your four-month-old baby demands to be placed on his back so he can see the world. Now, he's *interested* in the chaos . . . he's ready to play.

Your infant isn't the only one ready for this next chapter of life. I'm sure you too are ready for a little more play . . . and rest. For the past three months, you've unselfishly accepted pain, fatigue, and anxiety. Now, *you've* become one of the experienced parents on the block and you've learned enough to earn an advanced degree in "Baby-ology." It is my sincere hope that this book has been a useful part of that education in helping you see the world through your baby's eyes and in helping you master the ancient techniques of infant soothing and comforting.

At last, there *is* a light at the end of the arduous tunnel that was the fourth trimester and happily, far from being an oncoming train, that light is . . . a glorious rainbow. All your love and hard work have paid off and the real fun is just beginning. So congratulations! Your baby is now well on the way to becoming *one of the happiest babies on the block!*

Appendix A

Red Flags and Red Alerts:
When You Should Call the Doctor

Fortunately, most colicky babies aren't physically sick. Rather, they're sort of "homesick"—struggling to cope with life outside Mama's womb. But how can you know when your infant's cries *are* a sign of sickness?

Here's a primer of the ten red flags that doctors look for to decide when a baby's cry signals illness, plus a review of the ten red-alert medical conditions that these red flags may indicate.

The Ten Red Flags Your Doctor Will Ask You About

Whenever you're worried about your baby, you should, of course, contact your doctor for guidance. When you do, he'll likely ask you these two questions to help him decide if your baby has colic or something more serious:

1. Is your baby growing well and acting normal in all other ways?
2. Is your baby calm for long periods of the day?

If you answer no to either question, then your doctor will ask you how your baby acts when she isn't crying. He is looking for these ten red flags:

1. *Persistent moaning* (groans and weak cries that continue for hours)
2. *Supershrill cry* (unlike any cry your baby has made before)
3. *Repeated vomiting or any green or yellow vomit* (more than one ounce per episode and more than five episodes a day)

4. *Change in stool* (constipation or diarrhea, especially with blood)
5. *Fussing during eating* (twisting, arching, crying that begins during or shortly after a feed)
6. *Abnormal temperature* (a rectal temperature of more than 100.2°F or less than 97.0°F)
7. *Irritability* (crying all the time with almost no calm periods in between)
8. *Lethargy* (a baby sleeping twice as long as usual, acting "out of it," and not sucking well over an eight- to twelve-hour period)
9. *Bulging soft spot on the head* (even when your baby is sitting up)
10. *Poor weight gain* (gaining less than a half ounce a day)

The Ten Medical Red Alerts Your Doctor Will Consider

Whenever a doctor sees a crying baby who exhibits any red-flag symptoms, she tries to determine whether this indicates one of these ten serious—but treatable—medical conditions. Please remember, most of these conditions are *very, very* rare. (Excluding babies who cry because of food sensitivity or acid reflux less than one percent of infants with severe, persistent crying are affected by the problems listed below.)

1. **Infection: From Ear Infections to Appendicitis**
   You might think the best way to tell if your baby has an infection is to take her temperature, but many sick newborns don't get fevers. So even if your crying baby doesn't have fever, you should consider that her fussiness may be a sign of infection if she acts lethargic or irritable for more than a few hours. Call your doctor immediately. He may check her for:

   > **Ear Infection**—These babies may just get fussy and upset; they rarely pull on their ears.
   > **Urine Infection**—These babies can have smelly urine, but usually *don't*.
   > **Brain Infection (meningitis)**—These infants have bulging soft spots, vomiting, lethargy, and irritability that rapidly worsens over just a day or two.

Appendicitis—Extremely rare in infants, it may cause a hard stomach, poor appetite, and constant irritability.

Intestinal Infection—A baby with "stomach flu" vomits, has diarrhea, and usually has been in contact with a sick relative.

2. **Intestinal Pain: From Intestinal Blockages to Stomach Acid Reflux**

Some stomach problems cause pain and may explain crying in ten to fifteen percent of colicky infants (in descending order of seriousness):

Intestinal Blockage—This is an extremely rare medical emergency that may occur right after birth or weeks later. Babies suffer from waves of severe painful spasms plus vomiting and/or the cessation of pooping. With intestinal blockages, the vomit often has a distinct yellow or green tint. (During the first days of life, a breast-fed baby's vomit may also be yellow, because that is the color of colostrum. However, if your baby has yellow vomit, *never* assume it's from your milk. Immediately consult your doctor to make sure it isn't the sign of a more serious condition.)

Stomach Acid Reflux—This cause of burning pain occurs in approximately one to three percent of fussy babies.

A "Pain in the Rear": Can an Overly Tight Anus Block a Baby's Intestines?

In 100 A.D. the physician Soranus opined that a tight anus could block a baby's intestines, leading to spasms. He recommended stretching the anus to relieve a baby's crying. Over the next two thousand years, medical practitioners followed his advice and routinely stuck fingers up the behinds of crying babies. Today, however, we know this problem is extremely rare and probably never causes colic.

Food Sensitivity—Five to ten percent of fussy babies get better with a change in diet and so presumably have this condition. Besides crying, it may cause vomiting, diarrhea, rash, or mucousy blood in the stools.

(For a complete discussion of reflux and food sensitivities see Chapters 4 and 14.)

Crying before, during, and after feeding

Immediately before a feeding: hunger, thirst, challenging temperament

During a feeding: the gastro-colic reflex, the milk flow is too slow or too fast, the milk has a strange taste, stomach acid reflux

Immediately after a feeding: continued hunger, the gastro-colic reflex, needing to burp, needing to poop, wanting to suck more, food allergy, stomach acid reflux

---

3. Breathing Trouble: From Blocked Nostrils to Oversize Tongues

The most common cause of breathing trouble is a condition where a baby's tiny nostrils are blocked. Babies don't know how to breathe through their mouths, except when they're crying. That's why babies who are born with tight nostrils, or who have noses swollen shut from allergies or colds, get so frantic.

If you want to check for blockage, place the tip of your little finger snugly over one of your baby's nostrils, closing it off for a few seconds. She should easily be able to breathe through the open nostril. Then repeat this test on the other side.

If your baby can't breathe or gets agitated when you do this test, call your physician. If it seems the nostril is blocked from mucus, ask the best ways to clear it. And do your best to rid your home of dust, molds, sprays, perfumes, cigarette smoke, and anything else that might make her nose congested.

Very rarely, an infant will have trouble breathing if her tongue is too big for her mouth so it falls back into the throat and chokes her when she lies on her back. This problem is obvious from the moment of birth because her tongue will always stick out of her mouth.

4. **Increased Brain Pressure**

    When pressure builds up inside a baby's head, it also causes:

    - Irritability and crying from a headache
    - Vomiting
    - An unusual high-pitched cry
    - A bulging fontanelle (soft spot) even when the baby is seated
    - Swollen veins on the forehead
    - A head that's growing too rapidly (your doctor should measure your baby's head size at every well-baby checkup)
    - Sunset sign (a big-eyed stare with a crescent of the white of the eye displayed over the colored iris, making the eye look like a setting sun)

    If your baby fits the symptoms described above, contact your doctor immediately.

5. **Skin Pain: A Thread or Hair Twisted Around a Finger, Toe, or Penis**

    In years past, the sudden onset of sharp screaming in an otherwise calm baby made parents search for an open safety pin inside the diaper. Today, however, thanks to pin-less diapers, that no longer happens. Now a parent who hears that type of abrupt, shrill cry should look for a fine hair or thread wrapped tightly around their baby's finger, toe, or penis. This problem requires immediate medical attention. (Doctors often treat this problem by applying a dab of hair-removal cream to dissolve the hair.)

6. **Mouth Pain: From Thrush to Teething**

    Thrush, a yeast infection in the mouth, is easy to recognize because it causes a milky white residue on the lips and inside of the mouth that cannot be wiped away. Thrush may also cause a bumpy red rash in a baby's diaper area and/or itchy, red nipples in a breast-feeding mom.

Thrush rarely causes fussiness, but on occasion it can cause crying from an irritated mouth. Fortunately it is easy to treat, and recovery is rapid.

Many parents ask if teething causes their baby's crying. This is extremely unlikely, because teething two-month-olds are as rare as hen's teeth. However, if you think your baby is having teething pain, give her some acetaminophen drops and see if it gives any relief (ask your doctor for the correct dosage). This medicine won't help colic, but it may reduce mild teething pain.

7. Kidney Pain: Blockage of the Urinary System

A blockage of the kidney is a very rare cause of persistent crying that occurs any time, day or night. Unlike classic colic, which begins improving after two months, crying from kidney pain gets worse and worse.

8. Eye Pain: From Glaucoma to a Corneal Abrasion

Eye pain, also very rare, may come from glaucoma (high pressure inside the eyeball), an accidental scratch of the cornea, or even from a tiny, irritating object stuck underneath a baby's eyelid (such as an eyelash). Your doctor should consider these problems if your crying baby has red, tearful eyes and severe pain that lasts through the day and night.

9. Overdose: From Excessive Sodium to Vitamin A

Persistent, severe crying can result from giving babies excessive amounts of sodium (salt). This may occur when a parent mixes formula with too little water. It has also rarely been described after the first week of life if a breast-feeding woman is making so little milk that her breast milk becomes very salty. These babies are easily diagnosed because they are losing weight, not drinking any other liquids, and are both irritable and lethargic all day long.

Excess Vitamin A is an extremely rare cause of infant crying. It only occurs in babies who are given high doses of supplemental vitamins or fish oil.

10. Others: From Migraines to Heart Failure

Some extraordinarily rare conditions that have been reported as the cause of unstoppable crying in young infants include: a bone fracture, sugar intolerance in babies fed fruit or fruit juice, migraine headache, hyperthyroidism, and heart failure. These babies don't merely cry for three hours a day—they act poorly all day long.

Appendix B

A New Parents' Survival Guide:
The Top Ten Survival Tips for Parents of New Babies

Now that we've talked all about the baby's crying, let's talk about yours! All new parents know that if you ask five people for their advice (not that people even wait for you to ask), you'll get ten different opinions. So, even though you didn't ask *me* for my opinion, here is my list of ten sanity-saving survival tips to help you endure the challenges of your baby's first months a little more gracefully.

1. **Trust Yourself: You Are the Latest in the Unbroken Chain of the World's Top Parents**

    Leslie, still in her hospital bed with four-day old Gabriel, told me: "I'm usually such an optimist, yet I've had weird dreams of dropping him and leaving him places. My husband jokes that some special 'inexperienced-parent' alarm will go off when we take Gabe home from the hospital!"

    Trust yourself. You know more than you think you do.
    Dr. Benjamin Spock

    If you're like most new parents, you probably alternate between feeling like a major-league pro and an amateur. It's enough to give a person "parental whiplash!" And, the conflicting advice given by many baby experts can deepen the confusion.

But before you lose confidence, please remember this: You are part of an unbroken chain of successful parents that stretches all the way back to the beginning of time. You and your baby have survived because you are descended from the best mothers, most protective fathers, and strongest children in the world. That's why Dr. Spock's advice to parents to trust themselves is so correct.

Trust your feelings. Relax and remember that all your baby really needs from you is milk and your nourishing love. And all you really need is patience, support, a little information, and perhaps a massage every once in a while.

2. Lower Your Expectations

> *You'll see. Having a baby is like going to sleep in your own bed and waking up in Zimbabwe!*
>> Sonya to her daughter Denise a month before
>> Denise gave birth to Aidan

Becoming a parent is filled with all sorts of misconceptions and surprises. And perhaps the biggest misconception of all is

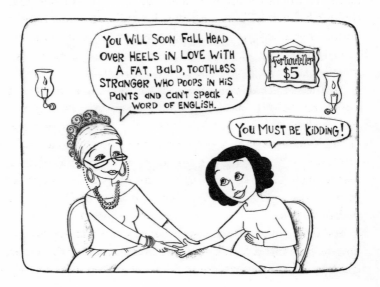

that you'll automatically know what to do the moment your baby is born. Yet even after giving birth to her third child, Beth quipped, "At the end of my first pregnancy about the only thing I was really prepared to do was filling out forms and buying maternity dresses!"

Parenting requires some practical experience (especially when caring for challenging babies). Yet many pregnant couples today have never even touched a newborn. Despite this lack of experience, they expect themselves to instantly be able to care for the babies *and* manage the household *and* have a job *and* be lovers.

Unfortunately, these unrealistic expectations have been growing in our culture for at least the past fifty years. Even though people warned you when you were pregnant, "Your life will never be the same!" you probably shrugged it off. Few believe *their* baby will be tough. For most women, being pregnant is so close to their regular life that they get lulled into a false sense of security. Before delivery, you can still linger in a hot shower and think, "I'm ready. I'm on top of this." It's so automatic that many women are tricked into believing that taking care of their newborns would be just as natural, but as you now know, that couldn't be further from the truth. It's only after your baby is born that you begin to see the demands of parenthood more accurately. Suddenly, that long hot shower you took a month before the baby came looks like a Caribbean vacation.

Another expectation that may not immediately materialize is loving your baby the moment you see her. Of course, many parents *do* instantly fall in love with their new infant; however, one of the little-told truths about becoming a parent is that many new moms and dads *don't* feel smitten right away. It makes sense that falling in love might take a little time. After all, few of us experience love at first sight. Don't worry, like the song says, "You can't hurry love."

And that's not all. You may soon notice your brain has also unexpectedly changed. Memory loss is one more proof that your life is temporarily out of your control. One new mom told me, "My best guess is that during the delivery a piece of my brain came out with the placenta."

Lots of moms feel that giving birth turns them into complete "boobs"—and in a way it does! Lactation makes your body awash with prolactin which, along with the other massive hormonal changes going on inside you, probably is the basis for this new forgetfulness. Finally, you'll notice your ditziness is made ten times worse by exhaustion. Clear thinking is terribly hard to hold on to in the face of prolonged sleep deprivation.

So be patient and kind to yourself. In a few short months you'll have your feet on the ground again and, what's more, you'll know your baby better than anyone else in the world!

3. Accept All the Help You Can Get

> When I moved to California from Florida, I was happy
> to be independent from my family. But when my baby
> was born, I missed them in a way I had never felt before.
> I suddenly wanted and needed my family around me.
>
> Kathleen, mother of two-month-old Ella Rose

Never in history were a mother and a father expected to care for their baby *all by themselves.* The idea of a nuclear family—one mother and one father to do it all—is one of mankind's most recent, and riskiest, experiments, attempted only over the last two or three generations. (That's a mere sixty years out of the 60,000 years since the modern human era began.) In the past, a couple's family and community always pitched in to help, and later the couple would return the favor.

> Sharon, mother of Noah and Ariel, was a work-at-home
> mom, a thousand miles away from her family, with no
> baby-sitters or nanny. Sharon's goal was to make sure her
> kids were happy and healthy—even if she was dead on
> her feet. She described feeling like an old tomato plant,
> where the fruit looks plump and delicious even though
> the plant that nourishes it looks scraggly and anemic.

I'm always telling the parents of my patients: Get help and don't feel guilty about asking—or paying—for it. Enlist your friends to bring you a frozen casserole, do some cleaning, or watch your baby while you nap. Just as you are giving so much of yourself to take care of your new child, lean on your support network to help take care of *you*—you'll pay it back later. The extra pair of "hands" of a niece, neighbor, nanny, or swing is neither an extravagance nor a sign of failure. It's the bare minimum that most new moms have had throughout time.

4. Get Your Priorities Straight: Should You Take a Break or Do the Dishes?

> *On the few occasions that my crying baby fell asleep before I did, I used the time for me! I soaked in a bubble bath, relaxed with a drink, read a book, and prayed that she would sleep a little longer.*
>
> Frances Wells Burck, *Babysense*

As I just said, I encourage you to get some help, but if you don't have access to help, don't worry: Your job is doable—as long as you put your priorities in order. The time will come to achieve everything you want, but that time isn't right after having a baby.

One of your top priorities is: Don't try to do too much. For example, the week after having your baby is not the time for you to host your family from out of town. As my mother used to say, "Don't be stupid polite!" A few well-wishers are fine, but only if they're healthy and helpful. Visitors who can't cook or clean take up your precious time and, what's worse, *they can carry germs into your home.* People you keep away may call you paranoid but, in truth, you never had a better reason for being neurotic and overprotective!

Another good idea is to leave a sweet announcement on your answering machine, giving your baby's important statistics and telling everyone that you won't be returning calls for a few weeks. Of course, you can always return calls if you want, but this at least frees up enough time to accomplish even higher priorities— like soaking in a hot tub.

Rest: The Essential Nutrient for New Parents

Sometimes the most urgent and vital thing you can do . . . is take a nap.

Ashley Brilliant

When we were teenagers, we were "dying" to stay up all night. Now, we're "dying" **if** we stay up all night!

The extreme fatigue that goes along with being a new parent can make you feel depressed, irritable, inept, and distort your perceptions of the world like a fun-house mirror. (Some countries torture people by waking them up every time they fall asleep!)

So please nap when your baby does, sleep when your mom comes, and, however you have to do it—get some rest!

5. Be Flexible: It's Much Better to Bend Than to Snap

You just have to accept that some days you're the pigeon and some days you're the statue.

Roger Anderson

There may be a few times in life when an unwillingness to compromise is admirable—but after becoming a new parent *isn't* one of them. That's why I believe the official bumper-sticker slogan for all new parents should read, *Be flexible—or die!*

Part of the fun, and responsibility, of being a mom or dad is to be able to choose which parenting options make sense to *you* and works for *your* child. However, it's also important to be able to throw your choices out the window and start all over again when things are not going the way you planned.

If you're a person who enjoyed being organized, on time, and having a spotless house, this new flexibility may require practice—and deep breathing. But you may as well take it all with a sense of humor because the time has come when your milk will gush down the front of your favorite blouse and when your little darling will empty her diaper load on your white sofa!

If you can, throw away your to-do list for a few months. Accept that the clock on your wall has been temporarily transformed from a time-management tool to a decoration. And know that for a while, day and night will cease to have any true relevance.

You've "bought your ticket," so let go and open yourself to the marvel, awe, and exhilaration of one of the greatest adventures of life!

6. Know Thyself: How Do Your Baby's Cries Make You Feel?

When your baby screams in your face, are you able to calmly think, *He must be having a bad day?* Or do you think, *Oh, my God, I'm doing something wrong!* or *I don't deserve to be a mother!* Or even, *Who the hell does she think she is?*

There's no question your baby's screams may trigger a flood of upsetting feelings from the past. You may suddenly remember voices of anger, criticism, and ridicule directed at you long ago. And you may begin to get angry or defensive. Of course, your newborn's cries can't possibly have a connection to your past traumas. She's much too young to feel anger or to be able to criticize or manipulate you. However, fatigue and stress can sometimes fool your mind and make these innocent cries feel like stinging attacks.

This, too, is a normal part of being a new parent. When these emotions well up inside you, take the opportunity to be brave and share your feelings with your spouse or someone else who truly cares about you. The more you discuss your past pains and your current fears, the more clearly you'll see how unrelated your baby's cries are to those old experiences.

7. Don't Rock the Cradle Too Hard: Babies, Frustration, and Child Abuse

> *David suddenly felt a wave of anger blow across him like a hot wind. After weeks and weeks of colicky screaming*

> by his twin sons, Sam and Ben, he got so angry he
> punched his hand through the door. "I was so frustrated
> and exhausted I couldn't control myself. I would never
> hurt my boys, but for the first time in my life I under-
> stood how a parent could be driven to such desperation."

Few things feel better than when we can easily calm our baby's screams, but when everything we do fails, few things can make us feel worse.

Remember, your baby can belt out a shriek that is louder than a vacuum cleaner. That's why it is so difficult to take when she's on your shoulder and blasting right next to your ear. The sound of her cry also sets off a "red alert" reflex inside your nervous system that makes your heart race and your skin cringe, creating an urgent desire to stop it. This crying can become almost intolerable when it's coupled with fatigue, depression, financial stress, hormonal chaos, family conflict, and a history of being abused. When these stressful forces combine, they can sometimes push even a loving parent over the edge into the dark abyss of child abuse.

A mild-mannered father I know told me that he once shocked himself, in the middle of the night, when his daughter's cries started to "get to him" and he found himself rocking her cradle "a little too hard." "I felt like such a terrible parent. My little Marlo was so unhappy, yet nothing I did seemed to help. I felt so incompetent."

Another great frustration for parents is when a technique that usually calms their baby suddenly does nothing. It's like getting mugged in broad daylight when you least expect it.

However, no matter how desperate you feel, always remember that there's a big difference between feelings and actions. When you are exhausted, you can joke all you want to about leaving your baby on someone's doorstep but, needless to say, you're not allowed to do it.

What should you do when you are feeling like you're near your breaking point?

- Lighten your workload and get some help to clean the house and watch the baby.
- Do something physical to vent your energy: dig a hole, hammer nails, beat the sofa, scream into a pillow, sob into a towel, or just go out and run!
- Talk to someone: a friend, a relative, or even a crisis hot-line. (The National Child Abuse Hotline—800 4-A-CHILD—has counselors available every day, all day.)

8. Keep Your Sense of Humor Handy

He who laughs . . . lasts! Mary Pettibone Poole

There are times when parenthood seems like nothing but feeding the mouth that bites you. Peter de Vries

The only normal families are the ones you don't know very well. Joe Ancis

Babies are always more trouble than you thought . . . and more wonderful. Charles Osgood

It's not easy for me to take my problems one at a time when they refuse to get in line. Ashley Brilliant

Raising a child is a constant series of tasks and challenges. You don't want to make mistakes, but you will. Remember, perfection is found only in the dictionary. So, forget dignity . . . forget organization . . . be gentle with yourself . . . and *laugh, laugh, laugh.*

Laughter is exactly what this doctor orders. Rent some funny movies or watch reruns of *I Love Lucy.* Try imagining Cleopatra burping her baby and getting a giant spit-up down *her* back.

Laugh at your hair, laugh at your baby, laugh at your messy house. Laugh at the fact that you are now one of those women you used to avoid who gets into heated discussions at parties about burping and the color of her baby's poop.

9. Take Care of Your Spouse (S/he Just Might Come in Handy Someday)

> When Curtis, Cheryl and Jeff's second child, was four
> weeks old, Jeff said "We haven't even had sex once yet."
> Cheryl shot back, "What do you expect? Every sexual
> part of my body is either oozing, bruised, or throbbing!"

Taking care of a new baby is so demanding and time-consuming that it's easy for a parent to start feeling like they're giving a hundred and ten percent effort (usually true) and their partner is giving only seventy-five percent (usually false).

- "I work all day and still come home and give the baby a bath." *vs.* "I take care of the baby all day and still make him dinner and scratch his back."

- "She's so lucky to lounge around the house, watch soaps, and hang out with the baby all day." *vs.* "He's so lucky to go to work and see different people."

The truth is, being new parents is a joint effort. There is so much to do that the only way to do it all, and still be friends, is to work as a team.

Your baby's world balances on the two of you. That's why she would never want to hear you say, "I gave up everything for you. I even put you ahead of my relationship with your father/ mother." In fact, if your baby could, she would sit you down and tell you, "Don't you worry about me. I'm fine, but I'm really gonna need you later. So, for right now, have some fun, see a movie . . . but please take care of yourselves."

Caring for your baby is only half your job; the other half is giving each other some TLC. Dads must support and adore their wives, moms must nurture and caress their husbands, and you both have to cut each other some extra slack and avoid harsh criticisms. (Of course, in any given situation your reactions will be different from your spouse's. You're separate individuals with unique life experiences.)

Make the time to take walks together, to give each other ten-minute massages, back scratches, or sexual pleasure. Try to never take your partner for granted and never go to bed angry. These first months are the hardest part of the first year, but the great news is, if you work together, your marriage can emerge from this period stronger than ever.

To Dads: Appreciate Your Wife—The Great Goddess of Creation

Can you imagine how embarrassed you would be if *your* "bag of waters" broke open in the middle of a business meeting? While a new dad has spent the past nine months going about his life in a fairly normal way, his wife has been stretched in a surreal kind of mind-body "taffy pull." Let's face it, any guy who has watched his wife give birth knows the real truth about who the weaker sex is.

Mothers are great heroes! When it comes to making babies, we men chip in a sperm while our wives essentially *pull a dog sled from Alaska to the Gulf of Mexico.* In fact, except for your 23 chromosomes, every single molecule of your baby was individually carried to her through your wife's body. It's almost as if each cell should carry a little tag that reads, *Inspected by Mom.*

And, after your child is born, your wife has another awesome responsibility on her shoulders. While you get to go to work, she's at home dealing with leaking breasts, sore nipples, an extra thirty pounds, and a frantic, red-faced person yelling at her—all after little or no training.

And then there's sex (or no sex)! You may be interested in having sex after abstaining for the last part of the pregnancy, but for many new moms, sex is the last thing on their mind. Women often have "pelvic exhaustion" after the delivery, and although your wife may look like she had a "boob job," she may not feel very erotic. (Remember those are really for the baby now.)

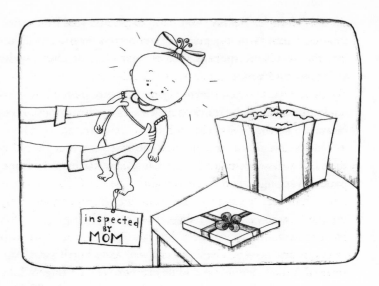

What should you do? Rethink your priorities. Remember, no one on his deathbed ever said, "My only regret is that I didn't spend more time at the office." Now is the time your wife needs your attention, support, and tenderness the most. (It's no accident researchers find the best predictor of breast-feeding success to be the spouse's support.) Bring home flowers, change some diapers, and give her a break to go out with friends—now, that's the type of "child support" she needs!

Another way to really help your wife is to take over the job of calming your baby. Men are superb at soothing babies when they learn the Cuddle Cure. Frank, a construction worker and father of colicky two-month-old Angela, said, "I love being able to soothe my screaming baby in seconds."

To Moms: Appreciate Your Husband—The Man Who Put the Us in Uterus

Okay, it's true: You *have* had to do all the hard work and "heavy lifting" so far, and you're so busy you barely get the chance to pee—but it's not easy being a new dad either.

Remember, your husband is descended from the world's most successful cavemen, and he probably has dinosaur-size expectations of himself. He may not have to protect you from saber-toothed tigers, but most men still feel a huge pressure to go out into the world and compete in order to provide for their families.

If your husband is quiet, don't think he doesn't feel things as deeply as you do. Men shown crying babies responded with less talking than their wives, but they had exactly the same sharp increase in sweating, heart rate, and blood pressure.

There's no doubt that many new dads feel as nervous handling their infants as the first time they asked a girl to the prom. So be patient with your sweetie. Be available if he needs you, but don't rescue him right away when he's fumbling around trying to figure out how to calm your baby—just remind him of the 5 "S's." He'll sense your confidence in him and he'll feel great when he can do it on his own. Then, rather than seeing himself as an outsider with the baby, he'll feel like a "star player on the team."

10. Don't Ignore Depression: The Uninvited Guest

> *My whole world suddenly turned black. My emotions jumped from guilt to rage to despair to such utter anxiety that I thought I would either jump out of my skin or lose my mind. I had terrible visions of hurting myself so I could be taken to the hospital and rescued from all this.*
>
> *I felt like I was being punished for thinking I could be a good mother. I felt like I didn't deserve to have a child . . . and I cried for hours.*
>
> Louisa, mother of three-week-old Georgia

As shocking as it sounds, approximately forty percent of new moms experience unhappy feelings intruding upon their joy during the days and weeks after the birth of their babies. You may notice yourself suddenly being tearful, worried, or exhausted yet unable to sleep—all of which may be early signs of postpartum depression.

Shortly after delivery, women may experience three different levels of depression: *the baby blues*—mild weepiness, anxiety, and insomnia; *true postpartum depression*—a bruising, more debilitating type of grief; or *postpartum psychosis*—a severe and rare condition including hallucinations, incoherent statements, and bizarre behavior.

The Baby Blues

The baby blues usually start a few days after the baby is born and last at least several days. No one knows exactly why they occur, but some scientists think they're triggered by the dramatic changes in a woman's hormones after delivery. In addition, the blues can certainly be worsened by all the other stressful situations going on in a new mom's life—including having a very fussy baby.

The blues are so common that many doctors consider them a normal part of giving birth. Nonetheless, the fatigue, fear, and unanticipated sorrow can be very distressing while you're experiencing them.

> *Feeling dejected and rejected Sarah called me. She had just about had it with her four-week-old daughter, Julie. Sarah said, "She's fussy and demanding all the time; I feel robbed of my joy. I dread her crying because I never know if it will last five minutes or four hours! And on top of that, I have insomnia. I'm a light sleeper by nature, but now I'm so attuned to Julie's cry that I can't sleep for longer than a cat-nap. I'm anxious, exhausted . . . falling apart.*
>
> *"I watched my babysitter act so calmly around Julie and I couldn't help but feel that I was making her worse with my awkward attempts at calming her."*

I asked Sarah and Tom to come in so I could teach them the Cuddle. I hoped much of Sarah's problem stemmed from her exhaustion, but I was also concerned about her having the baby blues. After teaching them the 5 "S's," I encouraged Sarah to make an appointment with a psychologist, just in case the techniques didn't help. Fortunately, the Cuddle made a dramatic improvement in Julie's screaming. Sarah quickly mastered the skills of calming her and getting her to sleep longer. As Julie slept more, Sarah began to feel like a better mom.

> "Yesterday, I calmed my little baby in less than five minutes! I was so proud! Within a week, I felt like the darkness lifted and my life had turned around."

True Postpartum Depression

One of the least discussed secrets about having a baby is depression. During the first weeks of what should be the greatest bliss of their lives, about five percent of normal moms (estimates range from three to twenty percent) experience strong feelings of sorrow and anxiety. If mild sadness after birth is called the baby blues, then this more severe depression should be called the baby "black-and-blues," because it is a bruising assault on a woman's psychological health.

Crashing waves of emotion knock these women off their feet and make them feel like they are drowning in sadness, shame, anger, anxiety, pain, fear, apathy, exhaustion, and hopelessness. It can take all the energy a mother has just to make a sandwich. Oftentimes they have fantasies of hurting themselves or their babies. These symptoms can occur at any time after delivery and last from a few weeks to several months.

A woman who feels this way can become so fragile that almost anything makes her think, *Every other woman would make a better mother.* Or, *I'm sure she's crying because she hates me.* No matter what words of support her loved ones offer, she feels totally adrift and thinks it's impossible for them to really understand how she feels.

This black hole sucks away a woman's optimism and self-confidence. Yet, at the same time, the shame and isolation accompanying postpartum depression lead most of these moms to keep their suffering a secret from their doctors.

However, depression *is* a medical illness. Although these mothers often feel responsible for their condition, they should have no more guilt than people suffering from allergies. Like its milder version, the baby blues, postpartum depression is believed to be caused by a temporary hormonal imbalance. It, too, is made worse by the stress of fatigue, financial pressures, family problems, and colic.

If you are feeling like this, you're not alone. Many women have experienced what you are going through. Fortunately, there are some very effective treatments that can help you feel better. Please, call your doctor. You may not even have postpartum depression—low thyroid levels after delivery mimic depression. And if you do have it, you can be greatly helped by any one of a dozen excellent new medicines, hypnosis, light therapy, or psychotherapy.

Postpartum Psychosis

This severe reaction to the physical, emotional, and hormonal shifts occurring around birth may affect as many as one in one thousand women (usually within two weeks of delivery). Typically, these distraught new mothers hear voices and see things that other people can't; their statements become irrational and preoccupied with bizarre trivia; and, they may refuse to eat and become frantically active and extremely confused.

Postpartum psychosis is treatable, but it's an absolute medical emergency! If you think you or someone you know may be suffering from this extremely serious condition, seek medical help *immediately.*

To get help with any level of postpartum depression, contact:

Postpartum Support International:
(805) 967-7636 or www.postpartum.net

Depression After Delivery:
(800) 944-4PPD or www.depressionafterdelivery.com.

Index

Page numbers of illustrations appear in italics.

Breast-feeding, (*cont.*)
  Supplemental Nursing System
    (SNS), 205
  supplementing, 205
  tooth-decay and, 182
  topping off the tank, 221
  underfeeding, 202–3
Burping
  GER and, 207
  how to, 34, *34*
  sleeping baby and, 226
Burping drops, 35, 193

C

Caffeine, 41–42
Calming reflex, 3, 10, 67, 92–103
  fetus and, 10, 92–93
  jiggling to trigger, 158
  side/stomach position and, 130
  sucking and, 174
  top ten ways you can imitate the
    uterus, 93
  turning on (5 "S's"), 3, 10–11,
    93–103 (*see also* 5 "S's")
  vigorous motion to trigger, 169
Care and Feeding of Children (Holt),
  155–56
Child Abuse. *See* Abuse
Colic, 25–32
  causes, top five theories, 32,
    33–60
  chiropractic, 208–9
  cultures where babies never get
    colic, 32, 39, 44, 53, 60, 68, 75,
    84–85
  fourth trimester (missing), 61–75
    (*see also* Fourth trimester)
  gas and poop and, 35, 36, 37, 74,
    105–6
  herbal teas, 207–8

homeopathy, 208
massage for, 194–97
medical problem, serious, 186,
  238–43 (*see also* Appendix A)
myths and ancient theories,
  28–29
osteopathy for, 208–9
pain and, 27–28, 31, 32, 48,
  73–74
preemies and, 31, 38–39, 44, 48,
  53, 60, 73
"Rule of Threes," 27
ten universal facts, 31–32, 43–44
timing of occurrence, 31, 39, 44,
  74
total hours of fussing, 26–27, *26*
walks outside, 197–98
warmth to soothe, 198–99
See also Gastro-esophageal Reflux
  (GER)
Constipation, 35, 36–7, 196, 201
  serious problem indicated, 202
Crying, 5–6, 17–24, 240
  cycles, 102–3
  distinct sounds of, 21–24
  emotional effect on parent,
    20–21, 251–53
  letting baby "cry it out," 30–31
  medical problem, 186, 200–7,
    238–43,
  myth of blowing off steam (or
    crying is good for baby),
    29–31
  overstimulation and, 11, 23, 50,
    51–52
  understimulation and, 52–53
  See also Colic; Cuddle cure; 5
    "S's"; Sleep
Crying reflex, 17–20, *19*
Cuddle Cure, 3, 11–14, 185–92
  keeping baby calm after you
    soothe crying, 189

D

Depression, 257–60
  baby blues, 258–59
  postpartum depression, 258–60
  postpartum psychosis, 260

E

Ear infections and pacifiers, 179
Efé tribe, Zaire, 133, 176

F

Fatigue or overtired cries, 23,
  221–22
Feces
  blood in, 41, 238
  normal appearance, 36
Feeding. *See* Breast-feeding; Bottle-
  feeding; Hunger
Fetal position, 9, 38, 130
Fetus
  calming reflex and, *9*, 10
  life in the womb, 62–63, 141
  missing fourth trimester, 8–9, 14,
    61–75, 194–95
5 "S's," 3, 10–11, *12*, 94
  finding your baby's favorite tech-
    nique, 187
  how to switch off your baby's cry-
    ing with, 126–27, *126–27*
  Shushing (shhhhing), 11, 12,
    93, 96–97, 100, 127, 139–51,
    217
  Side/Stomach position, 11, 12,
    93, 95–96, 126, *126*, 129–37,
    190, 216
  Sucking, 11, 12, 93, 98, 127,
    173–84, 191–92, 217

Swaddling, 11, 93, 94–95,
  105–26, 190, 199, 216
Swinging, 11, 12, 93, 97,
  127, *127*, 153–72, 191,
  217
  three reasons for a delayed
    response, 101–3
  vigor, 99–100, 169
  See also Cuddle Cure; Shushing;
    Side/Stomach position;
    Sucking; Swaddling; Swinging
Field, Tiffany, 195
Food sensitivity, 39–42, 72,
  199–201, 204
  bottle-fed babies (milk or soy
    allergy), 38, 40–41, 43–44,
    200–1, 207
  breast-fed babies, 39, 40–42,
    43
  caffeine, 41–42
Fourth trimester (missing), 8–9, 14,
  61–75
  colic and, 70–75, *71*
  parenting and, 67–70
  sucking and, 174, 175
  touch and, 194–95
  what it is, 62–67
  why baby needs, 66–67
Fussy baby, xiv, *xiv*, 5, 7, 9, 23, 54,
  89
  See also Temperament

G

Gala (milk), 175
Gas, 33–34, 38–40, 105–6
  colicky babies, 37
  massage for, 196
Gastro-colic reflex, 36–37, 240
Gastro-esophageal Reflux (GER),
  42–44, 72, 206–7, 239

S